EMPATHIC COUNSELING

SECOND EDITION

EMPATHIC COUNSELING

SECOND EDITION

Building Skills to Empower Change

JEANNE M. SLATTERY

CRYSTAL L. PARK

AMERICAN PSYCHOLOGICAL ASSOCIATION

Washington, DC

Published by
American Psychological Association
750 First Street, NE
Washington, DC 20002
https://www.apa.org

Order Department
https://www.apa.org/pubs/books
order@apa.org

In the U.K., Europe, Africa, and the Middle East, copies may be ordered from Eurospan
https://www.eurospanbookstore.com/apa
info@eurospangroup.com

Typeset in Minion-Pro/Gotham by Circle Graphics, Inc., Reisterstown, MD

Printer: Sheridan Books, Chelsea, MI
Cover Designer: Blake Logan, New York, NY

Library of Congress Cataloging-in-Publication Data

Names: Slattery, Jeanne M., author. | Park, Crystal L., author.
Title: Empathic counseling : building skills to empower change /
  by Jeanne M. Slattery and Crystal L. Park.
Description: Second edition. | Washington, DC : American Psychological
  Association, [2020] | Includes bibliographical references and index.
Identifiers: LCCN 2019033103 (print) | LCCN 2019033104 (ebook) |
  ISBN 9781433831225 (paperback) | ISBN 9781433832307 (ebook)
Subjects: LCSH: Counseling.
Classification: LCC BF636.6 .S59 2020 (print) | LCC BF636.6 (ebook) |
  DDC 158.3—dc23
LC record available at https://lccn.loc.gov/2019033103
LC ebook record available at https://lccn.loc.gov/2019033104

http://dx.doi.org/10.1037/0000171-000

Printed in the United States of America
Second edition

10 9 8 7 6 5 4 3 2 1

For the clients, students, friends, and family who patiently listened, supported, and guided me.

—J. M. S.

To my teachers.

—C. L. P.

BRIEF CONTENTS

Preface xix

I. Introduction to Empathy and the Mental Health Professional 1

Chapter 1   What Is Empathy, and Why Does It Matter? 3

II. Building a Framework for Understanding People 19

Chapter 2   Understanding Meaning Systems 21

Chapter 3   Understanding Culture, Identity, and Oppression 45

III. Developing Empathic Assessments 69

Chapter 4   Building the Therapeutic Alliance 71

Chapter 5   Communicating Empathy Verbally 91

Chapter 6   Assessing People in Context 111

Chapter 7   Thinking Critically to Ensure Empathic Assessments 143

IV. Facilitating Positive Change 157

Chapter 8   Developing Goals and a Treatment Plan 159

Chapter 9   Providing Empathic Interventions 187

Chapter 10 Ending Treatment 209

V. Professional Issues 225

Chapter 11 Ethics 227

Chapter 12 Writing Empathic Clinical Reports 253

Chapter 13 Self-Care 271

Glossary 291
References 299
Index 323
About the Authors 335

CONTENTS

Preface xix

I. Introduction to Empathy and the Mental Health Professional 1

Chapter 1 What Is Empathy, and Why Does It Matter? 3
Cases in Empathy: Did You Love Your Children? (Andrea Yates) 3
What Is Empathy? 4
Components of Empathy 6
    Understanding 6
Cases in Empathy: Looking Out His Window (Irvin Yalom) 7
    Acceptance 8
    Hopefulness 9
    Communicating Empathy 9
What Do Clinicians Do? 11
The Common Factors 12
Ethical Work 15
Our Model of Empathic Counseling 16
Summary 17
    Applying Concepts to Your Life 18
    Key Terms 18
    Learn More 18

II. Building a Framework for Understanding People 19

Chapter 2 Understanding Meaning Systems 21
Cases in Empathy: We Talk About Real Life (Doug Muder) 21
Meaning Systems 23
Components of Meaning Systems 24
Stability and Change in Meaning Systems 25
*Cases in Empathy: Building a Coherent Meaning System
   (Tara Westover)* 26
Meaning Systems in the Context of Therapy 28
    Interpersonal Relationships 29
        Authority 29
        Individualism–Collectivism 30

Sources of Information 30
Safety and Benevolence of the World and Other People 31
Why Bad Things Happen 32
Clinical Applications 33
Identity 33
Approaches to Problems and Problem-Solving 34
Responsibility and Control 34
Self-Efficacy 35
Time Orientation 35
Recognizing Values and Goals 37
Meaning Systems Inform Situational Meanings 39
*Cases in Empathy: Never Bothered to Consider the Consequences
(Reymundo Sanchez)* 40
When Clients and Clinicians Have Different Meaning Systems 42
Clinical Applications 43
Summary 43
Applying Concepts to Your Life 44
Key Terms 44
Learn More 44

**Chapter 3   Understanding Culture, Identity, and
Oppression 45**
*Cases in Empathy: You're Doing All of This for a Failure to Signal?
(Sandra Bland)* 45
Defining and Seeing Culture 47
Multiple Group Identities 51
Cases in Empathy: Learning to See Culture (Katy Robinson) 52
Impacts of Group Identity 54
The Role of Ethnic and Racial Identity in Treatment 55
Oppression, Discrimination, Prejudice, and Privilege 57
Cases in Empathy: Petty Tyrants With a Badge (Sandra Bland) 60
What Does It Mean to Be a "Multicultural" Therapist? 61
Problems Encountered in Working With Clients With
a Minority Identity Status 61
Clinical Applications 62
"Colorblind" Approaches to Clinical Work 62
Becoming Culturally Competent 63
The Cognitive Skills of a Multicultural Clinician 65
Using Culture in Therapy 66
Clinical Applications 67

Summary 67
>Applying Concepts to Your Life 68
>Key Terms 68
>Learn More 68

III. Developing Empathic Assessments 69

Chapter 4 Building the Therapeutic Alliance 71
>Cases in Empathy: Everyone Needs to Feel Understood and Supported
> (Anna Michener) 71
What Is the Therapeutic Alliance? 72
>Clinical Applications 74
Nonverbal Listening Skills 74
>Difficulties in Understanding Nonverbal Behaviors 76
>Responding to Both Content and Process 77
>Clinical Applications 80
Clients' Contributions to Treatment 80
Introducing New Clients to the Therapeutic Setting and Process 81
>Creating a Safe Setting for Treatment 81
>Clinical Applications 82
>Engaging Clients Through the Informed Consent Process 83
>Clinical Applications 85
>Collaborating on Goals and Methods 85
>Cases in Empathy: Conflicting Beliefs, Conflicting Treatment Goals
> (Lia Lee) 86
Summary 88
>Applying Concepts to Your Life 89
>Key Terms 89
>Learn More 89

Chapter 5 Communicating Empathy Verbally 91
>Cases in Empathy: "You Must Have Had a Very Good Reason"
> (Annie G. Rogers) 91
Barriers to Communicating Empathy 92
>Clinical Applications 93
Verbal Strategies for Sharing Understanding 93
>Paraphrases 94
>Reflections of Feeling 96
>Closed and Open Questions 97
>Cases in Empathy: Transcript of Confession (Andrea Yates) 98
>Clinical Applications 99

Encouragers 99
Summarizations 100
Cases in Empathy: It's Under Your Control (D'Ja Jones) 101
Accurate Empathy 102
Strategies for Understanding Others Deeply 104
Cases in Empathy: Understanding Anna (Anna Michener) 107
The Need for Validation and Hope 108
Clinical Applications 108
Summary 109
Applying Concepts to Your Life 110
Key Terms 110
Learn More 110

Chapter 6   Assessing People in Context 111
Cases in Empathy: Stupid and Crazy? (Raymond J. Corsini) 111
Recognizing Context 112
Developing Three-Dimensional Assessments 113
Clinical Applications 114
Psychosocial History 114
Cases in Empathy: Malcolm Little (Malcolm X) 118
Clinical Applications 125
Family Genogram 126
Timeline 129
Clinical Applications 130
Mental Status Evaluation 131
Case Conceptualizations 134
Taking Multiple Perspectives 136
Research Informs Treatment 137
Pulling Assessment Strategies Together 138
Summary 141
Applying Concepts to Your Life 141
Key Terms 141
Learn More 141

**Chapter 7   Thinking Critically to Ensure Empathic
               Assessments 143**
Cases in Empathy: I Call It Being Honest (Eminem) 143
Assumptions and Values in Clinical Practice 144
Social Psychological Processes Influencing Clinical Judgments 146
Critical Thinking 148
Clinical Applications 149

Choosing Among Alternative Explanations 149
    Clinical Applications 151
Countering Observer Biases 151
Recognizing Strengths and Exceptions to Problems 152
Cases in Empathy: Seeing Strengths and Weaknesses
   (Dylan Klebold and Eric Harris) 154
Summary 155
    Applying Concepts to Your Life 156
    Key Terms 156
    Learn More 156

IV. Facilitating Positive Change 157

Chapter 8 Developing Goals and a Treatment Plan 159
Cases in Empathy: "Jail Was My Saving Grace"
   (Reymundo Sanchez) 159
Change 160
    Clinical Applications 161
Stages of Change 161
    Precontemplation 162
    Contemplation 162
    Preparation 163
    Action 163
    Maintenance 164
    Clinical Applications 165
Good Goals 165
    Specific and Measurable Goals (SM) 165
    Achievable and Realistic Goals (AR) 166
    Time-Bounded Goals (T) 167
    Intrinsic Goals (I) 167
    Committed to Change (C) 168
Collaborative Goal-Setting Process 169
    Work From Where the Client Is 171
    Build Clients' Commitment to Change 171
    Address Obstacles to Change 172
    Respect Clients' Strengths and Contributions to Treatment 172
    Build Self-Efficacy and Mastery 173
    Focus on the "Forest" While Respecting Clients' "Trees" 173
    Clinical Applications 174
    Use Client Metaphors and Work Within Their Meaning
      System 174

Writing Treatment Plans *175*
    Attending to Strengths and Resources as Well as
        Weaknesses *176*
    Determining Services *180*
Revisiting the Treatment Plan Periodically *181*
    Clinical Applications 183
Summary *183*
    Applying Concepts to Your Life 184
    Key Terms 185
    Learn More 185

Chapter 9   Providing Empathic Interventions 187
Cases in Empathy: I Don't Drink Every Single Day
    (Beth Schneider) 187
The Process of Intervening *188*
    Listen *188*
    Share Your Understanding *189*
    Then, Introduce Change *192*
    Clinical Applications 194
Interventions to Help Clients Change *194*
    Interventions for Changing Behaviors *194*
    Clinical Applications 197
    Interventions for Changing Beliefs *197*
        Challenging Beliefs and Developing New Meanings *197*
        Developing More Adaptive Views of Themselves
            and Their Future *199*
        Reducing Rumination and Avoidance *200*
    Interventions for Changing Emotions *201*
Cases in Empathy: It Was All Too Much (Sandra Uwiringiyimana) 202
Identifying and Addressing Barriers to Change *203*
Evaluating Treatment *205*
Summary *207*
    Applying Concepts to Your Life 207
    Key Terms 208
    Learn More 208

Chapter 10 Ending Treatment 209
Cases in Empathy: I Felt Like I'd Been Beaten Up (Elyn Saks) 209
Normal Versus Premature Terminations *210*
    Normal Termination *211*
    Premature Termination *211*

Clinicians' and Clients' Feelings During Termination 212
> Clinicians' Reactions 213
> Clients' Reactions 213
> *Clinical Applications* 214

Goals for Ending Treatment Well 214
> Balancing Opposing Reactions to Termination 216
> Relapse Prevention 216
> *Clinical Applications* 217

Ethical Considerations During Termination 217

Managing Risk During Termination 219
> *Clinical Applications* 221

Strategies for Helping Clients Own Their Change 221

The Discharge Summary 222
> *Clinical Applications* 223

Summary 224
> *Applying Concepts to Your Life* 224
> *Key Terms* 224
> *Learn More* 224

V. Professional Issues 225

Chapter 11 Ethics 227

Cases in Empathy: A Band-Aid for Complex Problems (Dr. Helper) 227

The Aspirational Principles 228

The Ethical Standards 229
> Informed Consent 229
> *Clinical Applications* 230
> Competence 231
> *Clinical Applications* 232
> Confidentiality 232
> *Clinical Applications* 233
> Multiple Relationships 233
> *Clinical Applications* 234
> Sensitivity to Differences 235
> *Clinical Applications* 235

Balancing Client Rights With Ethical, Legal, and Other Requirements 236
> Legal Requirements 236
>> Mandated Reporting 236
> *Clinical Applications* 237
>> Duty to Warn 238

Cases in Empathy: How Could They Fail to Protect Our Family From Her? (Andrea Yates) 239

    Worksite Requirements 241

    Clinical Applications 241

    Financial Considerations 242

    Clinical Applications 243

    Limitations of Time and Energy 243

    Clinical Applications 244

    Supervisory Issues 244

    Clinical Applications 244

Making Decisions in Response to Ethical Dilemmas 245

    Risk Management 246

    Preventing and Responding to Ethical Problems 247

Toward a Positive Approach to Ethics 249

Summary 250

    Applying Concepts to Your Life 251

    Key Terms 252

    Learn More 252

Chapter 12 Writing Empathic Clinical Reports 253

Cases in Empathy: You Start Seeing Yourself as Deserving (D'Ja Jones) 253

What Do We Know? 255

    Clinical Applications 256

Why Clinical Writing Is Important 256

    Clinical Applications 258

Brief Reports 258

    What Should Be in a Report? 263

    SOAP Notes 264

    Recommendations for Guiding Clinical Writing 266

        Be Succinct 266

        Be Objective 266

        Be Strength-Based 266

        CYA 266

        CYCA 266

        Be Tentative About Those Things That Are Unknown 266

        Remember There Are Multiple Hypotheses for Any Single Observation 267

        Don't Be Afraid to Draw Reasonable Conclusions 267

        Be Respectful 268

Exclude Irrelevant Information 268
Consider the Audience 268
Choose Tense Thoughtfully 268
Proofread Carefully 269
Summary 269
Apply Concepts to Your Life 269
Key Terms 270
Learn More 270

Chapter 13 Self-Care 271
Cases in Empathy: "How Do You Do It?" (Sheila Carluccio) 271
Dangers in Providing Empathic Therapy 272
Blurred Boundaries 272
Clinical Applications 274
Compassion Fatigue 274
Cases in Empathy: How Can We Avoid Being "Institutionalized"?
(Michael Partie) 275
Vicarious Traumatization 275
Clinical Applications 276
Remaining Vigilant to Dangers in Providing Empathic Therapy 276
Other Stressors in the Life of a Clinician 277
Clinical Applications 281
Personal and Professional Identities 282
Aligning Personal and Professional Ethics 283
Coping Effectively With Empathic Hazards and Life Stressors 285
Preventing Stress-Related Problems 286
Cases in Empathy: My Clients Have Taught Me a Lot
(Anonymous) 288
Summary 289
Applying Concepts to Your Life 290
Key Terms 290
Learn More 290

Glossary **291**
References **299**
Index **323**
About the Authors **335**

PREFACE

Why Empathy?

This book introduces students to the fundamentals of counseling using empathy as a central theme because empathy is the foundation for effective clinical work. Understanding someone else's perspective can be difficult, especially when the other person's beliefs, values, or goals differ markedly from one's own. To work effectively with people of different backgrounds, cultures, and life experiences, clinicians must understand how multiple identities and contexts influence the client. They must be able to see the "whole person," including strengths and weaknesses. Contextualized in this way, clients become three-dimensional people, and case conceptualizations and treatment plans become more sophisticated and helpful.

Understanding, of course, is not enough. Empathic understanding must be communicated using the fairly simple, yet profound set of active listening skills that clinicians have honed over the years. This book explores not only how to understand clients but also how to communicate that understanding, and how to use it to guide assessment and treatment.

We have organized our book roughly to mirror the process of counseling. Part I introduces the basic concepts and issues that we will discuss further throughout this book. Part II provides a theoretical foundation for empathic counseling, emphasizing meaning systems and cultural context. Part III explores how to conduct an accurate, empathic assessment of clients, and Part IV explains how to help clients make positive change. Part V explores key issues that relate to every phase of therapeutic work, including ethics, empathic clinical writing, and self-care.

Pedagogical Features

Our students want a text that illustrates and applies theory, engages them in thinking about difficult ideas, and helps them develop the resources to perceive people more helpfully. We have written this text with our students in mind. Rather than only *talking* about counseling (low on Bloom's taxonomy), we have used case examples, sample clinical reports, and reflection questions throughout the text to help students perceive clients, therapists, and the treatment process differently. In particular,

- We approach course ideas from students' perspectives, considering their questions, not only our own. Our students have been invaluable resources for identifying key questions to address in this volume.

- We use real people and their own words throughout the text, often in multiple chapters that build on previous materials. We draw case material from memoirs, news reports, videos, and our own clinical practices to bring concepts to life and help students learn at a deeper level. Some of the cases are clinical, and others are nonclinical profiles of individuals with complex histories and lives.

- We often use especially challenging case material to help students shift their ways of thinking about people. It is easy to understand people who are similar to us but more difficult to empathize with people holding different meaning systems and making counterintuitive decisions.

- We encourage students to integrate ideas from the text using reflection questions at the end of each case, at transition points throughout chapters, and after chapter summaries.

- We provide a glossary with definitions of all key terms, which are boldfaced in the text when they are introduced (and sometimes boldfaced again later in the text if it has been a while since the student first encountered the term).

- We provide supplemental online materials for teaching, assessing, and studying the content.

New to This Edition

This edition is not only a revision of our original text but a thoroughly updated and contemporary take on introducing students to the field of counseling. We endeavored to retain and amplify those aspects that students and instructors praised in the first edition and to develop and implement additional pedagogical features to help bring the book alive. In particular,

- We added new case content, including material from high-profile news events, memoirs, a case in Jeanne Slattery's new psychotherapy demonstration video,[1] and several additional clinical applications.

- We updated the research throughout the book, leading to new and more sophisticated discussions of concepts (e.g., our discussions of race/ethnicity, culture, and oppression have been significantly revised).

---

[1]*Trauma and Meaning*, available from the American Psychological Association. See https://www.apa.org/pubs/videos/4310015

- We significantly reorganized the book to better mirror the process of therapy (e.g., emphasizing the therapeutic alliance and communicating empathy much earlier in the book).

- We broadened our discussion of worldviews into a more inclusive discussion of meaning systems, which emphasizes not only beliefs but also goals and values and reflects current psychological science.

- We streamlined and consolidated the material on case conceptualization, treatment plans, and ethics.

- We use a more modern, reader-friendly design to engage students.

- We added a companion website with student and instructor resources to facilitate teaching and learning (see http://pubs.apa.org/books/supp/slattery/).

Our mission remains that of guiding new clinicians in their development, and we continue to use a fundamental aspect of all good clinical work—empathy—as the unifying theme for our book.

Ethics and Pragmatics in Using Case Material

The extended case material in this book is from real people—pulled from published reports in the news, videos, memoirs, and other sources. Some, like Sheila Carluccio, Anna Michener, and Andrea Yates, gave their permission to talk about them in this context. Others gave their permission but asked that we disguise their identities. Some are dead (Malcolm X, Eric Harris, and Dylan Klebold). Their stories are by necessity incomplete, based on the information they—or their families, friends, or acquaintances—have been willing to share with the public. This is much like what happens in therapy, however, when clients and clinicians, together, tell some stories of their lives but not others.

We have tried to stay within the ethical aspirations of our profession in how we approached their stories. Writing and thinking respectfully about the people discussed in this book is consistent with the principles of beneficence and nonmaleficence (doing good while not causing harm). When we solicited case material, we acted in an open and honest manner, asking for permission to use materials in this book, sharing our writing with them, sharing the context in which it would appear, and making changes to correct errors (autonomy and fidelity). In some cases, people even talked about our interest and empathic understanding as empowering (beneficence). When possible, we also did these things with people who had previously published their memoirs or whose published interviews we used. If these were really our clients, highlighting the options that they had and have, would promote their autonomy. Finally, choosing people from a wide variety of contexts and cultural backgrounds, highlighting the contributions of these contexts, and encouraging you to do so furthers the ideal of social justice.

Acknowledgments

It's difficult to be complete in attributing influences on this book, as we believe that how we see things was a force set into motion from our early childhoods and by many interactions, large and small. Our lunch groups, family, and friends have been especially important to this process. Bea Slattery read many case studies beforehand, provided encouragement, and was generous in sending newspaper clippings and magazine articles. Friends and colleagues suggested a wide range of fascinating people to include here. Many of their suggestions ended up on the cutting room floor, partly because of space but also because of the limited information available on their lives. Nonetheless, these suggestions influenced the development of our ideas.

Anna Michener and Andrea Yates talked with us about our case material and helped us get it right. Don Finch wrote about his life and generously shared his experience. Others, like Rachael Busch, were willing to let us use things that they wrote for other sources. Others allowed us to disguise events from their lives for case material. Unfortunately, space limited what we could use but thanks to all who contributed.

Our students, friends, and family read drafts of this book in class. There are too many students to name individually (several hundred), although their careful and encouraging comments are remembered and appreciated. Jamie Aten, Carol Bolland, Mary Buchanan, Rachael Busch, Hope Cross, Julie Daniels, David De la Isla, Craig Esposito, Don Finch, Kathy Fleissner, Marité Rodriguez Haynes, LaDonna Hohman, Debi Jones, Deb Kossman, Niek-o, Allison Potter, Sandy Potter, Randy Potter, Rebecca Potter, Kahlid Qureshi, Jean Rumsey, and Dave Schlueter helped us in some way or contributed thoughtful comments and ideas about one or more parts of this book.

Finally, we appreciate our editors at the American Psychological Association. Susan Reynolds pushed us to write our previous book and was excited about this one. We appreciate that she held our toes to the fire when we would otherwise have stretched our deadline toward eternity. She was generous in her brainstorming and gracious when we chose a somewhat different direction. Beth Hatch worked extremely hard with us to make sure that we said what we meant to say and as strongly as we could. We have both worked with other editors, and with Susan and Beth, we recognize what a strong editor can do for a book and its authors. We owe much to both of them.

Part I

Introduction to Empathy and the Mental Health Professional

Empathy is foundational to change in psychotherapy. In this opening chapter, we explain what empathy is—and isn't—and why its presence matters to treatment. We begin by introducing Andrea Yates, a woman who drowned her five children. We discuss her case throughout this book and use it to illustrate the importance of understanding a person's experience from that person's unique point of view. You may find it difficult to empathize with people like Ms. Yates, but learning to do so will build your empathy skills and your success in helping clients make positive, meaningful change. This book presents our model of empathic counseling, a model that we briefly outline in this chapter. Empathic counseling includes having a strong framework for understanding people, the skills to apply that framework and build an empathic assessment of each individual client, and the expertise to apply interventions based on that assessment to help clients change.

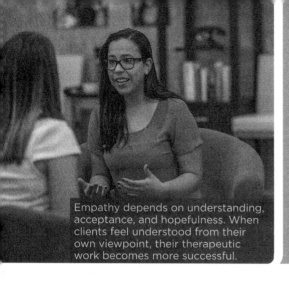

Empathy depends on understanding, acceptance, and hopefulness. When clients feel understood from their own viewpoint, their therapeutic work becomes more successful.

1 What Is Empathy, and Why Does It Matter?

Looking Ahead III➡

After reading this chapter you will be able to answer these questions:

1. Define *empathy*. Why is each part of this definition important?

2. What are *common factors*? What implications do common factors have for the fields of counseling and psychotherapy?

3. What do clinicians believe they are doing in the course of treatment? Why do they see these as important?

4. Describe the model of empathy-building that serves as the foundation of this book.

Cases in Empathy

Did You Love Your Children? **|** Andrea Yates

Andrea Yates (age 36) had five children: four sons and a daughter, all under age 8. On June 20, 2001, she drowned her children one at a time in the family's bathtub. The following transcript is from her interview with Dr. Phillip Resnick while she was at the Harris County Jail. Earlier in the interview she described herself as a "bad mother" because her children "weren't developing right . . . in an academic sense and a righteous sense." Here she describes what she means by this.

Dr. Phillip Resnick: You mentioned an aphorism from the Bible about a millstone. Would you say what that is?

Andrea Yates: It's better to tie a stone around your neck and throw yourself into the sea . . . than to cause . . . to cause a little one to stumble.

Resnick: Let me make sure I'm getting that. "Better to tie a millstone around your neck and throw yourself in the sea" rather than to do what?

Yates: Cause someone to stumble . . . stumble.

Resnick: Cause someone to stumble. Okay, uh, and when you say "stumble," you mean that, like on the path to righteousness.

Yates: Yes.

Resnick: And so you thought that your children, all five of your children, somehow because of what you saw as your defective mothering, were not on the path of righteousness and were stumbling. (Hmm) And did you feel then that it was good for them or bad for them, if you in fact threw them into the sea—or in a bathtub—in a very real sense? What were you trying to accomplish then when you did take your children's lives?

Yates: Maybe in their innocent years . . . God would take them up.

Resnick: It would be their innocent years and God would take them up? Is that what you said?

Yates: Be with him. Uh huh.

Resnick: God would take them up to be with Him in heaven? Is that what you mean? (Uh huh.) All right. And if you had not taken their lives, what did you think would happen to them?

Yates: Guess they would have continued stumbling.

Resnick: And where would they end up?

Yates: Hell.

(Andrea Yates Confession, clips 8 and 9, July 14, 2001)

What Do You Think?

1. How would you describe Andrea's beliefs about the world and her role in it? What motivates her?

2. How would you respond to Andrea given this understanding?

What Is Empathy?

What is a weed? A plant whose virtues have not yet been discovered.

—*Ralph Waldo Emerson*

Empathy is the ability to take the point of view of another person. This perspective taking can be difficult, especially when the other person's beliefs, values, or goals differ markedly from one's own. Nonetheless, empathy allows therapists, whom we also refer to in this text as **clinicians** or **counselors**, to understand and work effectively with someone like Andrea Yates. When clients do not feel understood *from their own point of view*—when they feel objectified or dismissed—they are less likely to self-disclose, work collaboratively and cooperatively, or remain in therapy (Elliott, Bohart, Watson, & Greenberg, 2011; Elliott, Bohart, Watson, & Murphy, 2018; Owen, Tao, Imel, Wampold, & Rodolfa, 2014). In contrast, when clients feel understood from their own viewpoint, their therapeutic work becomes more successful.

Thus, clinicians need to listen for their clients' attitudes and beliefs, recognize their clients' concerns and problems, and—importantly—also hear their clients' strengths. Clinicians who have negative attitudes about clients or a weak working relationship with them are more likely to identify problems as more severe, have clients report less symptom change across treatment, and have more clients terminate treatment before the treatment goals are met (K. N. Anderson, Bautista, & Hope, 2019; Coyne, Constantino, Westra, & Antony, 2019; Thompson, Chin, & Kring, 2019).

Although it may seem difficult or even impossible to understand someone like Andrea Yates, the good news is that people can become more empathic. Empathy is not a fixed trait but a set of active cognitive and emotional behaviors that can be learned and developed across time. But developing empathy requires more than just book learning and memorization (Pedersen, Crethar, & Carlson, 2008). One way to build empathy is to share similar experiences. This strategy can be useful, but empathy drawn solely from one's own experience would severely limit the types of clients with whom clinicians could work. Such clinicians could only treat clients with similar backgrounds and concerns. Furthermore, even if a clinician and client experienced the same event, each person might perceive the event very differently. In fact, while building empathy in this way can sometimes be helpful, assuming understanding based on similar experiences or shared group membership can also interfere with clinicians' abilities to see the world from their clients' points of view.

Thus, although life experience is one way of developing empathy, such experience generally must be supplemented in other ways. One of the most basic of these is cultivating an attitude of curiosity about others. Effective clinicians are curious about the values, beliefs, and goals that inform and motivate their clients' behavior. Empathy can be increased by sensitively observing clients' words and behavior. People reveal their beliefs about themselves and their world in many ways—what they discuss and choose not to discuss; their juxtaposition of topics and their manner of discussing them; changes in facial, postural, breathing, and spatial cues; and what they do within a session as well as patterns of change within and across sessions (Mozdrzierz, Peluso, & Lisiecki, 2009; A. G. Rogers, 2001).

Finally, empathy can be increased by sensitively observing one's own emotional and cognitive reactions. Changes in the *clinician's* breathing, mood, fantasies, thoughts, and activity might be important cues about a client. These physical, cognitive, and emotional cues can be difficult to interpret, however, without well-developed insight into one's own thoughts, feelings, dynamics, and motivations. Self-awareness increases the ability to use internal cues effectively and distinguish between reactions that are primarily due to the clinician's own issues and those that are the client's. Being self-aware can help clinicians distinguish between what is in the client's best interest and what instead serves the clinician's needs and purposes.

Components of Empathy

In a clinical context, empathy depends on three components: understanding, acceptance, and hopefulness. These three components are essential, but in addition, empathy is only effective when clinicians communicate it and their clients recognize it. Here we discuss this perspective on empathy and begin to outline strategies for building it.

Understanding

I do not ask how the wounded person feels. I simply become that wounded person.
—*Winston Churchill*

We tend to see others whom we know and like in favorable ways, perceiving the best in what they do (Hess, Cossette, & Hareli, 2016). We see their mistakes and problems as temporary conditions, or **states**, perhaps attributing them to situations rather than their own actions. In contrast, when we see flaws in people we dislike or don't know, we tend to see these flaws as enduring personality characteristics, or **traits**; those people are more likely to be seen as lazy, inconsiderate, or rude. Their behavior seems senseless, irrational, and unmotivated. However, they and their behavior make sense when seen in terms of their goals, values, and beliefs. Although clinicians may not agree with their clients' behavior because they recognize that their clients have other options, they can begin to understand it.

Self-injuring behaviors, tantrums, panic attacks, and aggressive acts may appear to happen "out of the blue" and "for no reason." We propose that these apparently senseless behaviors are motivated by factors outside of awareness—physical or emotional pain, fatigue, situational beliefs, feelings of being overwhelmed, and so on. Recognizing these factors increases empathy, facilitates the working relationship between client and clinician, helps clinicians develop effective interventions, and increases the effectiveness of those interventions.

One essential aspect of empathy is recognizing that different people often view the same situation differently. As we discuss in Chapter 2, people construct their experience of the world through their values, goals, and beliefs. They build **meaning systems**, or frameworks for understanding experiences, which includes their beliefs, values, and goals. These meaning systems are influenced by family, community, culture and context, but in turn they affect how family, community, culture, and context are perceived (Rigazio-DiGilio, Ivey, Kunkler-Peck, & Grady, 2005).

Empathy is like walking in someone else's shoes—experiencing the world like that person does. To be empathic, one must be aware of and willing to take other perspectives on the world. This ability to understand another's experience is built by developing curiosity about people and how they see the world, recognizing that there are multiple perspectives, and exposing oneself to them by traveling, reading memoirs and psychological fiction, meeting and listening to people from different cultural groups, watching international films, and eating foods and listening to music outside one's normal palate. Simple exposure is not enough, however, but must be combined with a willingness to really listen to another person.

Cases in Empathy

Looking Out His Window | Irvin Yalom

Irvin Yalom was born in 1931 of Russian Jews who had immigrated to the ghettos of Washington, DC. A psychiatrist, he is best known for his writings on existential psychotherapy and group therapy processes. One thread that he developed in each of these superficially different fields is to help people listen and connect despite their existential differences. He explores this idea here:

> Decades ago I saw a patient with breast cancer, who had, throughout adolescence, been locked in a long, bitter struggle with her naysaying father. Yearning for some form of reconciliation, for a new, fresh beginning to their relationship, she looked forward to her father's driving her to college—a time when she would be alone with him for several hours. But the long-anticipated trip proved a disaster: her father behaved true to form by grousing at length about the ugly, garbage-littered creek by the side of the road. She, on the other hand, saw no litter whatsoever in the beautiful, rustic, unspoiled stream. She could find no way to respond and eventually, lapsing into silence, they spent the remainder of the trip looking away from each other.
>
> Later, she made the same trip alone and was astounded to note that there were *two* streams—one on each side of the road. "This time I was the driver," she said sadly, "and the stream I saw through my window on the driver's side was just as ugly and polluted as my father had described it." But by the time she had learned to look out her father's window, it was too late—her father was dead and buried.
>
> That story has remained with me, and on many occasions I have reminded myself and my students, "Look out the other's window. Try to see the world as your patient sees it." The woman who told me this story died a short time later of breast cancer, and I regret that I cannot tell her how useful her story has been over the years, to me, my students, and many patients. (Yalom, 2003, pp. 17–18, italics in original)

What Do You Think?

1. Have you had the experience of looking out a very different "window" than someone else? How did each of you perceive the situation?

2. Did your responses affect your relationship? If there was a failure in understanding, what did each of you do to signal this failure?

Empathic understanding is both objective and subjective in nature. We need to be able to take a client's point of view while also remaining objective about his or her beliefs and values, symptoms, problems, and strengths—like simultaneously being inside and outside a circle. Effective counselors can enter a suicidal man's experience to empathize with his depressive feelings while simultaneously objectively viewing his experience from the outside, remaining aware of the severity and course of his depression, the lethality of his suicidal ideation, and the correspondence between the stressor and his response. In this way, empathy is like walking in someone else's shoes; however, clinicians retain their ability to step out of those shoes to adopt an external viewpoint. Although empathy and objectivity are equally important qualities, many clinicians have difficulty accessing both simultaneously. Effective clinicians foster both attitudes in their work.

What Do You Think?

Let's return to Andrea Yates. Imagine that she was court-referred into treatment with you after the drownings of her children. How would you apply these ideas here?

1. Think about your initial perception of Andrea. Did you like her? Were you sympathetic to her actions? Did her behavior make sense to you? Was your initial reaction more objective or subjective— or were you able to balance both perspectives?

2. Who is she? *From her point of view*, why did she do the things she did? What beliefs, values, and goals motivated her behavior? How would she describe her behavior?

3. How would this new viewpoint change the way you approached her? How would she respond differently to your approach based on your original viewpoint and this new one?

Acceptance

We cannot change anything until we accept it. Condemnation does not liberate, it oppresses.

—Carl G. Jung

Many people enter therapy because of a shame-invoking event (e.g., being molested, raped, or battered; committing a crime; questioning their sexual identity). Renowned psychologist Carl Rogers, an early advocate for the key role of empathy in counseling and therapy, argued that clinicians must provide **unconditional positive regard**, an attitude of caring, acceptance, and prizing that a clinician expresses toward a client irrespective of the client's behavior and without regard to the clinician's personal standards. To Rogers (1957/1992), this was one of three necessary and sufficient qualities for change in therapy; the other two were accurate empathy and genuineness. **Genuine** therapists are perceived as really listening and understanding, rather than only pretending to do so. Generally, words, behavior, and values are consistent across time. Later research has supported the importance of positive regard on treatment outcomes (Farber, Suzuki, & Lynch, 2018). Acceptance is not merely inhibiting actions or criticism. Instead, this sort of acceptance implies listening to a person without judgment or criticism.

Clinicians do not need to accept everything a client says or does but must find ways to accept the person. Judging clients can hook into their fears of being unacceptable or shameful, while listening and accepting can communicate that they are acceptable and worthy, thereby freeing them to change. Acceptance can be challenging. Taking the time to discover something likeable about clients and to recognize that their behavior made sense to them, given their meaning system and the specific context, can be helpful. Understanding and acceptance are related qualities, with understanding fostering acceptance.

Hopefulness

We must accept finite disappointment, but never lose infinite hope.
—Martin Luther King Jr.

Responding empathically also requires being hopeful about clients and their future. Clinicians may sometimes understand and accept clients but not see a possibility for improvement. A counselor can understand and accept a father's pain and suicidality following his child's death, but an effective one will see his pain as changeable. Hope—both the father's and the counselor's—can be built by recognizing the father's ambivalence about suicide inherent in his choosing to disclose rather than hide his suicidality, remembering that there have been both good times and bad, and acknowledging the healthy aspects of his response (e.g., his ability to connect with his son enough to grieve and with his counselor enough to disclose these feelings). This hopefulness can engage clients and help them to recognize their ability to change.

Hope is not blind optimism, but instead implies a real awareness of both the problems that a client is experiencing and the possibility that things can be different. Hope can be a creative process, allowing clinicians to search for new and creative solutions (Rosler, Cohen-Chen, & Halperin, 2017). Such hopefulness can be built by identifying situational factors affecting the problem behavior, recognizing variations in the behavior across time, working with other people with similar problems, and considering predictors of successful outcomes.

Communicating Empathy

Feeling empathy for clients is necessary, but effective clinicians must also communicate their empathy to clients so that clients can feel heard and understood (Elliott et al., 2018).

Clients may enter treatment expecting to be judged. Given their own feelings of shame, clients might expect that their clinicians will also see them as shameful, bad, and unable to change. A couple just learning that they will be unable to attempt another in vitro fertilization, for example, needs to have their mixed feelings of pain, regret, confusion, and relief heard. Their clinician's empathy needs to be shared both verbally and nonverbally. Furthermore, clients must recognize this understanding. In fact, clients' ratings of empathy are better predictors of the strength of the therapeutic relationship and therapeutic outcomes than are ratings by expert observers or the therapists themselves (Elliott et al., 2011, 2018).

Effective therapists can communicate empathy while also challenging clients about unhelpful behaviors or beliefs. In other words, doing effective counseling and psychotherapy takes a fair amount of assertiveness. Clinicians may behave nonassertively because they have never had an effective assertive model, because they learned that assertiveness is gender-inappropriate for them, or because they confuse assertiveness and aggression. Nonetheless, good therapists challenge their clients while maintaining a good therapeutic relationship. They can identify optimal times to assertively address problems. For example, a new client may have problems parenting well, be in an emotionally abusive relationship, and be acutely suicidal. Effective clinicians would recognize each of these problems but respond to the suicidality first, making sure the client is stable before challenging the client about other concerns (G. K. Brown, Jeglic, Henriques, & Beck, 2006).

Workers in some fields, especially juvenile justice and substance abuse, sometimes believe that aggressive responses are necessary and therapeutic. However, hostile-confrontational approaches are less effective and fail in their empathy or timing; they are less effective in creating change than are less confrontational approaches (Karno & Longabaugh, 2005; Norcross & Wampold, 2011a).

What Do You Think?

1. What could you say to Andrea Yates that would express your empathic understanding without missing the larger context (i.e., that she killed her children)?

2. How does your response demonstrate understanding, acceptance, and hopefulness? If you struggled with one or more of these qualities, what can you do to develop that quality further?

3. Which of your responses would best engage Andrea to work willingly with you?

4. What might happen if your response toward her was judgmental or angry?

What Do Clinicians Do?

Today there are hundreds of thousands of clean and sober individuals living productive lives only because, in a moment of truth, a counselor was there and made the difference.
—Patrick J. Kennedy

To understand the role of empathy in therapy, it is important to understand what clinicians do. Clinicians are mental health professionals who provide **psychotherapy** or **counseling**. We use these two terms interchangeably in this text, but the bottom line is that therapy and counseling are processes in which a professional (e.g., psychologist, counselor) uses interventions based on psychological principles and adapted for the client to help that client resolve a personal, psychological, or familial problem (Wampold & Imel, 2015). That "client" could be an individual, couple, family, or group, and although the strategies used in therapy often involve two people talking to each other in an office, therapy could include more people, little talking, or primarily play rather than talk.

Clinicians **empower** clients, which means they help clients to recognize, accept, use, and develop their personal and political power to meet their goals. Clinicians share a personal commitment to help clients and often work as active partners in the change process. They listen empathically, creating an atmosphere where changing is safe. Their authority and expertise inspire faith and hope. Clinicians encourage their clients to examine themselves, their lives and their problems differently; help them better express their emotions, and identify effective strategies for meeting their needs. Clinicians challenge their clients, engender hope, build strengths, and increase the number of options clients perceive.

Family and friends can be helpful and therapeutic, but counseling and psychotherapy are more purposeful and structured in their approach (Murphy & Dillon, 2015). Unlike conversations with friends, therapeutic interventions are based on the theory and science of the field (e.g., with an awareness of how an intervention might empower a client or address the avoidance seen with PTSD symptoms). Similarly, clinicians often reflect on how they present themselves, sometimes carefully considering the ways they dress or decorate their office and the messages their choices send clients.

Clinicians listen carefully and empathically to people's verbal and nonverbal communication. They listen to what clients say or do not say (i.e., the **content** of clients' communication) as well as how they say it (i.e., the **process** of clients' communication; Murphy & Dillon, 2015). Careful listeners can hear many layers in superficially simple statements, such as Evita's comment "*School* went well today."

- Why does Evita emphasize the word *school*? Did other things not go well?
- Evita's breathing became more rapid when she talked about family, and she broke eye contact at that point. What does that mean?
- Why did Evita shift the discussion from family issues to school?

Although empathic listening requires careful attention to the client's words (content) and changes in nonverbal behavior, style of relating, and shifts in content discussed (process), it also involves paying attention to one's own thoughts, feelings, and behavior. What happened as Evita began discussing school? Did you become more interested or bored? Understanding one's own and others' interests, values, and issues may be useful in decoding the meaning of her behavior. Boredom may reflect her avoidance of any real issues and difficulty connecting with someone else, but it could also reflect the therapist's own fatigue, feelings about school, distraction by stressors, or difficulties in connecting with others. As is emphasized throughout this book, understanding oneself and one's own reactions can increase a clinicians' effectiveness and empathy.

The counseling and psychotherapy relationship occurs in a valuing and cultural context. The client's and clinician's cultures and values influence their choices about what they identify as problems and treatment goals as well as how they agree to meet these goals. Culture and values influence what people choose to do, how they do it, and how they think and feel about what they do. Most clinicians do not directly solve their clients' problems for them but work to empower them to make change. They help clients discover ways of solving problems for themselves that are consistent with their clients' own values and that their clients will be able to continue doing after the counseling or therapy process is complete.

Although they share many commonalities, different clinicians use different therapy models in their work. A **therapy model** is a theoretical framework about what causes mental health problems and what will resolve them. Different models see the causes, treatments, and often assessments of a person differently. For example, cognitive therapists believe that psychopathology is related to beliefs that are **maladaptive**—that is, not conducive to adapting to one's environment. Accordingly, for cognitive therapists, treatment typically consists of identifying and changing problematic thoughts. In contrast, behavior therapists attribute psychopathology to maladaptive behaviors, and behaviors are learned through conditioning. Thus, for behavioral therapists, treatment focuses on observing clients' behavior—or having clients observe their own behavior—and then changing the environment and reinforcement schedules to "pull" more adaptive behaviors. Exhibit 1.1 highlights these and some other common therapy models.

The Common Factors

Very early in my work as a therapist, I discovered that simply listening to my client, very attentively, was an important way of being helpful. So, when I was in doubt as to what I should do in some active way, I listened. It seemed surprising to me that such a passive kind of interaction could be so useful.

—Carl Rogers

Exhibit 1.1 Common Models of Psychotherapy

Biological model. In this model, symptoms are attributed to an underlying biological predisposition, including genetics, neurotransmitters, or hormones. From the perspective of this model, symptoms are most commonly addressed through medications addressing neurotransmitters but also through other treatments including transcranial magnetic stimulation and electroconvulsive therapy.

Psychodynamic model. The psychoanalytic model focuses on the difficulties people have in handling anxiety-provoking stimuli. Unhealthy personalities may be overly rigid and demanding (superego) or indulge every impulse (id), and they may do so by distorting reality (using defense mechanisms such as repression, denial, or projection). Healthy personalities acknowledge needs and fears, then respond to these in flexible, health-promoting ways (ego). Problems in resolving psychic challenges such as trust, autonomy, initiative, or industry may make it more difficult to resolve future developmental challenges (fixation). From the perspective of this approach, the goal of treatment is to help people identify, work through, and face anxiety-provoking stimuli in psychologically mature ways.

Cognitive model. This model considers the roles that people's thoughts have in their emotions and behaviors. In general, people who are depressed hold rigid and unreasonable expectations and beliefs about themselves, the world, and the future (cognitive triad). These thoughts are often dichotomous, ruminative, and unrealistic. Treatment should help people identify thoughts that are maladaptive, challenge those effectively, and use healthier ways of thinking.

Behavioral model. From the behavioral perspective, problems are created through classical, operant, and observational learning. Treatment should assess for environments and reinforcement schedules that maintain problem and structure environments to create more adaptive behaviors. During systematic desensitization, therapists help clients substitute relaxation for fear and anxiety.

Person-centered model. This model is foundational for most other approaches and argues that people experience problems when, to feel accepted by others, they become alienated from their real selves. Relationships that are accepting (unconditional positive regard), empathic, and genuine are healing and allow people to begin to listen to and accept themselves as they are.

Multicultural model. This model understands people and communities in terms of context (e.g., race, gender, class, and religion) and the oppression and privilege associated with context. Identifying these factors can help clients feel heard, choose culturally appropriate interventions, and acknowledge barriers to change. Like the person-centered approach, this model is readily incorporated into other therapeutic approaches.

About 75% of clients with most diagnoses improve during counseling and psychotherapy (American Psychological Association [APA], 2012). Psychotherapy appears to be equal in effectiveness to antidepressants for all but the most severe depressions—and may be better at preventing **relapse**, which is the recurrence of a disorder or disease after a period of improvement or apparent cure (DeRubeis, Siegle, & Hollon, 2008). A recent analysis went even further, reporting that when both published and unpublished data are considered, antidepressants are no more effective than placebos, at least for mild to moderate depression (Kirsch, 2014). A **placebo** is a treatment without an inherently active ingredient. Lambert and Archer (2006) concluded that

> psychological interventions have been found to be equal to or to surpass the effects of medication for psychological disorders and should be offered before medications (except with the most severely disturbed patients) because they are less dangerous and less intrusive. . . . At the very least they should be offered in addition to medication, because they reduce the likelihood of relapse once medications are withdrawn. (p. 115)

Although it is difficult to compare therapeutic approaches because practitioners from each approach tend to work with different problems and have different goals, therapy models that have widely different theoretical frameworks generally appear to be about equally effective under most conditions (Wampold & Imel, 2015). In fact, as early as 1936, Rosenzweig famously noted the essential equivalence of therapy approaches, quoting the Dodo bird's line in *Alice in Wonderland*, "*Everybody* has won, and *all* must have prizes" (p. 412, italics in original). So, if the specific components of each model differ, what makes these therapy models work?

In explaining the essential equivalence of therapeutic models, many writers have suggested that although change may be partly attributable to the components of a specific therapy model, it is almost certainly due more to other factors, including the **therapeutic alliance** (i.e., the cooperative working relationship between client and therapist), the clinician's personality, clinician–client match, catharsis, or the receipt of an acceptable explanation of the problem.

Researchers have focused on four broad categories of change agents; the first three of which have been described as **common factors** because they are shared by all effective therapeutic interventions, regardless of the therapy model (Constantino, Ametrano, & Greenberg, 2012; Horvath, Del Re, Flückiger, & Symonds, 2011; Lambert, 2015; Norcross & Lambert, 2018; Norcross & Wampold, 2011a; Weinberger, 2014). These include the following:

- **Client variables and extratherapeutic events** (40% of treatment improvement is attributed to this). Client variables include symptom type and number, ego strength, psychological mindedness, and motivation for change (Norcross & Lambert, 2011). Extratherapeutic factors in clients' lives (e.g., family and social support, self-help books, spiritual support, and chance events) are believed to account for the large number of people who change without formal treatment.
- **Therapeutic alliance** (30% of treatment improvement is attributed to this). Factors that strengthen the therapeutic alliance are important to many effective treatments; these factors include empathy, alliance, soliciting client feedback, positive regard, goal consensus, and collaboration (Lambert, 2015).

- **Expectancies for change** (15% of treatment improvement is attributed to this). If the client and clinician believe that the client will get better, then the client is more likely to get better. This includes contributions to change that are attributable to a sense of hopefulness and an awareness of being treated. Although sometimes denigrated as placebo effects, expectancies are now seen as active contributors to the change process that clinicians should intentionally foster (Constantino et al., 2012; Weinberger, 2014). In fact, Fraser and Solovey (2007) concluded that restoring hope is the ultimate goal of psychotherapy and the common thread of all clinical interventions.
- **Therapeutic models and techniques** (15% of treatment improvement is attributed to this). A relatively small, but important, contribution to change has been attributed to therapeutic models and interventions. Therapeutic models organize interventions and provide a consistent direction for treatment, while creating expectancies for change and strengthening the therapeutic relationship (Fraser & Solovey, 2007; Norcross & Lambert, 2011).

Weinberger (2014) argued that different types of psychotherapy achieve their effectiveness through these common factors rather than the techniques and principles generally identified as their active ingredients. These common factors probably influence change made in fields as diverse as education, religion, and medicine. The factor most highly attributed to therapeutic change—client variables and extratherapeutic events—is beyond clinicians' control, but the second most influential factor is heavily based on empathy. Therefore, this book focuses on empathy as a foundation for effective therapy.

Ethical Work

Ethics is nothing else than reverence for life.

—Albert Schweitzer

Competent, respectful, and empathic work is by nature also ethical. A profession's code of ethics provides a framework for practicing in an ethical manner. Think of a profession's code of ethics as a safety net for clinical work. For example, the APA's (2017a) *Ethical Principles of Psychologists and Code of Conduct* (APA Ethics Code) provides a framework for ethical practice, research, and education. Exhibit 1.2 highlights common themes in the APA Ethics Code, which are described in greater depth in Chapter 11.

The APA Ethics Code provides enforceable **standards** (requirements involving specific behaviors) as well as nonbinding **aspirational principles** (broader ideals that should inform a clinician's ethical decisions).

Essentially, the aspirational principles are guiding values, encouraging clinicians to help without harming clients; behave in trustworthy ways while

Exhibit 1.2 Some Common Themes in the APA Ethics Code

Informed consent is both a formal process, whereby clinicians provide clients with information to make informed decisions about their treatment, and an ongoing discussion about treatment decisions over the course of treatment. This informed consent process involves clients in decision-making during treatment and acknowledges their autonomy.

Confidentiality means disclosing client information to others only when the client gives permission or when legally required to do so (e.g., duty to warn, mandated reporting), as a way of building trust in the clinician–client relationship.

Competence includes the knowledge and skills to perform treatment with a particular person or group at a particular point in time. Competence fluctuates across time as skills, understandings, and physical and mental health also fluctuate.

Multiple relationships should be avoided when possible. Multiple relationships occur when a clinician has additional relationships with a client beyond that of clinician alone (e.g., being both therapist and friend, being both therapist and business partner). These relationships have incompatible or competing expectations, goals, or needs and can undermine treatment.

Conflicts of interest should be avoided when possible. Multiple relationships are one kind of conflict of interest because other interests or relationships could reasonably be expected to impair a clinician's objectivity, competence, or effectiveness.

recognizing one's responsibility to the greater society; behaving fairly, honestly, and justly without bias; and supporting clients' autonomy (APA, 2017a). In contrast, the ethical standards help one avoid or navigate situations that would otherwise be high-risk, reminding clinicians to provide informed consent, offer only services that one is competent to provide, maintain confidentiality, and avoid relationships with inherent conflicts of interest

Although only APA members are required to follow the APA Ethics Code (and violating the code may result in revocation of APA membership), most mental health agencies follow an ethics code and require all of their clinical staff, even unlicensed staff, to meet the standards in it. Some other ethics codes commonly used in mental health settings are those of the American Association for Marriage and Family Therapy (2015), American Counseling Association (2014; APA, 2017a), and National Association of Social Workers (2017). Clinicians should read their agency's or association's code of ethics regularly to understand and apply them more fully and carefully.

Our Model of Empathic Counseling

I am a human being, so nothing human is strange to me.

—Terentius

We have described empathy as a multifaceted thread, including understanding, acceptance, and hopefulness, that underlies a range of therapeutic behaviors and that predicts therapeutic success (Norcross & Lambert, 2018). Empathy, as one of the common factors in successful therapy, can be learned and may underlie the effectiveness of clinicians from diverse theoretical approaches and professions, including education, religion, and medicine.

Empathic counseling requires three sets of tools, which we lay out in Parts II, III, and IV of this book:

- **A sufficiently complex framework to understand people (Part II).** We will focus on the foundational roles of meaning systems (Chapter 2) and culture and context (Chapter 3) in helping us understand clients.
- **Strong, empathic clinical assessments (Part III).** We will build the skills to develop a strong therapeutic alliance with clients (Chapter 4), communicate empathy verbally (Chapter 5), assess clients in context (Chapter 6), and think critically about those assessments to recognize alternate explanations for observations (Chapter 7).
- **Skills to facilitate positive change (Part IV).** We will describe the skills to listen to clients' goals and use these goals to guide treatment (Chapter 8), identify empathic interventions to help people change (Chapter 9), and end treatment (Chapter 10).

After exploring the three tool sets for empathic counseling, we conclude the book by discussing a few professional issues underlying effective work over the long run (Part V). These issues include ethics (Chapter 11), clinical writing (Chapter 12), and self-care (Chapter 13).

Summary

Empathy is an affective and cognitive understanding of a person's experience from that person's unique point of view. It is accepting and hopeful, without ignoring problems and symptoms, communicated both verbally and non-verbally, and recognized by that person.

Mental health fields share a common belief that healing and growth occur most easily in the context of a relationship in which one person listens to the other with empathy. In fact, although about 75% of people change during the course of counseling and psychotherapy, a relatively small amount of the change observed is attributable to therapeutic models and interventions (15%). The vast majority of the change that clients make is shared by the common factors: (a) client variables and extratherapeutic events (40%), (b) the thera-peutic relationship (30%), and (c) expectancies for change (15%).

We outlined a model of empathic counseling that is the focus of this book. Specifically, clinicians need a way to think about and understand people, tools for developing a strong clinical assessment of individual clients, and techniques for working effectively with this case conceptualization to help clients make positive changes in their lives.

For Review

Applying Concepts to Your Life

Almost everyone has attempted to change at one point. Think about an important change you made and what helped you change.

1. What made it easier or more difficult to change? Compare your experience with that of your friends or fellow students. What do you discover?

2. If someone—a parent, friend, minister, teacher, or therapist—helped you change, what did he or she do? What characteristics or behaviors seemed particularly helpful?

3. Compare your experience with that of your friends or fellow students. Which of these characteristics would you like to further develop? What steps could you take to make these changes?

4. How has it felt when someone really understood you? How has it felt when you were misunderstood, especially about something important?

5. How do you recognize when you are being treated respectfully? Would being treated respectfully in counseling be different than in a helping relationship in another part of your life? If so, how?

6. If you would like to be more respectful of others, especially in the counseling and psychotherapy process, what changes would you need to make? What steps could you take to make these changes?

7. Although this book emphasizes paying attention to all dimensions of another person—words, vocal cues, nonverbal behavior, dress and grooming, and posture, among others—it necessarily emphasizes the spoken word. What can you do to increase your understanding of someone else's words? What can you do that goes beyond the spoken word?

Key Terms

aspirational principles, 15
clinician, 4
common factors, 14
content, 11
counseling, 11

counselor, 4
empathy, 4
empower, 11
genuine, 9
maladaptive, 12
meaning systems, 6

placebo, 14
process, 11
psychotherapy, 11
relapse, 13
standards, 15
states, 6

therapeutic alliance, 14
therapy model, 12
traits, 6
unconditional positive regard, 8

Learn More

For more information about the concepts in this chapter, visit the *Empathic Counseling* companion website at http://pubs.apa.org/books/supp/slattery/.

Part II

Building a Framework for Understanding People

To have empathy for another person, you need to be able to shift your perspective and see the world differently from how you might normally. You must understand how the other person views the world. How, though? The chapters in this part discuss two factors that influence a person's worldview: meaning systems and culture. These concepts will guide our discussions throughout the rest of this book because they are fundamental to empathic counseling. To really understand a client, a clinician must be curious and ask questions about the client's meaning system and culture.

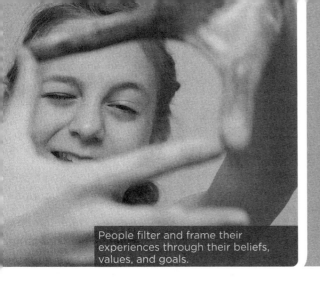

People filter and frame their experiences through their beliefs, values, and goals.

2 Understanding Meaning Systems

Looking Ahead III➡

After reading this chapter you will be able to answer these questions:

1. What are meaning systems?

2. How are meaning systems expressed in people's speech and behavior?

3. How can recognizing meaning systems strengthen clinical work and the therapeutic alliance?

4. How might failing to recognize your own meaning system interfere with treatment?

Cases in Empathy

We Talk About Real Life I Doug Muder

Doug Muder (born in the 1950s) is a lay minister in a very liberal Unitarian church. However, he was raised in a more conservative Lutheran church, which several of his family members continue to attend:

> I'm a Unitarian Universalist, but my Dad isn't. My parents seem quite happy in the same conservative branch of Lutheranism in which they raised my sister and me. It teaches the literal truth of the Bible, and its God is real, personal, and powerful. The God I met at home was more liberal than the God of my Lutheran grade school, but not by much. He was, at the very least, secure enough to be amused rather than threatened by my human attempts to be clever. At home, my heretical theological speculations

were always matters for discussion rather than reprimand. But nonetheless, God had spoken, and His word was law. If reason and conscience told me something different from what was written in the Bible, then I'd better think things through again. (Muder, 2007, p. 33)

Doug believes that social class and circumstance have influenced the form of religion that his family members have adopted and, through it, their meaning systems. For instance, his father was a factory worker who worked long hours making cattle feed, a smelly and noisy job that ruined his hearing. His was a harsh world. He went to work because he had to put food on the table.

In contrast, Doug's sister's world is easier. She went to college, entered a white-collar career, and married an engineer. Her husband, Ed, works long hours and travels. Ed's job is demanding but rewarding, and he also serves as finance chair of his church, which also seems to give him a sense of community and purpose. Their sons are in grade school and, although Ed loves them, he wishes he could spend more time with them. Doug describes attending the conservative Lutheran church with his sister and her husband, where the preacher's message seemed unrelated to their privileged life circumstances:

> I went to church with them. The sermon topic was "Resisting Temptation." In my mind I boiled the entire 20-minute sermon down to three words: Don't be bad.
> . . . Ed would have been so much better off in my church. We [preachers in my church] talk about real life, his real life. He didn't need to be told not to be bad. His issue wasn't Good versus Evil; it was Good versus another Good versus a third kind of Good. (Muder, 2007, p. 36)

Doug's religion helps him find purpose, solve the important questions in his life, and make decisions about what sort of Good to pursue. Although Doug believes his church would be more relevant to his brother-in-law's life, he cannot draw that same conclusion for his father: "The factory was not a competing Good. It was a necessary Evil" (Muder, 2007, p. 36).

Doug contrasts his father's life choices with those of his more privileged peers' children. Unlike his father, who has had limited choices besides working at the factory, many of Doug's peers encourage their children to find something in life that they love:

> [Among more privileged people], inspiration is the road to success. It's the way out of the maze. Or at least it's one way out, the bright way. . . . In the working class, the road to success is self-control. That's what you want to teach your children: Resist temptation. Walk the narrow path. Do the hard thing you don't want to do, so that you and the people who are counting on you won't be punished. (Muder, 2007, p. 37)

Doug worries about the harsh theology of more conservative churches, which "can justify harshness in this world" (Muder, 2007, p. 37). Nonetheless, for people living in a harsh world, a harsh theology can resonate with their experience of the world and address the real-world issues faced on a daily basis. He wonders whether choices of the kind that he wants for his own children are a luxury that ill-prepare working class youth for the harsh, very real world that they will face. He asks, what does church prepare one for, accepting where one is or searching for something better?

What Do You Think?

1. How does Doug Muder explain the differences between his church and the church his father, sister, and brother-in-law attend? How would these family members perceive his religious views?

2. Exhibit 2.1 lists some potential ways that religious and spiritual views might influence a clinician's work. If you become a clinician, how do you think your own beliefs might influence your work?

3. How might being aware of your meaning system and those of your clients influence your ability to be empathic with them?

Exhibit 2.1 Consider the Roles of Religion and Spirituality in Your Life and Practice

1. What kinds of experiences have you had with spirituality and religion throughout your life? Have they been primarily positive? Negative? Mixed?

2. What specific religious and secular beliefs and values are most important for you now? How might they be a source of connection or conflict between you and your clients?

3. How do you view human nature? Do you see people as good, evil, or able to become either?

4. Do you believe that people have free will? Can people make their own choices or are their thoughts, feelings, and behaviors determined by outside forces including God? How might this influence your work with clients?

5. Why do you believe bad things happen? Do you attribute bad things to God, evil spirits, poor choices, sin, karma, or chance? How might this influence how you see and work with clients?

6. In what ways do you believe religion and spirituality can be a source of strength for your clients? In what ways do you believe they can be a source of weakness?

7. What types of clients or problems involving religion or spirituality do you expect would be most challenging for you? Which would be the most engaging? Why?

Note. Data from Fukuyama and Sevig (1999).

Meaning Systems

> *We are what we think. All that we are arises with our thoughts. With our thoughts we make the world.*
>
> —*Buddha*

Far more occurs in one's experience than can possibly be sensed, understood, or remembered. People actively respond to this overwhelming amount of information by filtering and organizing it through their framework for understanding experiences—their **meaning system**, which includes their beliefs, values, and goals (Park, 2010, 2017a, 2017d). Meaning systems allow people to observe their current reality, imagine alternative realities, interpret the past, anticipate the future, consider their options and desires, and direct their energy and behavior accordingly. Because everyone's meaning system is unique, any two people—for example, Doug Muder and his father—can be in "the same situation" yet perceive and experience it very differently.

Meaning systems also limit what one can take in. Ideas and experiences that do not easily fit one's meaning system may be forced to fit into preconceived notions or even overlooked and excluded from awareness altogether. For example, people may be surprised when others do something apparently thoughtful or fail to notice it at all (because it does not fit with their beliefs about people as being unkind). Someone highly motivated by material wealth may be puzzled by someone's generosity or even attribute ulterior motives to it.

Paying attention to one's own meaning system and to those of others is important in many settings but especially so for clinical work. Recognizing meaning systems and their powerful and pervasive influences greatly enhances our ability to empathize. When clinicians understand their clients' meaning systems, they find it easier to create positive therapeutic relationships with them and can match interventions to their clients' beliefs, values, goals, and ways of thinking and behaving (Kim, Ng, & Ahn, 2005).

Components of Meaning Systems

We are usually convinced more easily by reasons we have found ourselves than by those which have occurred to others.

—Blaise Pascal

Meaning systems comprise people's beliefs about many aspects of the world, their values and goals, and their sense of meaning. Meaning systems have wide-ranging implications for people's lives. Throughout the day, everything we do reflects, to some degree, what we accept to be true, real, or valid (i.e., **beliefs**), what we see as important (i.e., **values**), and our purposes and desires (i.e., **goals**). These beliefs, values, and goals influence how we spend money, what material and nonmaterial goods we buy, how we dress, and whether we make eye contact. The next time you stand in a grocery line, look at your groceries. What do they say about your beliefs, values, and goals? Then look at the groceries of the people around you and consider this question.

Beliefs regarding control, for example, influence attempts and persistence at tasks (Bandura, 1997; Dweck, 2006). Many beliefs are unconscious or preconscious and might be available if deliberately focused on, but are rarely brought into awareness. The less available beliefs are to conscious awareness, the more difficult they are to recognize and challenge.

Values are also important aspects of meaning systems. Values are transsituational guiding principles in a person's life, influencing a broad range of their behaviors and choices and prescribing modes of conduct (e.g., being honest, helpful, or polite; S. H. Schwartz et al., 2012). Although values cannot be observed directly, they are reflected in behaviors, words, and thoughts. Values and goals do not translate perfectly into behavior, however, because of conflicting values and goals; lack of resources, time, skills, or opportunity; and other pressures.

Values direct goals, people's internal representations of desired processes, events or outcomes (Roberts & Robins, 2000). Goals refer not only to future aims but also to the maintenance of valued states or already-owned objects. Common life goals include relationships, work, wealth, health, knowledge, and achievement (Park, 2017a; Roberts & Robins, 2000). These goals are organized hierarchically, with higher level goals determining mid- and lower level goals (Vallacher & Wegner, 2012). Midlevel goals receive the most conscious attention and direct typical plans, activities, and behaviors. Feeling that one is progressing toward goals is an essential aspect of well-being; however, goal pursuits are often conflicted (Kelly, Mansell, & Wood, 2015; Klug & Maier, 2015). For example, many people report that career achievements and nurturing their families are both highly important goals but often struggle to direct enough time and energy to pursue both adequately (Shockley, Shen, DeNunzio, Arvan, & Knudsen, 2017).

Some goals are more **intrinsic**, important for their own sake, while others are more **extrinsic**, means for meeting some other sort of need such as belongingness, support, or prestige (Grouzet et al., 2005). People who choose more materialistic values and goals consume more products, incur more debt, have poorer interpersonal relationships, act in more destructive ways toward the environment, have weaker motivations for work and school, and report poorer personal and physical well-being (Kasser, 2016).

Extrinsic goals are less likely to be meaningful or congruent with the larger meaning system. Striving for personally meaningful goals is related to well-being, whereas striving for goals low in personal meaning can be pathogenic (Michalak & Grosse Holtforth, 2006). Of course, goals can be both intrinsic and extrinsic in nature. For example, reading and writing about philosophy can be intrinsically interesting and personally rewarding *and* put food on the table.

A well-constructed meaning system explains how and why things happen and promotes a sense that the world is coherent and understandable and one's identity within the world is clear (Heintzelman & King, 2014). Having a sense that one's goals are attainable and one is making good progress toward them promotes a sense of purpose. Collectively, such a well-functioning system of beliefs and goals produces a sense that life is meaningful (George & Park, 2016). People need a sense that life is meaningful to respond adaptively to their experiences (Heintzelman & King, 2014; Park, Edmondson, & Hale-Smith, 2013).

Stability and Change in Meaning Systems

Meaning systems are not static; they change during both normal development and following traumatic experiences (LoSavio, Dillon, & Resick, 2017). When confronted with information or situations that do not easily fit within their meaning systems, people experience change and uncertainty, anxiety, and distress. To defend against these negative feelings, people typically try either to assimilate or to accommodate the information. **Assimilation** means absorbing or incorporating the new information into one's existing meaning systems, whereas **accommodation** means radically reconceptualizing global beliefs and reconfiguring goals (Park, Currier, Harris, & Slattery, 2017). Nonetheless, meaning systems can shift with mere exposure to new people and ideas. For example, students going away to college may gradually perceive themselves as more capable and competent as a result of living independently and become more tolerant, open, and progressive through their interactions with a roommate from a different culture and exposure to new and different viewpoints (I. Gutierrez & Park, 2015).

The incidents that trigger large changes in meaning systems are often traumatic (Edmondson et al., 2011; Park et al., 2017). Trauma can violate fundamental global beliefs (e.g., "I am a good person so nothing bad can happen to me," "People are generally kind and benevolent") or confirm and strengthen maladaptive beliefs (e.g., "I am worthless, and bad things inevitably happen to me") and can render important goals unviable (e.g., "Being healthy and capable is important to me, but now I am permanently disabled"). Following such traumatic events, people may experience declines in meaningfulness (S. Y. Lee, Park, & Hale, 2016; Park, 2017c). However, trauma can also lead people to perceive positive changes; these perceived positive changes, sometimes called **posttraumatic growth**, may be experienced as changes in values, priorities, identities, and beliefs (e.g., "As a result of this experience, I have become stronger and more compassionate toward others' suffering"; Park, 2016, 2017b).

Although meaning systems are important to attend to in their own right, inconsistencies and conflicts in and among them are equally important. People may have competing values that are apparent in different contexts (e.g., at work and home) or may desire two apparently competing goals (e.g., parenting and career achievement). The desire to resolve or reduce discrepancies among beliefs, values, desires, and goals, as well as one's behavior and experiences, is often what brings people to therapy. Even flashbacks and ruminations associated with posttraumatic stress disorder may be attempts to resolve discrepancies (e.g., "I *should* trust him," and "I cannot trust anyone"; Gray, Maguen, & Litz, 2007; Price, MacDonald, Adair, Koerner, & Monson, 2016). Alternatively, such symptoms may reflect the inability of one's meaning system to respond to and keep anxiety symptoms at bay (Edmondson et al., 2011). Such discrepancies and conflicts are important to identify and work through in treatment (Park & Kennedy, 2017; Slattery & Park, 2011b, 2012).

Cases in Empathy

Building a Coherent Meaning System ▎ Tara Westover

Tara Westover (b. 1986) grew up in a White, Mormon family that was preparing for "end times" (the period leading up to Judgment Day, according to some religions). They withdrew from government services to the degree possible: They did not get driver's licenses or birth certificates, use medical services even in severe health emergencies, or attend school. Many people would identify her upbringing as emotionally and physically abusive, as well as physically neglectful, because her family repeatedly put Tara and her siblings in dangerous situations from a young age (e.g., having her work in the family scrapping business without safety gear) and failed to give her seriously ill siblings needed medical care.

From an early age, Tara sensed that her family's values were at odds with her own and, indeed, most of society's, although as a child she believed that her family's beliefs were the godly ones. She was homeschooled—more accurately, unschooled—because her parents didn't trust schools. She struggled to reject the messages she'd received about school, outsiders, and herself. In her memoir, *Educated*, she quotes her father as saying, "College is extra school for people too dumb to learn the first time around" (Westover, 2018, p. 41).

Because, as she matured, her beliefs and values began to conflict more and more with her family's, Tara faced some difficult ethical dilemmas. For example, when her brother Shawn had a motorcycle accident and incurred a second brain injury, her father told her to bring him home to be treated. She, instead, took him to the hospital. As she looked at her father's face in the hospital, she could tell he was disappointed in her.

> It hits me, a truth so powerful I don't know why I've never understood it before. . . . I am not a good daughter. I am a traitor, a wolf among sheep; there is something different about me and that difference is not good. . . . But wolf that I am, I am still above lying, and anyway he would sniff the lie. We both know that if I ever again find Shawn on the highway, soaked in crimson, I will do exactly what I have just done.
>   I am not sorry, merely ashamed. (Westover, 2018, pp. 147–148)

Sometimes her family gave her mixed messages, making it even harder to develop a coherent meaning system. One of the most damaging instances of mixed messages were those they gave her regarding her brother's abuse. Indeed, throughout her teen years, her brother had repeatedly pushed her head into the toilet; contorted her arm behind her back to force her into submission, once spraining her wrist in the process and threatening to shoot both her and her sister. Occasionally her mother named the abuse—she once said, "You were my child. I should have protected you" (p. 272)—but generally they blamed her.

> My parents said [Shawn] was justified in cutting me off. Dad said I was hysterical, that I'd thrown thoughtless accusations when it was obvious my memory couldn't be trusted. Mother said my rage was a real threat and that Shawn had a right to protect his [wife and son]. (Westover, 2018, pp. 291–292)

On the particular night in question, after Tara disclosed Shawn's threats against her and her sister, Shawn had killed his son's dog with a knife, then given Tara the bloody knife, encouraging her to kill herself rather than see what he would do to her.

Tara found it difficult to reconcile these conflicting family messages about her childhood, so she found herself revising her memory of events to be consistent with her meaning system. For example, in a later journal entry about one of Shawn's attacks, Tara denied her first interpretation of it: "It was a misunderstanding. . . . If I'd asked him to stop, he would have" (p. 196). Only when she was in college and on her own was she able to perceive her childhood as it had been. As she later said, "My life was narrated for me by others. Their voices were forceful, emphatic, absolute. It had never occurred to me that my voice might be as strong as theirs" (p. 197).

Later, in trying to understand her feelings about herself and her family, she wrote that

(TARA WESTOVER continued)

she now understood where her sense of shame came from:

> It wasn't that I hadn't studied in a marble conservatory, or that my father wasn't a diplomat. It wasn't that Dad was half out of his mind, or that Mother followed him. It had come from having a father who shoved me toward the chomping blades. . . . instead of pulling me away from them. It had come from those moments on the floor, from knowing that Mother was in the next room, closing her eyes and ears to me, and choosing, for that moment, not to be my mother at all. (Westover, 2018, p. 273)

What Do You Think?

1. What global beliefs and goals do you recognize in Tara's narrative?

2. In what ways did the abuse and neglect that she experienced violate her global beliefs about herself and her goals and create discrepancies? Consider the discrepancies that Doug Muder faces in his narrative.

3. In which aspects does she attempt to assimilate to close discrepancies and in which does she attempt to accommodate? What are the consequences of her strategies for closing these discrepancies?

4. If you had been referred by Child Protective Services to work with Tara Westover when she was a young teen, would you have challenged her beliefs about herself? Her family's beliefs about her? Why or why not?

5. What would you do to develop a therapeutic alliance with one or both parties? Why?

Meaning Systems in the Context of Therapy

> *You never really understand a person until you consider things from his point of view.*
> —*Harper Lee*

There is no consensus on the essential aspects of meaning systems. Some theorists have asserted that a small set of dimensions, such as benevolence and control, encompasses the critical elements of global beliefs (e.g., Ibrahim, 1985; Janoff-Bulman, 1989). Taking the opposite approach, Koltko-Rivera (2004) created a comprehensive model of 42 dimensions of global beliefs. Koltko-Rivera's model is far more complete but less useful in practice. Similarly, goals can be considered broadly (e.g., being motivated by intrinsic vs. extrinsic or self-transcendent vs. physical desires; Grouzet et al., 2005) or more specifically (e.g., achievement, spirituality, happiness, relationships, athletic performance; Park et al., 2016). The dimensions of global meaning discussed in this section are a compromise between these two extremes and chosen because of their relevance to the therapeutic process. Case material is presented to provide practice in understanding differing meaning systems.

Interpersonal Relationships

There is no such thing as society, only individual men and women and their families.
— Margaret Thatcher

Interpersonal relationships—with friends and family but also with clinicians—are often an important focus of treatment. How do clients treat their clinician, office staff, others in the office and in the balance of their life? Whom do they treat well? How are they treated? We describe two beliefs influencing interpersonal relationships: authority and individualism–collectivism.

Authority. How do clients expect to relate to the world and have the world relate to them? Some expect (beliefs) or want (goals) hierarchical relationships, with a clearly defined leader and chain of command, and others expect and want shared and egalitarian interactions with rotating or fluid leadership (Koltko-Rivera, 2004). In **egalitarian** relationships, the therapist and client share power over treatment decisions and goals. Cultures and individuals vary on this dimension. Asian Americans, Latin Americans, and Native Americans tend to prefer hierarchical relationships, with men having more power and authority than children, with women more intermediate (Sue & Sue, 2016). Nonetheless, whereas European Americans often value more assertive and egalitarian relationships, for example, others may be relatively cooperative, compliant with authority figures, and people-pleasing.

Clients differ in their preferences for **directiveness** in treatment, or the degree to which the clinician has control over treatment goals and direction. Those preferring more egalitarian relationships may resent being treated in an authoritarian manner because they may experience directive clinicians as implying that they are incompetent. Others may expect and prefer hierarchical and directive relationships. Asian Americans whose clinicians match and understand their more hierarchical and collectivistic beliefs, for example, are more likely to feel understood and to develop a more positive therapeutic alliance (Kim et al., 2005). Such clients may perceive clinicians who are not active and directive as incompetent.

When clients prefer hierarchical and directive relationships, clinicians must anticipate and address a potential downside. Clients may be reluctant to disagree with their clinicians or hide problems unless directly asked about them. Clinicians may see this behavior style as passive or resistant when it may, in fact, be culturally normative and respectful (Chen & Davenport, 2005; O'Connor, 2005). Although clinicians should acknowledge that they are the experts about treatment, Chen and Davenport encouraged clinicians to communicate to their clients, especially Asian American clients, that clients, themselves, are the experts on their own experience.

For many people, authority is also conflated with other factors: benign benevolence, power, perpetration and trauma, or unearned privilege

(D'Arrigo-Patrick, Hoff, Knudson-Martin, & Tuttle, 2017). These associated meanings of authority should be identified and, when appropriate, challenged in treatment when they cause or maintain problems. Identifying and addressing these meanings can be difficult, however because they might make a client such as Tara Westover unsafe. Further, validating abuses of power requires becoming aware of real social inequities and the privileges, authority, and power that clinicians enjoy but their clients do not (Miller, 2005).

Individualism–collectivism. Imagine: Sara wants to go to college to major in education, but her family needs her help to put food on the table. How is such a conflict between individual and group goals resolved? **Individualism** is a tradition, ideology, or personal outlook that prioritizes self-actualization, self-reliance, personal rights, personal privacy, competition, achievement orientation, emotional distance from family and group members, and individual pleasure (Triandis & Gelfand, 1998). **Collectivism** is a tradition, ideology, or personal outlook that prioritizes group goals ahead of individual ones and emphasizes interdependence over independence, family connections over emotional distance, and sociability over individual needs. Individualistic cultures emphasize self-reflection, whereas collectivistic cultures deemphasize it and focus on attending to and maintaining social norms. When making a choice between school and work, Sara would focus on her family's needs and deemphasize or ignore her own needs and desires if she were more collectivistic in orientation. If she were more individualistic, she would tend to assert her individual beliefs, values, and goals over those of her family and community.

Although the distinction between collectivist and individualist has been useful and frequently cited, Voronov and Singer (2002) observed that people from collectivist cultures behave more individualistically in some situations than in others. Many individuals and cultures show a mix of both individualistic and collectivistic attitudes (e.g., being cooperative yet self-reliant). Voronov and Singer suggested that people from collectivist cultures may sacrifice their self-interest for the group's benefit in the short term when they can reasonably expect rewards for doing so in the long run.

Sources of Information

People differ widely in the ways they go about understanding the world. Some focus primarily on their own sensory data, and others on authority figures, science, or spiritual sources to learn about the world (Slattery, 2004). They may resist or be openly antagonistic to other types of information or explanations. Assessing their clients' style of understanding the world can help clinicians find effective ways to frame clinical interventions (Shafranske, 2005).

For example, the following people consider their depressive symptoms differently:

Cheryl: I am depressed each fall as the days get shorter. My depression seems to be especially bad each year right around the time that my mother died [sensory observation].

Justin: Depression is a genetic disorder that seems to run in families and affects neurotransmitters in the brain. There is strong evidence that drugs increasing the availability of catecholamines decreases depression. What is the evidence for the antidepressant that you're suggesting [scientific information]?

Tosha: My mother says the women in our family get depressed at menopause [familial authority].

Marjane: I have been praying for an end to my depression. I will take my Prozac because you tell me to, but the depression will end when it's God's will [religious authority].

These explanations are not mutually contradictory; Marjane, for example, listens to medical authorities, although is skeptical about their advice. Nonetheless, people often rely on some approaches at the expense of others. People may also rely on a particular source of information in some situations but use a different source in situations when it seems more relevant (e.g., a scientist who relies on observations and the scientific method at work, but uses her mother's advice for parenting decisions). Tara Westover, for example, sometimes listened to religious and familial authorities and their explanations of behavior but listened to her professors at other points.

Safety and Benevolence of the World and Other People

Safety and benevolence of the world is an important aspect of clients' global beliefs (A. A. Cooper, Zoellner, Roy-Byrne, Mavissakalian, & Feeny, 2017). Do they see the world as a safe and benevolent place? Is their world dangerous, with others out to hurt them? Clients like Tara Westover, who have had a defining experience in which others were perceived as unsafe or hurtful, often have difficulty trusting others and seeing them as reliable (Price et al., 2016). These perceptions can cause problems in relationships.

People may reveal their beliefs about the benevolence of the world by their behaviors. How big is their personal space? How far do they sit from others in the waiting room? When do they make eye contact and when do they avoid it? What happens when they are accidentally touched? Such observations can provide important cues about clients' interpersonal trust and their beliefs about the world's—and other people's—benevolence.

Why Bad Things Happen

People entering therapy often wonder why bad things happened to them (Janoff-Bulman, 1989). They may become more depressed and pessimistic, concluding that the world has no meaning, or believe that life is capricious. For example, trauma can shatter previously hopeful and optimistic views of the world, even though many trauma survivors can recover and some may even experience a greater sense of meaning (Park et al., 2017).

Many people subscribe to the belief that they get what they deserve and deserve what they get (i.e., the **just-world theory**; Lerner, 1980). For example, Anna McCloy, in talking about her husband, the only survivor of the Sago mining disaster, made the following statements while she waited to discover her husband's fate:

> He's always told me that no matter what, he knew he was in a dangerous job, and if something happened, he said, he would survive *because he had two kids and a wife that he loved and he would take care of.* (Gately, 2006, para. 11, italics added)

Others attribute events to the person's *behavior* rather than to their personality (Janoff-Bulman, 1989). From this perspective, events happen because of factors that we either set into motion or that we failed to prevent. Like the just-world theory, this belief leads victims (and their families and friends) to blame themselves (or the victim). This blame is for different reasons, however, and is often of the "should have, could have" type rather than because clients see themselves as bad, and behavioral self-blame tends to be less associated with posttraumatic stress than does characterological self-blame (Peter-Hagene & Ullman, 2018). This difference in causal attributions can be an important clinical distinction. An **attribution** is a belief about the cause of behavior, or a person's quality or trait. Attributing problems to behavior rather than to personality provides a sense of control and prevents depression (Shapiro, 1995). It also provides clearer behavioral change targets when planning treatment goals.

When describing what happened in the Sago mining disaster and what they would have to do to get back on track, Ben Hatfield, CEO of International Coal Group, made both just-world attributions (i.e., "good people") and focused on the miners' and the company's behavior (i.e., "to do the right thing"):

> We are hardworking people that count on good people to do their job. And we believe we attract skilled miners that want to make this company successful. We want to make this company successful. And so we will do all we can to motivate efforts to that end.
>
> But the people that work for this company and know us, know the management team and know that our intentions are to do the right thing and to protect our people as best we can in what is a fairly dangerous business. (News Conference with CEO of International Coal Group, 2006, para. 62–63)

Finally, others may believe their fate is due to chance events, that life is random, and that there is no way of making sense of why things happen (Janoff-Bulman, 1989). Hatfield's statement included a sense of that when he observed mining was "a fairly dangerous business." The following comments focus on life's randomness and unpredictability:

> Rick Caskey (runs a mining technology program at a community college): There's always things that you don't foresee. You know, methane is odorless, colorless, and tasteless. (Samson, 2006, para. 14)

People often use their religious or spiritual beliefs to explain why trauma happens, although people may give very different explanations and draw different meanings based on their religious views (Park, 2013; Park et al., 2017). Major life events, however, can shatter the meaning-making systems of clients, regardless of how religious they are (S. Y. Lee et al., 2016). Religious clients may ask, "Why me, God?" and lose their faith. Nonreligious clients may challenge previously held assumptions about the world and begin searching for meaning, spiritual or otherwise. Trauma can change or foreshorten expectations about the future (Ai & Park, 2005) or, as with Viktor Frankl's (1946/1984) experiences in Auschwitz, deepen a sense of meaning and commitment to new goals or a rededication to already-held ones.

Clinical Applications	Jade recently lost her job at a local human services agency and has been increasingly depressed. She said, "It feels like nothing matters any more. All I can do is think about what I've lost. I think that everyone sees me the way that my boss saw me." What is she saying about her past sense of meaning? What is she saying that she needs? How might you want to respond? Why?

Identity

Men often become what they believe themselves to be. If I believe I cannot do something, it makes me incapable of doing it. But when I believe I can, then I acquire the ability to do it even if I didn't have it in the beginning.

—Mohandas Gandhi

Self-perceptions influence the degree to which people see the world as safe (Hart, Shaver, & Goldenberg, 2005; Janoff-Bulman, 1989). For example, clients may both believe that people get what they deserve (Lerner, 1980) and also see themselves as good, moral, and worthy, and thus relatively safe from hardship.

Trauma or significant illness can redefine a client's sense of identity and self-worth in a variety of ways (Bernard, Whittles, Kertz, & Burke, 2015). For example, Randal McCloy, the lone survivor in the Sago mining disaster, might conclude that good things happen to him (because he alone survived), that bad things happen (because he was injured and so many others perished), or that he was lucky or unlucky in the disaster and his subsequent treatment. Although some of his interpretations depend on his preexisting meaning system, the meaning-making process that he and others take in the period after the disaster will also influence it.

Approaches to Problems and Problem-Solving

How people perceive problems influences whether they believe that they can change and how. Do they see a problem? If so, what sort? Do they believe it can change? If so, under what circumstances? What do they believe caused the problem? Something inside themselves? Something outside? Do they believe they can do things to change, or does the change have to come from elsewhere? Or is change simply impossible?

Responsibility and control. Perceiving control for past and future events have different implications for therapy and can be usefully distinguished. People who believe that they could have prevented something bad (and did not) are more likely to be depressed; people who believe they can control their recovery and prevent future trauma are less likely to become depressed (Frazier, Mortensen, & Steward, 2005). **Locus of responsibility** is the degree to which a person believes she is responsible for past events and conditions in her life, whereas **locus of control** is the degree to which a person believes she can control future events and conditions in her life.

People can be described as having either an internal or external locus of responsibility and an internal or external locus of control (Sue & Sue, 2016). People with an **internal locus of responsibility** take responsibility for past problems and blame themselves; those with an **external locus of responsibility** blame others or environmental factors. For example, rape survivors who blamed themselves for the assault withdrew from others, leading to more distress (Frazier et al., 2005). Conversely, people with an **internal locus of control** believe that they can control recovery and prevent future trauma; those with an **external locus of control** attribute control over future outcomes to others (or society) and recognize little control for themselves.

People with an internal locus of control believe they are able to control their lives and prevent problems. They are more self-confident and socially engaged and more frequently use cognitive restructuring to cope with stressors (Frazier et al., 2005). They are also less likely to be depressed than are people with an external locus of control (Culpin, Stapinski, Miles, Araya, & Joinson, 2015; Sue & Sue, 2016). People who have low self-esteem and feel that the world is random experience more distress and more negative outcomes (Ginzburg, 2004).

People differ in their general perceptions of control, but specific control appraisals they make in a given situation vary widely. For example, a client may feel she is in control of her health but that she can do little to influence the behavior of her children. Even within a given situation, people may feel they have control over some aspects of the situation and not others. For example, people with cancer can identify positive ways of controlling some aspects of their health or well-being and participating in their treatment while also coming to terms with the notion that they do not have total control over treatment outcomes (Carney & Park, 2018).

Self-efficacy. Another dimension on which people vary is their **self-efficacy**, or belief in their ability to perform a task or make changes. This sense of efficacy increases with perceived success and decreases with perceived failure (Bandura, 1997; Dweck, 2006). Self-efficacy can be domain-specific, so a woman may feel confident in her ability to become a better athlete but believe her mood swings are genetically caused and unchangeable (Bandura, 1997). Word choice can signal a person's level of commitment to change (e.g., "I'm not sure I want to do this," "That's it; I'm done using") and can usefully predict outcomes in substance abuse work (Amrhein, Miller, Yahne, Palmer, & Fulcher, 2003; Norcross, Krebs, & Prochaska, 2011; Thomas, 2005). Self-efficacy is related to adaptive coping, whereas feelings of helplessness are related to depression (Brennan, 2001).

Continuing in the face of failure requires a shift in meaning. Inaction might be due to expectations of negative consequences (C. J. Anderson, 2003). Failing to initiate change could be a defensive strategy to protect oneself from regret, anxiety, or other anticipated consequences associated with change. Helping clients gather more information; reevaluate their values, goals, and beliefs; and address perceived obstacles can foster change and increase self-efficacy in that realm (Norcross et al., 2011).

Time Orientation

Psychological theories vary in their **time orientation**, or preference toward past, present, or future thinking. Psychoanalysis has traditionally focused on childhood events. Gestalt therapy, family therapy, and behavior therapy are more present-focused and less interested in the ultimate cause of problems than in what maintains them. Career counseling is more future-focused, attending to present behaviors as a means of meeting future goals.

Cultures also vary in their time orientation. Buddhist-influenced cultures emphasize living mindfully in the present. Some Eastern cultures honor ancient tradition and ancestors who died centuries earlier. Upper-class and upper-middle-class members of Western cultures tend to worry about the past and anxiously plan for the future, whereas people from lower class groups often have a foreshortened view of the future and are more fatalistic (Zimbardo & Boyd, 1999).

Native Americans, Latin Americans, and Hmong typically see time as more elastic and punctuality as relatively unimportant relative to European Americans (Slattery, 2004), whereas European Americans more typically see time as a commodity to be saved and spent wisely, earning important dividends in the future. Punctuality is important and tardiness is often seen as a passive aggressive statement about an activity's perceived value. Clinicians and clients holding different orientations about time can easily misinterpret each other's actions and become frustrated or angry. For example,

Harris: You're late. Again. It doesn't seem like you really value our time together. I wonder whether you really want to get better.

Dafne: Where do you get that? My car is just so unreliable. I'm here, aren't I?

Harris's interpretation might have been on track (although certainly not tactfully expressed). In failing to acknowledge that Dafne does not have the same objective level of control over her time as he has, nor the resources and ability to plan ahead, he acted out and damaged their relationship. Imagine if he had instead reacted like this:

Harris: You're late again. It seems like you're having a hard time getting here so we have our full hour together. I wonder what that's about.

Dafne: I *am* having a hard time. My car is just so unreliable. (pause) It's hard thinking about working on what I'm going to do when I get off Welfare when, frankly, I just don't see it. I just feel like all I can do is get by from day to day.

Time orientation can differ on the dimension of productivity ("doing-future") versus spontaneity ("being-present"; Koltko-Rivera, 2004). People with doing approaches tend to be more interested in earning worth through productivity, whereas those with being approaches experience more flow, find tasks more intrinsically interesting, and are more self-aware and absorbed in the task at hand (Csikszentmihalyi, 2014). On the other hand, engaging in higher levels of temporal distancing—imagining how one might experience a negative experience in the future—is associated with greater confidence in one's coping resources, experiencing less intense negative emotions and more positive emotions, less rumination, and greater well-being (Bruehlman-Senecal, Ayduk, & John, 2016).

Time orientation influences a wide variety of behaviors, including goal-setting and achievement, sensation-seeking and risk-taking, and guilt and rumination. Even health behaviors, body mass, choice and number of sex partners, use of safe sex practices, and substance use are all, to some extent, influenced by time orientation (J. Adams & White, 2009; Zimbardo & Boyd, 1999). Students from a fatalistic, present-oriented culture might run into problems in school, for example, a setting that rewards people for engaging in sometimes tedious or boring activities for anticipated, but uncertain, positive consequences (Zimbardo & Boyd, 1999).

Our actions derive from past experiences, present appraisals, and expectations about future options. People may differ in which time frame they emphasize and why (Bandura, 1997; Zimbardo & Boyd, 1999). Some might

Table 2.1 Successful and Unsuccessful Past, Present, and Future Time Orientations

Time orientation	Unsuccessful	Successful
Past	Focused on past harm or victimization. May be unable to see the present clearly or anticipate a positive future.	Has a sense of tradition and roots that create a sense of positive identity.
Present	Either engages in hedonistic activities that have a high risk of self-harm or fatalistically withdraws. Is self-focused or self-absorbed. Time drags.	Approaches daily life through genuine, joyful or playful interactions. Lives in present rather than postponing satisfaction for future rewards. Loses self-awareness and becomes absorbed in task at hand. Time flies.
Future	Is worried or anxious about the future; puts off present needs in favor of future goals.	Sets goals and plans for the future. Future orientation gives meaning to current work and strivings.

Note. Data from Csikszentmihalyi (2014) and Zimbardo and Boyd (1999).

focus on the present, for example, as a way of avoiding the future or because they do not see one. They may tell stories about past and anticipated victimizations or "what might happen if . . ." Most people spend at least some time in each time frame, however. The important issues are how much time is spent in each as well as how that time is spent. Table 2.1 describes positive and negative aspects of each time orientation.

Recognizing Values and Goals

People may be unable to directly articulate their values and goals in therapy. Sometimes, as in the following excerpt, values and goals can be inferred through topics avoided, language used, juxtaposition of topics discussed, and nonverbal behaviors displayed (Mozdrzierz et al., 2009; A. Rogers, 2001).

Bonnie 1: (eyes averted) I can't feel anything but empty toward Ben. I know staying with him is the wrong thing. I just can't get past the abuse, no matter how much he says he's changed. (long pause while wringing her hands) I just don't want to hurt my children . . .

Jon 1: It sounds like you're of two minds. You feel used and abused in your marriage but also want to do the right thing by your children. You don't see how you can be happy—and you've tried to make the marriage work for a long time—and also be a good mom.

Bonnie 2: (looks up, hands still) Yes. Exactly.

Jon 2:   It feels like you're setting this up as a choice—your happiness or your children's.

Bonnie 3:   (looks down) Yes. I don't know what else to do.

Bonnie perceives a goal conflict (B1), which Jon identifies (J1). Her values are revealed in several other ways—hand movements and physical activity, points at which she makes and breaks eye contact, and pauses. Values are also communicated by other nonverbal behaviors (e.g., smiles, grimaces, gestures), paralanguage (e.g., intonation, cadence, speed, and volume of voice), and actions. Values and goals are expressed differently in different contexts, depending on their salience at the time. Bonnie might be calmer when her husband has been out of town (able to focus on her needs, while feeling like a good mother) but anxious when he is back in town and critical of how her "selfishness" affects their children.

People may avoid, distract, project, or otherwise distort their experience, depending on their own self-perceptions, the listener's reactions, and the context (Mozdrzierz et al., 2009; A. G. Rogers, 2001). When discussing personally meaningful issues, people often talk about value conflicts and unsettled aspects of their lives. For example, when Bonnie complained about her "emptiness" toward her husband (B1), she was both describing a problem and identifying what she expects and wants in relationships (i.e., warmth and closeness). If she were to fail to see emptiness as a problem—perhaps because that was what all relationships in her family were like—she would not discuss it.

Nonverbal behaviors can have several meanings, so throughout this book, we emphasize that clinicians' initial hypotheses should be tentative and supported by careful observations. For example, people break eye contact during conversations for at least two reasons: because of embarrassment or shame and because breaking eye contact allows focused thought on difficult ideas (Doherty-Sneddon & Phelps, 2005). As a result, Jon started his paraphrases with "It sounds" and "It feels."

What Do You Think?

1. What do you value most in your life? What is less important or unimportant to you?

2. How well do those values translate into your goals? Do you spend time, money, and effort in proportion to your goals' importance? How can you make your values and goals align better?

3. Imagine that you only had the outcomes or qualities on your list of goals. Would you be satisfied? If not, what else would you need to be happy?

4. Does your context influence your values and goals? Have there been times when a value may have been particularly important and other times when it was less important?

Meaning Systems Inform Situational Meanings

Individuals' meaning systems inform the **situational meanings** that they assign to their experiences (Park, 2010). These situational meanings are appraisals of a specific event or situation as a loss, threat, or challenge; causal attributions for why the event occurred (e.g., God's will, coincidence); determinations of the extent to which the events or situations are discrepant with one's global goals; and decisions regarding what can be done to cope. Global meaning and situational meanings differ in the breadth of their implications, and thus in their effects on treatment. For example, a woman who has been fired from her job might believe that she is to blame and that her job loss will be a devastating blow to her future. Treatment may need to address her self-blame and her tendency to catastrophize about the job loss and its ongoing effects. Others may draw a different situational meaning, focusing on the shaky financial footing of the agency and newfound freedom to pursue more satisfying and lucrative career opportunities. Loss of a job that is deeply connected to one's calling and profession could be devastating and threaten a person's central identity and purpose, whereas loss of a temporary and easily replaceable job may barely register as stressful.

By influencing how people interpret specific situations, meaning systems can have many influences on behavior. For example, a person who believes that others cannot be trusted might withdraw from others and put on a happy face, while avoiding all but superficial relationships, or the person may attack first, as Reymundo Sanchez (Lil Loco), described shortly, often did. Understanding our clients' meaning systems helps predict their behavior; recognizing the role of situational and contextual directives and constraints, as well as their beliefs about appropriate and effective action in a particular situation, makes those predictions more accurate and useful. A man who withdraws may believe that contact with others will leave him hurt (low trust, low self-efficacy, external locus of control). Lil Loco, however, seemed to believe he could only stay safe by attacking first (low trust, high self-efficacy, internal locus of control).

Although meaning systems may be important determinants of action, particular situations, such as a church service, a family dinner, or a party, can elicit different behaviors. People can also perform the same behavior for different reasons. They can enter therapy because they were court-mandated to do so, because they see it as the most expedient thing to do, or because they truly choose to be there. Effective interventions must be based on (a) a strong assessment of an individual's meaning system, but also (b) interactions among relevant aspects of his or her global beliefs and goals, (c) perceptions of the applicability of values and goals to a given situation, (d) beliefs about options in that situation, and (e) the situational context.

Clinical work often directly or indirectly addresses conflicts in goals, beliefs, or values. Bonnie may be unhappy in her marriage but stay because she is afraid of disappointing her family and hurting her children (valuing her family's happiness and children's welfare more than her own). Her husband may be outraged that she wants a divorce because it is "the influence of the devil" or "a sin" (reflecting religious beliefs and the goal of living within religious teachings). Identifying and findings ways to work through these discrepancies in beliefs or conflicts in values or goals is often a central aspect of helping clients move. Why hasn't Bonnie moved out? She may experience a goal conflict preventing her from acting on her stated intentions, but she may also lack the requisite skills and resources to change. Clarifying her goals can help her feel more fully heard and identify strategies for working through the conflict.

Cases in Empathy

Never Bothered to Consider the Consequences |
Reymundo Sanchez

Reymundo Sanchez was born in Puerto Rico in 1963. His father, who had married a woman more than 40 years younger than he, died when Reymundo was 4. With the death, Reymundo lost his father's advice and support. Soon after his father's death, his mother remarried. While his mother and stepfather honeymooned, Reymundo stayed with his aunt and cousins. He was brutally beaten by his aunt and cousins and raped by his oldest cousin; the sexual abuse continued until his family moved to Chicago when he was 7. There, his mother gave birth to a daughter and, when her second husband disappeared, she remarried, giving birth to a son. His life got considerably more difficult with each new child.

> [My stepfather] became an asshole. He would do things like padlock the refrigerator so that only his daughter could drink milk. He would hang a box of crackers from a rope high up on the ceiling so that we couldn't have any. All of his anger was taken out on us. (Sanchez, 2000, p. 5)

He had hoped that his mother would protect him, but, at best, she stood back from the abuse. As he got older, she also became physically abusive. His friend Papo called her a bitch for beating him, but Reymundo came to her defense because he believed he should honor his mother no matter what. His mother's name and actions were above question.

When his mother became pregnant again, his stepfather moved the family back to Puerto Rico. Reymundo lived there for 6 months until his mother sent him back to Chicago because she was tired of breaking up fights between her husband and son. There he briefly lived with Hector, his stepbrother, who dealt drugs but largely left Reymundo alone. When Hector moved, Reymundo was again homeless and scrambled for a place to stay—sometimes with a girlfriend, sometimes with a surrogate mother (who was sometimes sexual with him), sometimes with the gang, and sometimes on the streets.

Against this background of abuse and neglect, Lil Loco, as he came to be called, internalized his parents' attitudes about him and looked for ways to feel better. He said,

> All the problems of the world were unimportant compared to mine. Feeling sorry for myself also became an excuse for accepting failure. Like my mother, I blamed everything and anything. Nobody felt the

pain I felt. Nobody else suffered but me. That way of thinking became imbedded in my mind and became my way of life for a long time. (Sanchez, 2000, p. 33)

Some things helped, at least for a while. One of these was sex. A 35-year-old woman seduced him when he was 13 (only later did he see this as abuse), and Lil Loco began turning to sex to fill the emotional void. Drugs, at first only marijuana, also helped:

> When I was high I could think about doing evil things and feel good about it. I would imagine killing Pedro and my mother over and over again, and be forgiven. . . . Marijuana became my way out of the horrible reality that was my life. (Sanchez, 2000, p. 31)

Finally, his membership with a gang gave him a feeling of belonging and respect.

> I enjoyed the way crowds . . . would part when I walked through. No matter how long the cafeteria line was, I could be first if I wanted to. I could sit in the stairway, smoke a joint, and be warned of any authority figure coming. It never crossed my mind that it was others' fear that made me popular. I never bothered to consider the consequences. (Sanchez, 2000, p. 167)

Lil Loco was expected to perform hits on other gangs and was lauded and given special privileges when he acted bravely and violently. Signs of weakness or cowardice were punished. He quickly learned what he needed to do to stay in the group's best graces. Initially, his gang involvement was mostly positive, but when he was set up to be murdered, saw his friends killed, and had nightmares about murders he had performed, his involvement felt more negative, and he stayed in the gang out of fear: "I was too scared to face the world as the person I really was. Being a King gave me a role to play, friends, a lifestyle—everything I wanted." (Sanchez, 2000, p. 181). Besides, there were lots of perks to being a King:

> [Cocaine] got me accepted in places I had never dreamed of entering. I got just about every woman I desired and had many Kings willing to lose their lives for me. I was so busy manipulating others that I didn't realize I was also becoming a cocaine junkie. (Sanchez, 2000, p. 256)

What Do You Think?

1. Describe Lil Loco's meaning system. What are his core beliefs, values, and goals? How did Lil Loco justify his actions? How are these justifications related to his beliefs? What were his values and goals? To what degree did Lil Loco experience a sense of purpose and meaning? How do you know?

2. How are his global beliefs and goals related to his early experiences of poverty, physical and sexual abuse, and neglect? Consider how cultural factors such as *respeto*, *machismo*, and *familism* influenced how Lil Loco responded to these risk factors. See Exhibit 2.2.

3. If you were assigned to work with Lil Loco and did not speak Spanish, would you see that as an ethical problem? Why or why not? Would it matter that he had learned English and could speak it relatively fluently?

4. If Lil Loco reported having murdered someone of another gang, what would you do? Why? What if he instead had said that he was *planning* on killing someone? Frame your response in terms of our discussions of ethics.

5. Would there be any conflict between your personal and professional ethical standards with regard to these questions? How would you resolve these questions?

Exhibit 2.2 Latinx Cultural Values and Norms

Collectivism. Group needs tend to supersede individual needs. In addition, people are expected to sacrifice their needs for the greater good of the group.

Familism. Reflects strong identification with and attachment to the nuclear and extended families, including feelings of loyalty and reciprocity among family. This is a special case of collectivism, with people expected to sacrifice individual needs for needs of the family (e.g., taking a job that will provide better for the family, even though less individually satisfying).

Personalismo. Preferring personal relationships over impersonal ones. Expects that knowing someone will be personal rather than primarily based on external factors, such as occupation or socioeconomic status (e.g., may perceive helper as a family member or friend).

Respeto. Requires deferential and respectful treatment of a powerful person or person in authority. Conversely, personal power is derived from being treated respectfully.

Simpatía. Behaviors promoting pleasant, harmonious, and conflict-free relationships (e.g., withholding HIV status to maintain harmony).

Machismo. Emphasizes manly courage and honor. Signs of power and virility include exaggerated male stereotypical behaviors (i.e., aggressiveness, stubbornness, and inflexibility with men and arrogance and sexual aggressiveness with women).

Marianisma. Values traditional roles and idealizes women's work caring for the home and family. Women are seen as morally superior and needing protection (a manifestation of *respeto*). Can include an acceptance of fate and of men's *machismo* as the will of God.

Bien/mal educado. *Bien educado* is a compliment, indicating that parents raised children to become well behaved and respectful. Conversely, *mal educado* implies that the family members did not fulfill their responsibility to teach a child to behave well.

When Clients and Clinicians Have Different Meaning Systems

Clients who see their global beliefs and goals as being more similar to their clinicians' meanings systems perceive more empathy from and stronger therapeutic alliances with their clinicians (Kim et al., 2005; Lilliengren & Werbart, 2005). This perceived empathy facilitates change. However, clients and clinicians often differ in their beliefs, values, and goals, which can affect treatment (Farnsworth & Callahan, 2013).

No one would suggest that clinicians must hold or endorse the same beliefs, values, and goals as their clients. In this regard, it can be helpful to differentiate between respect and uncritical agreement. Clinicians must be able to recognize their own meaning system, then respectfully step outside of it to understand their clients' meaning systems, but not necessarily agree with or support them (Farnsworth & Callahan, 2013). Clinicians must also help their clients question the status quo and their own standard assumptions. Although this process may be more difficult for clinicians who are unaware of, uncomfortable with, or insecure in their beliefs, many value conflicts can be successfully negotiated with supervision, diversity training, and self-reflection.

People can respond very differently to the same objective situation. Understanding clients' meaning systems can help clinicians recognize and understand these differences. Many people open up when they feel deeply understood, but others may be threatened by this degree of empathy. Paying close attention to clients' verbal and nonverbal responses can suggest when empathic responses are perceived as helpful, off track, or intrusive.

Clinical Applications	Imagine that over the course of your day as a clinician, you saw Doug Muder and his father, Reymundo Sanchez, Tara Westover, and Andrea Yates. Each has a very different meaning system. How would their differing meaning systems influence how you talked and worked with them? Why? How could you remain genuine even if you concluded that you needed to respond differently to match each of their meaning systems?

Summary

Global beliefs can be difficult to recognize (Ivey & Ivey, 2014; Koltko-Rivera, 2004). Further, people actively seek out information to support their beliefs and may fail to take in information that does not fit. Similarly, global goals can be difficult to discern from individuals' behavior given the complexity and potentially conflicting motives and values they express and the other constraints on their behavior. Assuming there is only one right way of doing things interferes with a therapist's ability to help clients find solutions that fit them well. These considerations are especially important for therapy, where stressed clients may be less articulate than usual about the ways that they see their world and pursue their goals.

Although beliefs, values, goals, and situational meanings are similar in many ways, we have distinguished among them here. Beliefs refer to core assumptions about reality. Values reflect relative rankings of the worth of different qualities, activities or goals and guide future behaviors. Global meaning systems comprise a wide range of assumptions, values, and goals that filter perceptions of self, others, and the world. They affect a broader range of behaviors and are less flexible and less easily altered than are situational meanings. Situational meanings are more discrete than global meanings, more accessible to awareness, and more easily changed.

For Review

Applying Concepts to Your Life

1. Describe your meaning system, including your beliefs, values, and goals. How is your meaning system characterized by both major and minor themes? With what contradictory themes do you struggle?

2. How have you felt when someone failed to acknowledge your own beliefs or values? Why?

3. How is your meaning system similar to or different from the meaning systems described in this chapter?

4. How might your meaning system affect your work with others? Which issues and problems would be most difficult for you to respond to? Which might be easier?

Key Terms

accommodation, 25
assimilation, 25
attribution, 32
beliefs, 24
collectivism, 30
directiveness, 29
egalitarian, 29
external locus of
    control, 34

external locus of
    responsibility, 34
extrinsic goals, 25
goals, 24
individualism, 30
internal locus of
    control, 34

internal locus of
    responsibility, 34
intrinsic goals, 25
just-world theory, 32
locus of control, 34
locus of
    responsibility, 34

meaning systems, 23
posttraumatic
    growth, 26
self-efficacy, 35
situational meaning, 39
time orientation, 35
values, 24

Learn More

For more information about the concepts in this chapter, visit the *Empathic Counseling* companion website at http://pubs.apa.org/books/supp/slattery/.

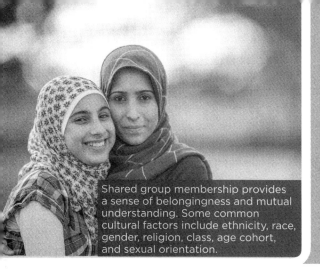

Shared group membership provides a sense of belongingness and mutual understanding. Some common cultural factors include ethnicity, race, gender, religion, class, age cohort, and sexual orientation.

3 Understanding Culture, Identity, and Oppression

Looking Ahead ⮕

After reading this chapter you will be able to answer these questions:

1. How do cultural perceptions, experiences, and meaning systems contribute to group identity?

2. What does it mean to have multiple group identities, and how might this intersectionality influence clinical work?

3. What are oppression and privilege?

4. How can one become multiculturally competent?

You're Doing All of This for a Failure to Signal? ▎ Sandra Bland

In July 2015, Sandra Bland, a 28-year-old African American woman, was stopped by police officer Brian Encinia for failing to signal a lane change. The subsequent heated encounter, which drew national attention, was videotaped by the police car's dashcam and her cell phone. The following excerpt is a transcript from the police car dashcam, which was released to the public by Texas police officials:

Officer Encinia: You okay?

Sandra Bland: I'm waiting on you, you, this is your job. I'm waiting on you. Whatever you want.

Encinia: You seem very irritated.

Bland: I am. I really am, because I feel like it's crap for what I'm getting a ticket for. I was getting out of your way. You were speeding up, tailing me, so I move over, and you stop me. So, yeah. I am a little irritated, but that doesn't stop you from giving me a ticket, so.

Encinia: Are you done?

Bland: You asked me what was wrong, and I told you. So now I'm done, yeah.

Encinia: Okay. You mind putting out your cigarette please? If you don't mind?

Bland: I'm in my car, why do I have to put out my cigarette?

(SANDRA BLAND continued)

Encinia: Well, you can step on out now.

Bland: I don't have to step out of my car.

Encinia: Step out of the car.

Bland: No, you don't have the right.

Encinia: I do have the right, now step out or I will remove you.

Bland: I refuse to talk to you other than to identify myself and—

Encinia: Step out or I will remove you.

Bland: I am getting removed for a failure to signal?!

Encinia: [raises voice] Step out or I will remove you. I'm giving you a lawful order. Get out of the car now or I'm going to remove you.

Bland: And I'm calling my lawyer.

Encinia: I'm going to yank you out of here. Get out!

Bland: Okay you're going to yank me out of my car? Okay. All right. Let's do this.

Encinia: Yeah, we're going to. [reaches in to grab her]

Bland: Don't touch me!

Encinia: Get out of the car!

Bland: Don't touch me! I'm not under arrest, you don't have the right to take me!

Encinia: You *are* under arrest!

Bland: No, I'm not! I'm under arrest for what? For what? For what?

Encinia: Get out of the car! [pauses] Get out of the car! Now!

Bland: Why am I being apprehended? You trying to give me a ticket for a failure—

Encinia: I said get out of the car!

Bland: Why am I being apprehended? You just opened my car door—

Encinia: I am going to drag you out of there—

Bland: You just opened my car door. So you're threatening to drag me out of my own car.

Encinia: [pulls out a stun gun] Get out of the car!

Bland: And then you're going to stun me?

Encinia: [points the stun gun at Bland] I will light you up!

Bland: Wow.

Encinia: Get out of the car!

Bland: Wow. [gets out of the car] Wow. For a failure to signal? You're doing all of this for a failure to signal.

Encinia: Get over there! [points to the sidewalk]

Bland: [walks to the sidewalk] Right, yeah. Yeah, let's take this to court. Let's do it.

Encinia: Go ahead!

Bland: For a failure to signal? Yep, for a failure to signal?!!!

Encinia: Get off the phone! [pauses] Get off the phone!

Bland: [who has been holding up her phone recording the encounter] I'm not on my phone. I have a right to record.

Encinia: Put your phone down!

Bland: This is my property. This is my property. Sir?

Encinia: Put your phone down! Right now! Put your phone down!

Officer Encinia ultimately arrested Ms. Bland for assaulting a public servant (i.e., elbowing him while in handcuffs and kicking him), although there had been no physical contact until after he initiated the arrest, and he was the person who had initiated the physical contact by grabbing her. Ms. Bland, who may have had a history of depression and posttraumatic stress disorder, committed suicide in jail 3 days after being arrested.

When Officer Encinia was investigated by his agency regarding his decision to use force against Ms. Bland, he argued that he had feared for his safety (Ohlheiser & Philip, 2015). Others, however, have argued that his interactions with Ms. Bland were driven by **racism**, or negative attitudes about a person based on race. Ms. Bland's sister, Sharon Cooper, stated, "My sister died because a police officer saw her as a threatening Black woman rather than human" (S. Cooper, 2019, para. 2).

What Do You Think?

1. How do you think Officer Encinia and Sandra Bland each perceived this arrest? Why?
2. What, other than racism, could explain Officer Encinia's decision to arrest Ms. Bland?
3. Why might Sharon Cooper appraise her sister's arrest as an oppressive event, part of a larger cultural pattern? Why might Officer Encinia see his arrest differently?

Defining and Seeing Culture

Culture is the shared attitudes, values, beliefs, habits, traditions, norms, arts, history, institutions, and experiences of a group of people that, together, define their general behavior and way of life. Ethnicity, race, gender, class, age cohort, and sexual orientation, among other demographic groups, are frequently identified as cultural groups. Race and other cultural aspects (e.g., ethnicity, gender, social class, age, sexual orientation, spirituality) are important to consider when building empathy, which is essential for effective therapy. Members of a cultural group generally have a shared identity, with similar values, beliefs, assumptions, goals, patterns of behavior, preferences, and norms. See, for example, Exhibit 2.2 and Exhibit 3.1. Although such meaning systems may be difficult to identify from within a group, shared group membership provides a sense of belongingness and mutual understanding (Nelson, Englar-Carlson, Tierney, & Hau, 2006).

People ask about who they are and where they belong, both as individuals and as group members with shared perspectives and goals (Verkuyten, 2016). Group identities inform one's meaning-making system in diverse ways: influencing beliefs, values and goals; shaping perceived meanings and values associated with group membership; and guiding or directing thoughts, emotions, and behaviors associated with group membership (or believed to be associated with it; Oyserman & Destin, 2010). People tend to perceive the world through identity-congruent lenses and prefer behaviors more congruent with their identity over those that are less congruent. In general, group identities (e.g., race, ethnicity, gender, social class, age, sexual orientation, spirituality) help people feel good about themselves, competent, and connected to others; recognize their world as meaningful; and experience a sense of continuity. Group identity can help "you know what you are and where you come from, what the right thing to do and to think is, where you belong, what makes you proud, and what makes life meaningful" (Verkuyten, 2016, p. 1802).

Groups and individuals are embedded in a cultural context that may have unique defining historical events and figures (American Psychological

Exhibit 3.1 Asian American Values and Norms

Collectivism. Focus on the needs of the group and family rather than the individual (e.g., thus the family name is given first). Group and family obligations are emphasized over individual wishes, thoughts, and feelings. Self-reliance and independence are deemphasized relative to group responsibility and obligation. Individualism is a flagrant social norm violation.

Filial piety. Children are expected to respect their parents, feel obligated to them, and obey their wishes. Parental authority is often difficult to question.

Hierarchical structure. Older individuals and men generally have more power. Authority figures often have broad scope and power to make decisions. People are expected to obey and defer to rather than challenge authority figures and those with more status.

Harmony. Reflects the emphasis on connections among apparently unrelated events. Polar opposites are seen as part of the same entity, with one's existence depending on the other.

Interpersonal harmony. Because of the emphasis on the family and group, maintaining group harmony is important. Actions that "save face" foster harmony, whereas disclosing problems shames the group. Modesty supports the group, whereas announcing successes undermines it.

Restraint of strong emotion. Expected to restrain both positive and negative emotions. Sharing emotional problems shames the family. Love is not shown directly, although it may be demonstrated by performing actions benefiting family. Thinking decisions through is valued, impulsive actions discouraged. Stress and psychological distress may be expressed in somatic complaints rather than verbal descriptions.

Academic achievement. Families expect children to do well and enter careers with high social status. Individual success brings pride to the family and is primarily valued as such.

Note. Data from Chen and Davenport (2005).

Association [APA], 2017b). **Context** is a broad range of influences on a person, including culture, family, history, political environment, trauma, and life events. For example, many Jews' self-concepts and beliefs have been shaped by the Holocaust, the Diaspora, their view of themselves as God's Chosen Ones yet also outsiders, and their fight for homeland (Carmel, Granek, & Zamir, 2016; D. Greenberg & Wiesner, 2004). The civil war in Bosnia and earthquake in Turkey defined and organized the memories of people living through these catastrophes (Brown et al., 2009). Historical slavery, ongoing racism and oppression, and the high rates of poverty and community dysfunction common in many urban neighborhoods influence all African Americans to greater or lesser degrees (Verkuyten, 2016). However, events must be personally relevant rather than only historically important to influence memories of one's life (N. R. Brown et al., 2009).

Although group differences are important, differences among individuals within a group may be much larger than differences between groups. See Figure 3.1. For example, my male and female students are different, on

FIGURE 3.1 Differences Between Groups Versus Differences Within Groups

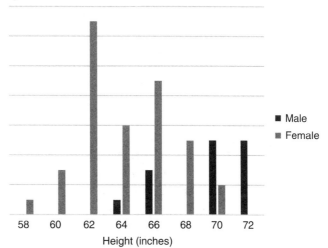

average, from each other in height, but the distributions of male and female heights considerably overlap with each other, such that the tallest women are more similar to the male average and the shortest men are closer to the female average. We need to remember both the differences and the overlap as we think about group identities.

People within a given culture may perceive the same defining event or experience differently. For example, one study reported that many Holocaust survivors (45%) reported that the Holocaust made their own aging and impending death more difficult (Kahana, Harel, & Kahana, 1998). On the other hand, 55% reported that the Holocaust either made no difference or made growing old and dying easier. Although Native Americans have rates of binge drinking and heavy alcohol use that are similar to those of Whites (and higher than other racial and ethnic groups), they have higher rates of both alcohol use disorders and abstinence than do Whites (Substance Abuse and Mental Health Services Administration, 2017, 2018).

We should consider the meaning individual people draw from their identities. Group identities shape the options people perceive, the choices that make sense and those that are ignored or feel awkward, and their well-being across time (Oyserman & Destin, 2010). Does surviving the Holocaust, for example, empower a person or induce guilt and hopelessness?

Group members can also share issues and concerns. African American women's concerns about racial discrimination influence how they parent, including enforcing household rules for sons less frequently and monitoring girls more closely (Varner & Mandara, 2013). Lesbian, gay, bisexual, and transgender (LGBT) teens have significantly higher rates of suicidality, especially when they live in a community with more hate crimes directed at LGBT individuals (Duncan & Hatzenbuehler, 2014; Taliaferro & Muehlenkamp, 2017).

Groups may differ in how they express themselves and view the world. African Americans are often relatively more assertive, self-reliant, resourceful, and achievement-oriented. African American children are often supported by extended families with strong kinship bonds (D. W. Sue & Sue, 2016). Religion plays an important role for African Americans, with 75% identifying religion as "very important" in their lives compared with 49% of Whites (Pew Research Center, 2014). African American youth are relatively more expressive and confrontational than are White youth, which may cause White teachers to perceive them as more aggressive and noncompliant (D. W. Sue & Sue, 2016). As a result, they are more likely to be expelled from school and receive harsher consequences than their White peers, despite not acting out more (Rudd, 2014).

Bernal and Sáez-Santiago (2006) proposed seven dimensions to consider when first meeting clients:

1. **Language.** What is the client's preferred language? What is the client's fluency with it?
2. **Identity.** What impact will group similarities and differences between clinician and client have on treatment?
3. **Metaphors.** What concepts and ideas are salient for the client and the client's culture?
4. **Content.** How can cultural values, customs, and traditions be used in treatment?
5. **Context.** What social, economic, and political factors should be considered in treatment?
6. **Case conceptualization.** How might the client's global beliefs, values, and goals affect presenting concerns?
7. **Methods**. What culturally congruent interventions and strategies can tailor treatment to the client?

Of course, we believe clinicians should consider these issues with all clients (Allan, Campos, & Wimberley, 2016).

What Do You Think?

1. As you read case material throughout this book, pay attention to the unique concerns of each person's group identity(s). What unique issues do men, women, gifted children, Deaf adults, and so on face in their lives? In what ways are their experiences similar to each other?

Multiple Group Identities

People belong to, identify with, and are influenced by multiple cultures and contexts (e.g., ethnicity; race; gender; class; religion; sexual orientation; physical ability; and family, neighborhood, school, and work contexts; APA, 2017b; Bronfenbrenner, 1989; Butler, 2015). See Figure 3.2. These **multiple identities** can profoundly influence the individual in ways that interact with each other (Bowleg, 2008). The experience of a White male is often quite different from that of a White female (the former often feeling less comfortable expressing emotions, more expected to achieve than to nurture, and less vulnerable in sexual situations). The experience of a gay White male can be very different from that of a straight White male (the former often feeling less accepted and safe in daily life). The experience and meaning system of a gay, White, male, fundamentalist Christian is different from that of an agnostic, gay, White male living in a supportive gay community (the former often having more **internalized homophobia**, which is the negative beliefs and attitudes about homosexuality and LGBT people that a person with same-sex attraction turns inward on themselves, whether or not they identify as LGBT).

As Danny Brom describes here, different contexts can highlight different group identities:

> When you live in Holland, certainly if you lead an Orthodox Jewish life, you feel Jewish all the time because you're not able to eat with people in restaurants, for example. And then when you move to Israel, that is not a problem. But then suddenly you feel more Dutch. (quoted in Beauchemin, 2004, para. 5)

FIGURE 3.2 Multiple Identities

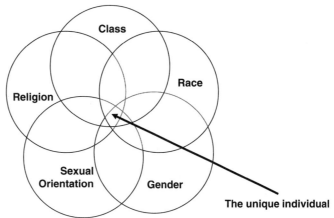

From *Counseling Diverse Clients: Bringing Context Into Therapy* (p. 32), by J. M. Slattery, 2004, Belmont, CA: Cengage. Copyright 2004 by South-Western, a part of Cengage, Inc. Reprinted with permission.

As Danny Brom suggested, different group identities can also have differing and conflicting expectations and demands, meanings, loyalties, and allegiances, which can make it difficult to identify with more than one group at a time (Oyserman & Destin, 2010; Verkuyten, 2016). These multiple identities may shift in salience across time and contexts and lead to different thoughts, emotions, and behaviors depending on the situation and salient identity (APA, 2017b; Oyserman & Destin, 2010; Umaña-Taylor et al., 2014; Verkuyten, 2016).

This complex way in which multiple identities overlap is known as **intersectionality**, which influences how people perceive the world and how they are seen by others. Although Ms. Bland and Officer Encinia were different races, they also had different levels of education and different amounts and kinds of power. Consider how these factors contributed to Ms. Bland's arrest and her response to Officer Encinia.

Because context is a "normal" part of a person's background, it is easily overlooked, especially for members of the **majority culture**, the group in a society possessing greater power and whose language, religion, behavior, values, rituals, and social customs are seen as normative (Pedersen, Crethar, & Carlson, 2008; D. W. Sue & Sue, 2016). But even those who typically overlook the role of their own culture may learn to "see" it when they change contexts, such as when traveling to a foreign country.

Cases in Empathy

Learning to See Culture | Katy Robinson

Kim Ji-yun was adopted from Korea when she was 7 years old, moved to Salt Lake City, and was renamed Katy Robinson. With her adoption, she gained three older brothers and two new parents, becoming, in her words, an "Honorary Irishman" overnight. In her transition to the United States and her new family, she had to give up what it meant to be Korean, including her language (now using English rather than Korean), where she slept (in an American-style bed rather than at the side of her parents' bed), and what she liked to eat (coming to prefer blander American foods and chocolate rather than fruity desserts).

At seven, with her *halmoni* (grandmother) and birth mother on another continent and unreachable, Katy did not have the luxury to hold on to both cultures. At 28, however, she went to Korea to search for her birth parents and *halmoni*, saying to her adoptive mother, "Why didn't you teach me about my Korean heritage? Why didn't you help me keep my name or language?" (Robinson, 2002, p. 35).

In the United States, she had always looked and felt different. In Korea, her hairstyle, dress, gestures, values, and viewpoint identified her as American. She assimilated more easily into the Korean adoptee community, with whom she shared the search for a blood connection and concerns about the adoption process, even though other adoptees were often from Canada or Europe rather than from the United States. She also became more aware of her femaleness in a society where gender restricted access to some settings, required some behaviors and prohibited others, and placed her near the bottom of the social hierarchy in most interactions.

Each of Katy's families—Korean and American—were similar. In both families, her parents were no longer a couple: Her adoptive parents divorcing when she was a young adult and her birth parents never marrying. In both families, she had difficulties with her fathers, whom she saw as brusque, domineering, and insensitive to her needs. She got along well with her adoptive mother and idealized her birth mother, whom she never found.

However, the two cultures were very different. Katy learned some Korean habits easily: covering her mouth when laughing, bowing rather than shaking hands, filling her Korean half-brother's glass correctly, and behaving in a self-deprecating manner to protect relational harmony. However, she made mistakes: giving gifts such as chocolate and cake, which were embarrassingly inappropriate in Korea. U.S.-typical habits and behaviors had different meanings in Korea (e.g., wearing bangs covering her forehead was seen as disrespectful to her husband). She recognized different perspectives: She saw her decisions as personal choices, while her half-brother framed decisions in terms of family obligation. Discipline, obedience, and diligence were emphasized in the Korean culture and school system and led to her academic success in the United States.

Other differences frustrated her at every turn. Because Katy was born during an affair supplanting her older half-brother's mother, her Korean siblings indirectly refused to help with her search, sometimes telling her outright lies in the process. She was hurt when she discovered that they had lied in saying that her birth mother was dead, although later was able to think about their actions as a way of protecting their mother (who had become very upset when faced with information about her ex-husband's affair). As Katy became "more Korean," she also was able to understand behaviors that had seemed unnecessary subterfuge to the American part of her. She was also able to understand why her Korean family was indirect in their responses (to maintain harmony) rather than directly refusing to help her.

After Katy and her husband had spent almost a year in Korea, her adoptive mother came to visit her. They joined her Korean half-brother for dinner. Katy noticed the obvious physical differences (e.g., freckles, round eyes, red hair, jewelry) that set her mother apart from her Korean family, but also her American mannerisms. Her mother was confident rather than demure and acquiescing. She fed herself first, accepted the best morsels of meat, and did not refill her host's glass. She lounged casually and talked to their translator, rather than to her host. Katy thought, "Didn't she notice the break that caused in the harmonious flow of the group?" (Robinson, 2002, p. 266). She noted, however, with surprise that

> it was not with mounting criticism that I observed these subtle gestures. What I felt was more like a dawning revelation that I had, perhaps, become more Korean during the past year. One culture was not necessarily better than the other, and for the first time I could see that I contained qualities of both. But the differences were fascinating. With my [adoptive] mother, for instance, what you saw was what you got. Every emotion and thought lay open and exposed on her face, ready to slip from her tongue and make instant contact. She embodied the American declaration of individuality: if she had a craving, she satisfied it. If she found herself in the seat of honor, she happily claimed it. My brother, on the other hand, was concerned, foremost, with the harmony of the group at the expense of self-comfort and moments of frivolity. His was a life of self-restraint, as I had come to understand. Gracious and selfless host that he was, one had to guess and pull at the thoughts behind his masked face, subtle gestures and unspoken words. (pp. 266–267)

Katy also noted the differences within each culture. Her brother, as head of his family, had more power than other members of his family and was doted on by his mother and wife. His sister was single, planned never to marry, and turned her income over to their mother, giving her sister an unusual amount of power for a woman. Their father, a man who had married twice and fathered at least five children by three women, did not fit in with her brother's family and was as uncomfortable with them as they were with him. Her aunt, also 28, also born out of wedlock, lived in Australia for 8 years and flouted social norms almost as much as they bound Katy's brother.

What Do You Think?

1. Why might Katy find it easier to recognize her cultural values as an outsider rather than in her adoptive culture?

2. Although Katy primarily discusses ethnicity, she also alludes to her gender and adoption status. How do these contexts influence her?

3. Compare the case example with the values and norms described in Exhibit 3.1. How are they similar or different?

4. Think about a situation in which you entered a new culture—either for a long period (e.g., studying abroad) or for a shorter one (e.g., watching an international film, dining out, meeting with a visitor from another country). How did you feel in that setting? Were you comfortable or uncomfortable? Judging or accepting? Why?

Impacts of Group Identity

I do not understand this squeamishness about the use of gas. I am strongly in favour of using [it] against uncivilised tribes.

—Winston Churchill

All I demand for the black man is, that the white people shall take their heels off his neck, and let him have a chance to rise by his own efforts.

—William Wells Brown

A heavy guilt rests upon us for what the whites of all nations have done to the colored peoples. When we do good to them, it is not benevolence—it is atonement.

—Albert Schweitzer

Each of these statements makes different attributions about other races and recommends different responses to them. Churchill objectifies "uncivilised tribes," Brown asks that Whites step back and allow Blacks "to rise by [their] own efforts," while Schweitzer describes "heavy guilt" necessitating atonement. Each response reflects **racial identity**, an individual's sense of being defined, in part, by membership in a particular racial group. The strength of this sense depends on the extent to which an individual has processed and internalized the psychological, sociopolitical, cultural, and other contextual factors related to membership in the group. Racial identity influences a wide range of thoughts, emotions, and behaviors both inside and outside of mental health treatment and should be considered during treatment planning and implementation.

Although attitudes and beliefs about one's group, that group's relationship to other groups, and its position in society depend on historical, social, geographic, and political contexts, group identity also changes with age

(Umaña-Taylor et al., 2014). Young children generally accept the status quo and, as they enter adolescence and emerging adulthood, begin to think less dichotomously, more complexly, and more abstractly (Umaña-Taylor et al., 2014). Teenagers and emerging adults, for example, may begin to consider their identity in more complex ways in which the status quo is one of several possibilities, changeable, and unfair (Verkuyten, 2016). They may actively think about their race or ethnicity, talk about it with friends and family, and participate in activities associated with their racial or ethnic group, ultimately leading to successful identities where they struggle as well as celebrate with their group and work to maintain the group's culture (Umaña-Taylor et al., 2014). Group identity can also vary by social context. For example, a mixed-race person might identify as mixed race in one context and Black in another.

Positive group identities are associated with psychological adjustment and other positive indicators of wellbeing (Rivas-Drake et al., 2014). For example, positive ethnic and racial identities are associated with positive social functioning, well-being, academic achievement, and attitudes about school; people with such identities are less likely to report depressive symptoms, health risk attitudes and behaviors, and externalizing and internalizing symptoms.

The Role of Ethnic and Racial Identity in Treatment

Considering ethnic and racial identity in treatment can be helpful for several reasons: Identity is often central to our clients' meaning systems (Trimble, 2007). People identifying more positive aspects of their identity tend to have better psychological and physical health (Rivas-Drake et al., 2014). Having a sense of positive connectedness to one's group, as well as the psychological resources and structures to identify and challenge discrimination, can improve adjustment following discrimination (Quintana, 2007). Failing to attend to clients' ethnic or racial identity could mean missing significant aspects of their meaning system (Trimble, 2007).

A clinician's race does not necessarily make someone either an effective or ineffective clinician for racial and ethnic minorities, but paying attention to race and culture does improve treatment outcomes (Worthington, Soth-McNett, & Moreno, 2007). Especially for White clinicians, effective work with ethnically and racially diverse clients includes identifying as a racial being, recognizing oppression and privilege, overcoming racism, and accepting the sociopolitical impacts of race and ethnicity—in addition to possessing other clinical skills. In general, White clinicians with more "mature" or "sophisticated" attitudes about race have stronger self-reported multicultural counseling competencies (Cokley & Vandiver, 2011).

Clients with strong ethnic and racial identities may be frustrated with clinicians who ignore racial identity issues or are uncomfortable addressing them.

Similarly, clinicians with strong ethnic and racial identities may be frustrated when working with clients who deny or minimize the impact of racial or ethnic discrimination (Cokley & Vandiver, 2011). As you read the following examples, consider how racial identity might affect a clinician's work. When might a clinician not be competent to work with clients of a different race or ethnicity?

- A White caseworker acknowledges the historical reality of racism but dismisses its current reality. She attributes problems to her clients' lack of motivation for change. Her Latinx client, who feels significant discrimination at her job, became angry and refused further treatment from her and any other caseworkers, saying, "They're all like that!"

- A Black client accepts negative stereotypes about his race and is self-blaming. His White psychologist is well intentioned and struggles to understand the discrimination her client faces but lacks confidence in her ability to identify discrimination correctly.

- A Muslim woman entered treatment seriously depressed and suicidal. Her Chinese American counselor hypothesizes that her depression may be related to microaggressions experienced in her new job. She is initially resistant to this suggestion, but because they have developed a good relationship—and because he is interested in understanding her perspective—they work together to consider this and other viewpoints.

With greater self-awareness and understanding of other cultural groups, clinicians can respond more effectively to identity-related issues. Admitting mistakes, validating concerns, and processing them with clients can be helpful (Owen, Tao, et al., 2014).

> We got off on the wrong foot when I wondered what you were doing that your coworkers responded to you in this way. It seems that I jumped to conclusions and misunderstood the situation and you. Will you tell me if you feel I'm not understanding you—all of you?

What Do You Think?

1. What multiple identities influence you? What do they mean to you? How do they influence your meaning system, perceptions of the healing process, and relationships with others?

2. Consider some of the people discussed in this book (e.g., Andrea Yates, Lil Loco, and Sandra Bland). What identities are most important to them? When do these identities shift in importance?

Oppression, Discrimination, Prejudice, and Privilege

Counseling and psychotherapy may serve as instruments of cultural oppression rather than therapeutic liberation.

—D. W. Sue and Sue (2016, p. 23)

Oppression is a system of institutional power that marginalizes and discriminates against some groups (often called "target groups") while benefitting others (often called "dominant groups"). Oppression can take many forms (e.g., racism, sexism, heterosexism, ableism), such that people can experience several kinds of oppression at the same time, while not experiencing others.

Oppression is **systemic**, meaning that it operates on individual, interpersonal, institutional, and cultural levels.

- **Individual.** People have beliefs, values, and feelings about groups that are different from them.

- **Interpersonal.** Individual attitudes may influence that person's actions, behaviors, and language toward members of another group. A person may feel that other people's misfortunes are due to their own poor choices and then lecture or shame them about those choices.

- **Institution.** An institution may have written or unwritten rules, policies, and practices that welcome some groups and prevent other groups from fully participating.

- **Cultural.** A culture shares messages about right and wrong, truth, and beauty. These cultural messages and norms are arbitrary; can influence individual, interpersonal, and institutional decisions; and can serve to maintain power and privilege for those in dominant groups (e.g., men, middle class, Whites).

- **Privilege** is unearned advantages that come solely or primarily from group membership.

To illustrate the systemic nature of oppression, consider race-based housing discrimination. **Discrimination** is unfair treatment of a group based on group membership or the perception of such treatment. In the 1930s, various federal programs were created to lift Americans out of poverty. One such program refinanced home mortgages at low interest rates to prevent foreclosures. The entity that administered this program created maps that highlighted in red (or "redlined") neighborhoods that it deemed poor investments and thus not "safe" enough to refinance loans in. Every single Black neighborhood in these maps was redlined, even upscale ones (institutional oppression).

Furthermore, banks began using these same redlined maps to guide their decisions about loans and refinancing (Harriot, 2019).

Thus, at the same time that segregation laws prevented African Americans from buying homes in White neighborhoods, redlining also prevented African Americans from buying homes in Black neighborhoods. In effect, African Americans were denied home ownership at a time when White Americans were given financial assistance for buying homes. Home ownership was, and remains, one of the main ways for individuals and families to build wealth, and families tend to pass their wealth on to subsequent generations. Although redlining was instituted more than 80 years ago and has long since become illegal, its enduring effects continue to economically disadvantage African Americans (Harriot, 2019). This system of individual, interpersonal, and institutional oppression was justified on the basis of cultural beliefs, values, and norms (cultural oppression).

Discrimination, of the kinds described in the preceding paragraphs, is usually the behavioral manifestation of **prejudice**, which is a negative attitude toward another person or group formed in advance of any experience with that person or group (individual oppression, which may be informed by cultural oppression). Prejudice typically includes an emotional component that can range from mild nervousness to hatred; a cognitive component including assumptions, beliefs, and stereotypes about groups; and a behavioral component, such as negative behaviors and violence. As a result, discrimination often involves negative, hostile, and injurious treatment of the members of target groups.

Some oppression, like being denied a mortgage or access to buying a home, is overt. **Microaggressions**, however, are more subtle. D. W. Sue and colleagues (2007) defined these as "brief and commonplace daily verbal, behavioral and environmental indignities, whether intentional or unintentional, that communicate hostile, derogatory, or negative racial slights and insults to the target person or group" (p. 273). These include stigmatizing messages, stories, or jokes in the media, from family and friends, or during casual conversations; assumptions of group-related problems; sexualized comments about a person's dress or looks; being ignored as a result of one's group membership; and observed discrimination against other group members. Even the results of a Google search for "attractive people" and "successful people," including the images of some people but not others, can be a microaggression (Abdulrehman, 2018). Microaggressions can be ambiguous, leaving people wondering whether they misinterpreted what someone else did or said and, as a result, can make people feel unsafe and undeserving (D. W. Sue et al., 2007).

People from oppressed groups have more difficulties accessing and using quality mental and physical health services (U.S. Department of

Health and Human Services, 2014). These problems can be cumulative in nature (Berkman, 2009). Having a parent who abuses or is addicted to substances, for example, puts children at risk for a variety of negative outcomes in adolescence, including increased mortality (APA, 2017b). People living in resource-poor environments experience numerous difficulties relative to those living in resource-rich environments: more dangerous neighborhoods, poorer and less accessible health care, lower quality school systems, fewer easily accessible nutritious foods, more exposure to air and environmental pollution, and transportation barriers (APA, 2017b). Unfortunately, people experiencing discrimination or other barriers are more likely than Whites to live in resource-poor areas (Williams & Jackson, 2005). Living in such environments can create other barriers later, including difficulties accessing social resources to obtain employment, health care, and housing.

Oppression has many effects. Values and opinions belonging to the less powerful group or person are suppressed and performance is impacted. Children who are excluded or bullied, for example, tend to withdraw from classroom activities, perform poorly academically, and avoid school (Buhs, Ladd, & Herald, 2006). Simply highlighting race or gender during a task with task-related stereotypes can cause a drop in performance (Oyserman & Destin, 2010; Steele, 1997).

Another effect of oppression is underrepresentation in positions of power. In the United States, men and Whites comprise about 80% and 78% of the members of Congress, 66% and 82% of full professors at universities, 95.2% and 95.4% of CEOs of Fortune 500 companies, and 93.3% and 94.5% of principal owners of professional sports teams, respectively (Bump, 2017; Garcia, 2018; National Center for Education Statistics, 2017; Szczepanek, 2017; Zarya, 2018; Zillman, 2014). Given that men comprise 49.2% and Whites 76.6% of the U.S. population (U.S. Census Bureau, 2018), this underrepresentation suggests unequal opportunity.

Privilege is an advantage based on one's group membership. Just as there are many forms of oppression, there are many forms of privilege (e.g., White privilege, male privilege). Often people are unaware of the ways in which their privilege benefits them. For example, able-bodied people may not even notice that a space is inaccessible to wheelchairs. Thus, privilege can be described as "the unearned assets which I can count on cashing in each day, but about which I was 'meant' to remain oblivious" (McIntosh, 1989, p. 11). Being denied jobs or housing because of sexual orientation, for example, is discrimination, while being listened to and taken seriously because of group membership alone, rather than intellectual or technical expertise, is a type of privilege. The freedom to walk down the street holding hands with your partner or buy a greeting card depicting people who look like you are forms of privilege.

Empathic counseling involves learning about a client's multiple identities, including those that confer privileges *and* oppression. Most people have privilege associated with at least some parts of their identity (e.g., being male, able-bodied, and well-educated) and oppression associated with other parts (e.g., being African American and poor; APA, 2017b). When a clinician fails to identify systemic and environmental constraints that affect clients, instead focusing only on individual behaviors, then the clinician may empathize less well with clients and may inappropriately blame them for their problems. Moreover, empathic clinicians are able to examine society and challenge the systemic barriers that affect different groups. It takes courage to acknowledge oppression in one's own society because this acknowledgment challenges a core belief that many people share: the belief that life is fair (i.e., the **just-world theory**). Thus, it takes courage to acknowledge that opportunities to work, go to a good school, and live well may be unavailable for some for arbitrary and unfair reasons (D. W. Sue, 2004). Clinicians must recognize their own privileges (APA, 2017b; Neville, Awad, Brooks, Flores, & Bluemel, 2013) and challenge the systemic factors that maintain oppression.

Cases in Empathy

Petty Tyrants With a Badge ❙ Sandra Bland

The arrest and subsequent suicide of Sandra Bland sparked widespread outrage. Some people defended Officer Encinia's actions, arguing that his use of force was justified because he had felt threatened and, besides, Ms. Bland had been unnecessarily argumentative. But many critics have pointed out that being argumentative is insufficient reason for arrest, let alone use of physical force and the threat of tasering.

Even among those who agree that Officer Encinia's actions were unacceptable, there is disagreement about whether this arrest was an isolated incident or part of a broader problem with police brutality, particularly against African Americans. Was this just one bad apple, or is the whole system rotting?

In an editorial titled "Why, Yes, Sandra Bland Was 'Irritated,'" columnist Eric Zorn (2015) relates Ms. Bland's arrest to systemic violence. According to Zorn, police brutality is such that merely obeying the police is insufficient; one must do so with a humble, submissive attitude or risk brutality:

> You must always defer meekly to the police. Even when they're acting like bullies, goading you or issuing you preposterous orders like to put out your cigarette as you sit in your own car, don't challenge their authority. . . . Comply. And if you feel your rights are being violated, take it up later with a judge.
>
> [However,] the scandal to this case is the same as the lesson: that you must always defer meekly to the police. That even in an age of dashcams and omnipresent smartphone video cameras, and even in a nation that prides itself on freedom and a Constitution that explicitly limits the power of government, a petty tyrant with a badge still feels comfortable choosing to escalate a minor traffic offense into a major confrontation. (para. 23–24)

What Do You Think?

1. What do you think about Zorn's criticisms of the police force, especially Officer Encinia?

2. Why might good, well-intentioned people behave in ways others perceive as racist or otherwise oppressive?

3. Why might many Whites have difficulty understanding the Black Lives Matter movement?

What Does It Mean to Be a "Multicultural" Therapist?

All mental health counseling [can be] multicultural. If we consider age, lifestyle, socio-economic status, and gender differences.

—Paul Pedersen

Traditionally, most theories of counseling and psychotherapy have focused on European American–specific values and the needs of **YAVIS** clients (Young, Attractive, Verbal, Intelligent, Successful), especially insightful, upwardly mobile professionals. Counseling and psychotherapy approaches have traditionally emphasized rationality, analysis, introspection, insight, individualism, and autonomy rather than intuition, action, collectivism, and interdependence.

However, this traditional emphasis often does not work with clients who are racial and other minorities. Norcross and Wampold (2011b) identified culture and religiosity/spirituality as two of four patient characteristics that were demonstrably effective to use to adapt therapy to clients (the other two were reactance/resistance and client preferences). In general, psychotherapies that have been adapted for a cultural group—for example, using cultural stories, metaphors, or resources—are significantly more effective for ethnic minorities than are unadapted psychotherapies (Benish, Quintana, & Wampold, 2011). Cultural adaptations for their own sake can be empty political rhetoric, whereas evidence-based practice without cultural sensitivity can be irrelevant (Morales & Norcross, 2010). Cultural adaptations and evidence-based practices should go hand-in-hand. Successful collaborations often require behavioral flexibility from clinicians to create a good working relationship (Lazarus, 2002), especially with clients from minority groups (D. W. Sue & Sue, 2016).

Problems Encountered in Working With Clients With a Minority Identity Status

Despite their good intentions, clinicians may have biases that negatively influence their ability to understand and empathize with clients, especially clients with different cultural backgrounds. Clinicians may have "great difficulty

Clinical Applications

Sherae has been talking about her anger about being turned down for a position that a less experienced White man received. Marta became more and more uncomfortable listening to Sherae and found herself excusing the decision. How might she handle her response once she recognizes this pattern of discomfort and avoidance?

✳ ✳ ✳

In the weeks after a recent police shooting of a young Black man, Marta had two clients with very different responses to the shooting: one who perceived it as a racist act and another who did not. How should she respond to a client who perceived this shooting as racist? How should she respond to one who did not? How might Marta's responses differ if the client is African American rather than White or another race? Why?

freeing themselves from their cultural conditioning. . . . They are, in essence, trapped in a Euro American worldview that only allows them to see the world from one perspective" (D. W. Sue, 2004, p. 762). The multiple contexts and identities of both client and clinician influence their behavior and perceptions of each other, what is discussed and what is omitted—even though some identities and contexts may be invisible to observers. Thus, to be most effective in their work, clinicians must learn about other cultures, recognize their clients' multiple identities, identify aspects that are salient at that point in time, and reflect on their own multiple identities, assumptions, preferences, and meaning systems (APA, 2017b). Such a reflective process facilitates considering that "what might be therapeutic (effective) to one group may be harmful to another" (D. W. Sue, 2015, p. 361).

It is impossible to know everything about all of the client groups you work with. However, it is helpful to approach clinical work with an attitude of **cultural humility**—a willingness to listen to a client and learn about that client's cultural heritage with respect, openness, and curiosity (Owen, Jordan, et al., 2014). Actively listening to sociocultural issues allows clients to feel safe and comfortable in exploring painful experiences related to their identities and experiences of oppression and predicts positive therapeutic outcomes when race and religion, at least, are considered (APA, 2017b; Owen et al., 2016).

"Colorblind" Approaches to Clinical Work

Some clinicians try to approach their work by ignoring cultural differences: "People are people," "We're all the same under our skin," "I don't look at color; I look at the person." Clinicians using a colorblind approach apply assessments and interventions without considering the roles of culture and oppression and how these influence behavior (Pedersen et al., 2008). A colorblind approach may be a well-intentioned attempt to be fair; however, in denying differences, clinicians dismiss the very real role culture has on their clients (APA, 2017b; Neville et al., 2013). Such an approach interferes with accurate assessments of problems, inhibits disclosures in treatment, and leads to increased rates of **premature termination**, which is when treatment ends before treatment goals are met and generally against the clinician's advice (K. N. Anderson et al., 2019; D. W. Sue et al., 2007).

Microaggressions in treatment, like avoiding discussions of race and racism, may leave clients feeling "crazy" or invalidated and actually reflect racial intolerance and prejudice. In one survey, about half of the university counseling center clients reported such a microaggression (Owen, Tao, et al., 2014). When clients and therapists did not discuss microaggressions occurring in treatment (73% of the time), the therapeutic alliance was negatively affected, but when clients successfully discussed that microaggression, there was no negative impact.

Other studies have found that clinicians who endorsed more colorblind attitudes generally denied or minimized the role of racism and had poorer multicultural knowledge, skills, and understanding (Johnson & Jackson Williams, 2015). They showed lower levels of empathy than did those with greater racial awareness and attributed greater responsibility for reported problems to the client (Burkard & Knox, 2004). When clinicians examine their own and others' meaning systems regularly and on an ongoing basis, they are less likely to impose their beliefs, values, or goals in their professional work (APA, 2017b; D. W. Sue & Sue, 2016).

What Do You Think?

1. Observe your own and others' responses to race-related incidents (personal or in the media) for several days. If you (or someone else) ignore the effects of race and racism, how do you feel? If you dismiss the role of race and racism, consider your intentions in doing so.

2. Imagine that you say something in therapy that your client identifies as a microaggression (e.g., "Family is really important to Chinese people"). How might you respond? Why?

Becoming Culturally Competent

I come from the East, most of you [here] are Westerners. If I look at you superficially, we are different, and if I put my emphasis on that level, we grow more distant. If I look on you as my own kind, as human beings like myself, with one nose, two eyes, and so forth,

then automatically that distance is gone. We are the same human flesh.
I want happiness; you also want happiness. From that mutual recognition, we can build
respect and real trust of each other. From that can come cooperation and harmony.

—The Dalai Lama

Traditional Western psychotherapies see psychiatric problems as residing in individuals and as statistically deviant from "normal." They tend to assume that principles derived from the dominant group are universally applicable and that diagnosis and treatment can be performed without considering the cultural context (D. W. Sue, 2015).

In contrast, multicultural treatments attend to systemic issues as well as individual ones, noting cultural contexts, oppression, and sociopolitical constructions. Clinicians who have **cultural competence** have the skills and knowledge that are appropriate for, and specific to, treating a given culture. Culturally competent clinicians recognize there is no absolute reality and that knowledge is socially constructed. They perceive similarities across people as well as the differing experiences and contexts shaping their world and their perceptions (Pedersen et al., 2008). As a result, "all interactions are cross-cultural . . . all of our life experiences are perceived and shaped from within our own cultural perspectives" (APA, 2003, p. 382).

Multicultural clinicians increase treatment effectiveness by recognizing and accepting differences in cultural values, beliefs, and preferences; developing multicultural sensitivity, knowledge, and understanding; identifying attitudes, biases, and beliefs that affect their perceptions of and interactions with clients of other cultures; and using culturally appropriate skills in their clinical practice (APA, 2017b; Berlinger & Berlinger, 2017). They recognize and address cultural and structural barriers that can make clients appear resistant to or noncompliant with treatment (Berlinger & Berlinger, 2017) and use cultural strengths (e.g., social support and insight about cultural oppression) to help clients respond with resilience (Clauss-Ehlers, 2008).

Clinicians who are knowledgeable about, interested in, and appreciate their clients' ethnicity and culture have more positive client outcomes (Worthington et al., 2007). Similarly, clinicians who consider their clients' problems in a cultural context, rather than only perceiving individual causes, have more positive results, are evaluated more positively by clients and have better client outcomes and fewer dropouts from treatment. Therapies that have been tailored to a client's culture appear to be more effective because they provide a "language" that offers a useful and meaningful explanation of their suffering (Benish et al., 2011). This language interprets symptoms subjectively experienced, explains the etiology of the disorder, reflects assumptions about the course of disorder, and identifies acceptable treatment options: "psychotherapy is not simply the vehicle for the delivery of psychological ingredients but is, rather, a highly entwined system that uses language to construct or, better said, *re*construct the client's interpretation of the world" (Wampold, 2007, p. 862, emphasis in original).

What Do You Think?

Consider the roles of ethnicity, race, and context in your life and practice (Exhibit 2.1, adapted from Fukuyama & Sevig, 1999).

1. What kinds of experiences have you had with your own and other ethnicities, races, and contexts throughout your life? Have they been primarily positive? Negative? Mixed?

2. What specific cultural beliefs and values, if any, are most important for you now? How might they be a source of connection or conflict between you and your clients?

3. In what ways do you believe your clients' ethnicity, race, and context can be a source of weakness? In what ways do you believe they can be a source of strength?

4. What types of clients or problems involving ethnicity, race, and other contextual issues do you expect will be the most challenging for you? Which will be most interesting? Why?

The Cognitive Skills of a Multicultural Clinician

Multicultural work is facilitated by knowledge of other cultures, critical thinking, self-reflection, and the ability to step back and look at situations from different perspectives (S. Sue, 1998). Skillful **multicultural clinicians** understand their own meaning systems, are knowledgeable about the particular cultural groups with which they work, and possess the intervention techniques and strategies that are uniquely suited to work with clients from different cultural groups (APA, 2017b). Obviously, no one can know everything about all cultural groups, but culturally competent clinicians possess cultural humility, reflect on what they do not yet know, and build skills when needed.

Clinicians use multicultural research to guide treatment but think critically and test hypotheses guiding their interventions (S. Sue, 1998). How would they recognize whether a client's paranoia is a psychotic symptom, an acute and normal response to stressors, or a healthy cultural response to a threatening situation? What evidence can they gather that will help them differentiate among these hypotheses? Such perspective-taking helps minimize bias and builds multicultural competence. Treatment outcomes are more positive when clients feel understood.

Culturally competent clinicians use research on group differences to guide assessments and therapy but avoid stereotypes by flexibly applying knowledge of cultural meaning systems to individual clients (Hwang, 2016). This flexible application facilitates generalizing from a clinician's experiences to build empathy with clients. For example, a Latina clinician can understand a gay man's reactions to being discriminated against based on her own experiences with discrimination, while recognizing that being discriminated against on the basis of ethnicity might feel different from being discriminated against because of one's sexuality. D. W. Sue (2015) concluded, "avoiding harm does not occur through simply eliminating behavioral or non-verbal manifestations of microaggressions but requires major personal change and self-reckoning" (p. 363). Considerable evidence indicates that we may be unaware of our own biases and that these biases can have negative consequences. One summary of the research in medicine concluded that health care providers communicate more effectively with White patients than those from other groups, affecting the nature and extent of diagnostic assessments, the number of questions asked and tests ordered, and the range and nature of treatments offered; the author suggested that bias is associated with higher rates of complications, morbidity, and mortality (Alspach, 2018). Clearly, we should know ourselves and challenge the biases we carry.

What Do You Think?

1. In what ways does your demeanor and typical way of communicating indicate an openness to people of other groups?
2. In what ways does your office space and decor (or your home or apartment if you don't have an office) indicate an openness to people of other groups? Which groups? How?

Using Culture in Therapy

Although understanding a person's identities can help contextualize a client, build empathy, and individualize treatment, some styles of referring to cultural information can be perceived as stereotyping clients and, rather than facilitating treatment, interfere with it (Hwang, 2016). Sensitive approaches to treatment use contextual information to individualize treatment rather than to stereotype clients. For example, rather than saying, "Family is really important to Chinese people," clinicians can say, "I can tell that you really care a lot about your family and that family is really important to you." Similarly, research can inadvertently stereotype clients and create barriers. Rather than telling an educated, acculturated Asian American, "Thought records don't work with Asian Americans," clinicians can use more specific and tentative language, such as, "Thought records work better with more educated and more acculturated Asian Americans" (Hwang, 2016, p. 295). We can engage clients by giving them immediate direct benefits from treatment. For example, we can use the data on race and other contextual variables to normalize experience: "I understand that there is a lot of stigma about mental illness and its treatment in the Chinese American community" (p. 295).

As we discussed in Chapter 2, it is helpful to work within a client's meaning system and translate clinical concepts into ideas that clients know and understand, using their favorite music, books, or movies, for example. Similarly, cultural metaphors, teachings, stories, and figures can be used to enrich treatment and personalize therapeutic stories. Hwang (2016) suggested that we might ask, "Chinese people have a long history of strength and resilience; are there any cultural metaphors or stories that can help you find a solution to this problem?" (p. 296). Accessing positive cultural metaphors and images can make options that are not currently "like me" possible and more likely (Oyserman & Destin, 2010).

| **Clinical Applications** | Da'Janae has been talking about feeling depressed and hopeless. Rana remembered that Da'Janae wore a Black Lives Matter T-shirt to last week's session. How might Rana use this knowledge in her work with Da'Janae (e.g., as a way of understanding her meaning system or to reframe her depression)?

✳ ✳ ✳

Rana discussed her work with Da'Janae with her supervisor, who dismissed the role of race in Da'Janae's depression. How might Rana respond to this dismissal? Why? |

Summary

All people are racial and cultural beings, with multiple group identities (e.g., race, ethnicity, gender, social class, religion, sexual orientation). Group identity influences values, goals, habits, preferences, beliefs, and the ways people perceive the world and are perceived by others. Attending to culture helps clinicians contextualize clients' experiences, recognize the meanings they draw, and listen empathically.

Clinicians can generate hypotheses about the impacts of culture by considering a variety of sources, including examining research on a cultural group's typical beliefs, values, goals, customs, expectations, and challenges. The group's historical context and typical group experiences can influence how clients in that group see themselves and are seen by others, their meaning making in response to a stressor, and their coping strategies. Multicultural therapies attend to oppression and privilege—respectively, the ways life is less than fair and the role of unfair opportunities. Identifying oppression and privilege builds the therapeutic alliance and promotes individual and community change. Multicultural approaches use empowering interventions within an egalitarian relationship, when culturally appropriate.

Cultural competence is related to greater treatment satisfaction and **therapeutic alliance** strength and fewer premature terminations (K. N. Anderson et al., 2019). Becoming culturally competent is an ongoing process requiring cultural knowledge, critical thinking skills, self-reflection, and situational applications. Culturally competent therapists test their hypotheses rather than assume stereotypes; they consider cultural differences and the degree to which stereotypes apply to individual clients. They reflect on the role of culture in their own lives and respect how it affects clients' lives, attend to differences in values and goals, and use culturally appropriate assessment tools and therapeutic approaches (APA, 2017b).

For Review

Applying Concepts to Your Life

1. Most people experience both oppression and privilege. How is your life privileged? What are you less able to do, feel, say, or be as a result of your group identities? What do you believe you should do, feel, or be as a result of your group identities?

2. Think about a time when you felt like you were on the outside. How did you feel? How was your functioning influenced, positively or negatively?

   What would happen if you felt this way much of the time?

3. How your experiences similar to those of Katy Robinson? How could you use these similarities to understand yourself—or someone else—better?

4. Develop a plan for expanding your own multicultural competencies. What might you do?

Key Terms

context, 48
cultural competence, 68
cultural humility, 62
culture, 47
discrimination, 57
internalized homophobia, 51

intersectionality, 52
just-world theory, 60
majority culture, 52
microaggressions, 58
multicultural clinician, 65
multiple identities, 51

oppression, 57
prejudice, 58
premature
    termination, 63
privilege, 59
racial identity, 54

racism, 46
systemic, 57
YAVIS, 61

Learn More

For more information about the concepts in this chapter, visit the *Empathic Counseling* companion website at http://pubs.apa.org/books/supp/slattery/.

Part III

Developing Empathic Assessments

Before attempting to help clients change, clinicians need to assess the problem on the basis of their therapeutic model. That assessment requires a strong therapeutic alliance, which is a cooperative working relationship between the client and clinician. We therefore begin this section by reviewing strategies frequently used at the beginning of treatment to build a therapeutic alliance, especially nonverbal listening strategies. But listening and feeling empathy isn't enough; clinicians also need to communicate that empathy so that clients feel understood. Thus, the next chapter covers strategies for expressing empathy verbally. After that, we explain how to assess a client and build an empathic case conceptualization that takes into account the client's context. A case conceptualization explains what the client's presenting problem is, where it comes from, what factors maintain it, and what interventions will alleviate it. To ensure that a case conceptualization is accurate, clinicians must be aware of cognitive biases that may interfere with assessment. Thus, we conclude this section by reviewing critical thinking strategies to minimize the effects of cognitive biases and strengthen an empathic assessment.

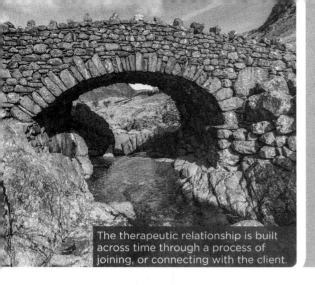

The therapeutic relationship is built across time through a process of joining, or connecting with the client.

4 Building the Therapeutic Alliance

Looking Ahead III➡

After reading this chapter you will be able to answer these questions:

1. What strategies do clinicians use to develop their ability to be empathic?

2. Why is the therapeutic alliance important?

3. How do effective listeners express empathy nonverbally?

4. In what ways do clinicians structure treatment to build the therapeutic alliance?

Cases in Empathy

Everyone Needs to Feel Understood and Supported ▌
Anna Michener

Anna Michener was hospitalized for long periods as a teenager and felt taken advantage of and misunderstood by the adults in her life. She now feels

> very glad to have reached a point in my life where I feel fairly secure and comfortable with my beliefs about myself, and no one who disagrees with me can seriously impact my life or my sense of self anymore.

Nonetheless, she remains angry at the events that led to her earlier hospitalizations:

> I can't help also considering it very important to point out the inescapable differences between dealing with two adults with such conflicting viewpoints and dealing

with an adult and a child. What child has more personal capabilities, more external resources, more options with which to deal with such conflicts than an adult? Everyone needs to feel understood, validated, and supported, but children most of all. . . . Of course caretakers deserve empathy for and support with their monumental task of raising children, but can't this be done in a way that also helps, rather than harms, an inherently less powerful and more needy child?

> I believe the first step to such an achievement would be to actively seek and consider, in all cases, other views of a child in question than that of the primary caregivers—especially the view of the child. Anyone who reads

[this] has more information about my viewpoint and has considered it more carefully than almost everyone involved in my case as a child. If only they had at least consulted my teachers or other adults who knew me they would have received an entirely different picture of me than that provided by my family. And now I have the starkly contrasting experience of seeking psychological counseling for myself as an adult and seeing exactly how listening to me and considering my viewpoint valid results in strikingly different, and actually helpful, diagnosis and treatment than that which I was given in my childhood. (A. J. Michener, personal communication, January 17, 2005)

What Do You Think?

1. Anna felt misunderstood and objectified by her family and clinicians. How might these feelings have affected her treatment? Why? How might she have indicated whether she felt understood and accepted (or not)?

What Is the Therapeutic Alliance?

Let us watch well our beginnings and results will manage themselves.

—*Alexander Clark*

Clients entering treatment are often unsure whether their new clinicians will be able to understand and help them and may feel ambivalent about change. The degree to which a client perceives empathy from the clinician determines, in part, the extent to which a therapeutic alliance is formed. A **therapeutic alliance**, also called a **therapeutic relationship**, is a cooperative working relationship between client and therapist. The therapeutic alliance is considered by many to be essential for facilitating positive change (cf. Wampold & Imel, 2015). Developing a strong therapeutic alliance can help clients resolve their ambivalence and increase their likelihood of change. Clients who have weak alliances with their clinicians and do not share their clinicians' treatment goals or believe in the treatment approach are less attentive and involved in treatment, and more likely to drop out (K. N. Anderson et al., 2019; Olivera, Challú, Gómez Penedo, & Roussos, 2017; Swift & Greenberg, 2015). In fact, a statistical analysis of several separate but similar studies, called a **meta-analysis**, concluded that therapeutic outcomes were moderately strongly related to the quality of the therapeutic alliance (Horvath, Del Re, Flückiger, & Symonds, 2011).

The importance of the therapeutic alliance seems to hold true across a range of treatments and client diagnoses (Goldfried, 2019; Horvath et al., 2011), but it may be especially important for clients who have difficulties forming relationships (Zilcha-Mano, 2017). For example, adolescents with callous and unemotional traits—sometimes described as adolescent psychopathy—who reported stronger therapeutic alliances had greater reductions in delinquent behaviors across treatment (Mattos, Schmidt, Henderson, & Hogue, 2017). In another example, for people in the course of a first or second psychotic break, a strong therapeutic alliance predicted recovery, an association that strengthened across time (Goldsmith, Lewis, Dunn, & Bentall, 2015). However, with weak alliances, attending more sessions actually increased the number of psychotic symptoms reported.

The therapeutic relationship is built across time through a process of **joining**, or connecting with the client. To build this relationship, therapists listen carefully, inquire about client strengths as well as weaknesses, offer choices, check in with clients to see how they are doing, respect clients' cultural values, and attend to nonsymptomatic parts of clients' lives (Slattery & Park, 2011a). Joining with new clients can be difficult because clients and clinicians may enter the treatment process with diverging agendas, goals, and values. As Anna Michener described, this divergence is especially true for children and teens, who are often mandated into treatment by parents, Child Protective Services, or Juvenile Justice agencies. Criticism, confrontation, and judgment undermine the therapeutic alliance (Serran, Fernandez, Marshall, & Mann, 2003). Clients respond to such approaches by discrediting their clinician or the issues raised or superficially agreeing to change. By listening to and working with—rather than on—clients, clinicians powerfully and directly communicate that they are on the same side and want the same goals (Fraser & Solovey, 2007).

Clients must feel their clinicians are genuinely listening, understanding, and accepting them rather than only pretending to do so. They may attend to discrepancies between a clinician's statements, nonverbal listening, and actions to identify whether their clinician's support of them and their growth is genuine. Further, clinicians who are rigid, self-focused, blaming, belittling, aloof, distracted, bored, exploitive, critical, moralistic, or defensive have difficulty forming strong therapeutic alliances (Ackerman & Hilsenroth, 2001). For example, imagine a clinician checking the time while saying, "I get what you're saying." The words convey empathy, but the nonverbal communication (checking the time) suggests that the clinician's statement may not be genuine.

Although a strong therapeutic alliance is almost certainly an important and even necessary precondition to change during counseling and psychotherapy (C. R. Rogers, 1957/1992), significant individual and cultural differences mean that what people want in a clinician can vary widely. Some clients prefer their clinicians to be authority figures, while others prefer more egalitarian ones. Some prefer a businesslike consultation, while others want warmer and more empathic relationships (Lazarus, 2002). Otherwise skillful clinicians can be ineffective when they fail to match their style to individual clients.

A strong alliance can be formed in many ways. The listening and structuring aspects of this process (i.e., setting safe boundaries, getting informed consent, and collaborating on treatment goals and methods) are described later in this chapter. However, clinicians can also take small steps to help their clients recognize that they are being heard and understood and that their contributions to treatment are valued. They inquire about strengths, offer choices, respect their clients' personal and cultural values, and attend to and inquire about nonproblematic parts of clients' lives. The following are some examples:

- Clinician A: "I know that next week is Yom Kippur. Do you still want to meet at this time, or is there a better one for you?"
- Clinician B: "We talked about a lot of things this week. What was most important to you?"
- Clinician C: "What do you want to work on here?"

People often become entrenched in old problems, preferring old solutions and avoiding new ones (Fraser & Solovey, 2007). Clinicians must do two apparently contradictory things in treatment: They must simultaneously validate the client's concerns and rationale for choosing a particular approach to solving a problem while also helping them identify a new approach (Fraser & Solovey, 2007; Ivey & Ivey, 2014). Listening to clients' global beliefs, values, and goals and responding to them can help clinicians join well, build a therapeutic alliance, and intervene effectively.

Clinical Applications	Lin found herself bored during her first session with Bohai, who seemed to be rambling on about meaningless things. She considered whether she was otherwise distracted, hungry, or tired and decided that these did not play a significant role in her reactions. Instead, she thought the problem might be that she had not joined well with Bohai. What might she do at this point?

Nonverbal Listening Skills

Only when the clamor of the outside world is silenced will you be able to hear the deeper vibration. Listen carefully.

—*Sarah Ban Breathnach*

An important part of listening is nonverbal. Nonverbal listening strategies serve three functions in treatment situations: They (a) help clinicians focus and listen well; (b) communicate interest, respect, and empathy; and (c) build and strengthen the therapeutic alliance.

What do effective listeners do? In Western cultures, effective listeners share several qualities. Smiling, head nods, an interested facial expression, eye contact, and a relaxed and open posture with arms and legs uncrossed are related to client perceptions of clinician trustworthiness, expertise, and attractiveness (Ivey & Ivey, 2014). See Figure 4.1. Effective listeners are relaxed and relatively still and avoid fidgeting or other nervous habits. The physical space between clinician and client is relatively small, reflecting the intimacy of the relationship.

Strong listening skills can help clinicians listen to clients more effectively. A particularly effective way of listening nonverbally is **mirroring**, which is reflecting or emulating clients' posture, movements, breathing, language use, and paralanguage to indicate comprehension of what is being said or to reflect bonding. Many people do this naturally—speeding up their speech when talking to someone who is excited, for example, and speaking more slowly and quietly when talking to someone who is depressed and silent. Although mirroring too closely can make some people uncomfortable, observing breathing and other nonverbal behaviors can be an important route to both gaining and communicating empathy (Blum, 2015).

Culture influences how nonverbal behaviors are interpreted. European Americans generally see eye contact as respectful and its absence as a failure

FIGURE 4.1 Closed (left) and Open (right) Postures

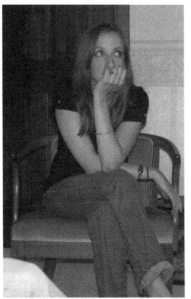 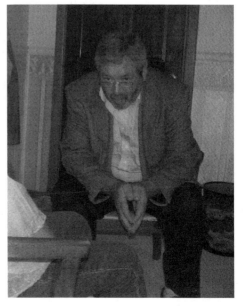

to listen, but people from other cultures, especially Asians, Native Americans, and older African Americans, may see eye contact as disrespectful under some circumstances, especially with authority figures, as it may be seen as impolite (Paniagua, 2014). Touch can be comforting or anxiety-provoking, depending on a client's history of abuse and violence. Native Americans may see a firm handshake as a sign of aggression (Paniagua, 2014). Some clients and cultures are comfortable with long silences; others, especially adolescents, find them uncomfortable. Effective clinicians monitor their behavior and observe its impact on their clients, modifying their listening style so that it is effective with that particular client.

Difficulties in Understanding Nonverbal Behaviors

As seen in the following example, poor listening skills can have a negative impact on the therapeutic process. Notice how, despite treatment being very good in other ways, this clinician's behavior influenced the client's feelings about her clinician, what and how she discloses, and whether she will return to treatment.

> I have a question regarding a therapist I have seen three times. He's definitely good at what he does and in a short time has displayed good insight. He has managed to get me to think about certain things [which have] led to some important revelations. Basically, I am very happy with him. The only problem, and it's leading to an apprehension on returning for another session, is I feel that he is displaying signs that he either doesn't like me or is offended in some way. I make sure not to use foul language and I have not discussed anything of a sexual nature. Yet, I have noticed that he sits with his legs crossed at the knee, pointed away, and will at times cross his arms over his chest. I tend to have an open posture as I want him to know I am open to his thoughts and/or suggestions. I don't know if I'm reading too much into this or not. It's not that I'm looking for a therapist who totally likes me, but I really don't want to see one who has a strong dislike either. It's kind of uncomfortable and not really conducive to revealing innermost thoughts and feelings. (Anonymous, 2008)

One difficulty in displaying or interpreting nonverbal listening cues effectively is that cues can be at odds with each other. A person who has an otherwise relaxed and inviting posture may have dry skin that causes fidgeting. Another may listen well but look away while thinking. Even when nonverbal behavior is clear and consistent, communications may be misinterpreted. For example, people diagnosed with borderline personality disorder or paranoid disorders may have difficulty trusting others regardless of the effectiveness of the other person's listening style. They may be much more aware of and reactive to signals of problems in relationships (e.g., fidgeting, poor eye contact) than to signals of effective listening.

Some clinicians believe that they listen better using other styles of listening; nonetheless, many clients in the West find it difficult to believe that people who are fidgeting, doodling, looking away, sitting in a closed posture, or failing to mirror them are listening and taking them seriously. Their rate or level of disclosure can be affected by their perception of whether they are being heard. As counseling and psychotherapy are about the client rather than the clinician, clinicians need to find ways to communicate their understanding genuinely and in ways in which their clients will perceive, even when those ways may initially feel awkward to the clinician.

Responding to Both Content and Process

The most basic of all human needs is the need to understand and be understood.
The best way to understand people is to listen to them.

—Ralph Nichols

One of the difficulties of using nonverbal behavior to understand another person or to communicate one's own understanding is that nonverbal behavior is ambiguous and can mean many things. Is a client's failure to make eye contact due to feelings of shame or discouragement about ever being understood, to poor social skills, or to low self-esteem? Is silence due to embarrassment, a failure to find words to respond, or respectfully giving the other person space to speak? Collecting other kinds of information can help answer these questions.

Paying attention to the client's **content**, the overtly expressed thoughts and feelings, is one important path for developing an empathic understanding. In what follows, we offer one possible paraphrase of Anna Michener's verbally expressed concerns from a hypothetical therapist whom we call Robbie.

Robbie: It sounds like you wish they had asked people other than just your mother to get a fuller, more valid picture of you. If they had really *listened* to you, they would have developed a more helpful diagnosis, and you would have received more helpful treatment than you ever received.

Robbie's paraphrase both communicated his understanding and facilitated further disclosures by demonstrating she can be understood rather than judged.

Although overt content is important, clients embed indirect messages in their statements. Anna Michener used few feeling words; however, her statement had a passionate and emotional tone. When she said, "Everyone needs to feel understood, validated, and supported, but children most of all," she implied she had not felt understood, validated, or supported. When she asked, "Can't [supporting parents and caretakers] be done in a way that also helps, rather than harms, an inherently less powerful and more needy child?" she suggested that she felt harmed by the support her mother and grandmother received. Perhaps Robbie would respond to these indirect messages like this:

Robbie: It sounds like you felt alone, misunderstood, and unsupported during that period. Their support of your mother and grandmother might have been helpful to *them*, but you were *hurt* by it.

If this reflection of feeling was effective, Anna might have listened, relaxed, nodded, and expanded on what she had been saying, perhaps, "Yes, I felt like no one cared." If it had been off-track, she might have stopped, held her breath, broken eye contact, and—if Robbie had been lucky—corrected him, "Well, I really felt *guilty* asking for any help." If Robbie had been less lucky, Anna would have changed the subject or made a relatively superficial response. As seen in this example, the client's **process**—changes in nonverbal behaviors across time and juxtapositions of content, emotional and behavioral reactions, and so on—can be very helpful in successfully understanding a client and communicating that understanding.

Anna's ability to label the harm that she experienced and her contrast between her past and present experiences suggest that it was not only "strikingly different" but also more positive. Robbie might continue by saying,

Robbie: While you felt very alone then, being heard and understood now seems to be both helpful and also *healing*.

Robbie's responses rely not only on Anna's words but also on the unverbalized emotions that are below the surface. His observation of the discrepancies between one aspect of what she said and another allowed him to communicate a fuller, more complete, and more accurate picture of her experience.

What clients say is modulated and modified by process variables, including changes in nonverbal behaviors and discrepancies between words and nonverbal behavior. How was Anna sitting as she talked? Did she use an open posture with a forward lean, or was she turned away with a tense, closed posture? What was her tone like? Flat? Expressive? Tentative? If her tone or posture changed during a session, when did it change? What was she talking about at that point? Perhaps if Anna had had a tense, but open, posture and spoke tentatively, without obscuring her ideas, Robbie would have instead responded somewhat differently:

Robbie: While you felt very alone then, it sounds like you're feeling heard and understood now. It is scary to believe that you'll be understood, yet you're willing to take some small risks.

Finally, earlier client statements and nonverbal behaviors can contextualize and illuminate later ones, changing interpretations of their intentions and meaning. For example, imagine if Anna had said, "*Of course* caretakers deserve empathy for and support with their monumental task of raising children . . ." (italics added). Is she saying this is obvious, or is she criticizing the mental health system? Her meaning can be deciphered by considering her typical use of verbal underlining, her previous use of sarcasm, and earlier discussions of this topic. However, although knowing someone well can help one make more sophisticated and useful inferences, it also increases the tendency to fit new observations into preexisting hypotheses. **Expectancy confirmation** is the natural tendency to see what one expects to see. Clinicians who understand expectancy confirmation can take steps to avoid getting stuck in old and unhelpful thinking patterns (Lidén, Gräns, & Juslin, 2018).

This section discussed the multiple modes that clients use to communicate. Additional verbal and nonverbal behaviors contributing to understanding are outlined in Exhibit 4.1. When clinicians listen carefully, recognizing the layers of messages inherent in clients' speech, clients are more likely to feel understood in a way that builds the therapeutic alliance.

Exhibit 4.1 Verbal and Nonverbal Behaviors That Can Help Clinicians Develop Empathic Understanding

Content. The overt message communicated by the client's words alone. When contradicted by other indicators, content may indicate what they believe or would like you to believe.

Word choice. Provides overt clues to emotional tone and meaning (e.g., "I feel so alone").

Verbal underlining. Words that are emphasized (e.g., "*He* is important to me," "He is *important* to me") to modify a sentence's meaning.

Paralanguage. Changes in speed, volume, and intonation (e.g., speaking rapidly and dropping the volume at the end of the sentence).

Discrepancies. Can occur between words, among nonverbal behaviors, or between words and nonverbal behaviors. Discrepancies "fatten" the client's meaning by hinting at two poles of a client's beliefs or feelings (e.g., "Well, it's time to go now," while hesitating and not moving, or "I like you," while leaning back and looking away).

Rate and volume of breathing. Reflects autonomic nervous system activity and associated levels of stress or anxiety. Slow and deep breathing generally signals relaxation; more rapid and shallow breathing generally indicates stress or anxiety. Increases in breathing rate within a session may indicate anxiety-provoking topics.

Eye contact. Eye contact can indicate many emotions, including interest, challenge, respect, disrespect, or anger. Breaks in eye contact can signify shame, poor self-esteem, respect, guilt, boredom, disinterest, or the need to gather one's thoughts.

Facial expressions. Raised eyebrows, smiles, wrinkled foreheads, and other facial expressions, although ambiguous, modify and change the meaning of verbal and nonverbal behaviors.

Posture. Open posture is characterized by less body tension, uncrossed limbs, and often a slight forward lean. Closed posture is characterized by greater body tension and crossed limbs. See Figure 4.1.

Personal space. Larger personal space suggests a more formal or less intimate relationship. Smaller personal space suggests greater trust and intimacy or a less formal setting.

Touch. Can express intimacy or reassurance, be soothing, send sexual messages, or demonstrate power or aggression depending on speed, pressure, size, and speed of gesture.

Clinical Applications

Lin began carefully noticing what Bohai discussed as well as how he talked about it. Bohai continued to discuss acculturation issues raised by living with his traditional parents who had immigrated from China, but his speech had become more halting, and he had become more reserved as he surveyed Lin's office and noticed a number of traditional Chinese decorations, some of which were rather expensive. What might Bohai be thinking? What might Lin do at this point?

Clients' Contributions to Treatment

I know that you believe you understand what you think I said, but I'm not sure you realize that what you heard is not what I meant.

—Robert McCloskey

Clinicians make an important contribution to the therapeutic change process, but change is not done *to* clients, but with and by clients. Clients' assessments of their clinicians and the change process is perhaps more important than the clinician's intent or actions (Fraser & Solovey, 2007).

> [The client] is determining whether he can trust the clinician with his assumptive world. . . . Before he will allow the therapist to be admitted into his inner sanctum, the part of him that is within his self-protective system, he needs to have a sense of the therapist's personhood. Is the therapist a person who is capable of understanding his problem? Does the therapist genuinely care about him and respect him despite his problems? Is the therapist genuine and congruent, or is there the hint of a hidden agenda? Does the clinician seem competent? Does the therapist know what [to] do about the client's problem? (Fraser & Solovey, 2007, p. 89)

Clients must be hopeful and believe that they can change, as opposed to only wanting to change (Frank & Frank, 1993; Norcross & Lambert, 2011). Although clinicians can act in ways that provoke hope, clients must believe that they can change. Clinicians can care about their clients, but clients must *feel* cared for (Goldfried, 2004). Clinicians must accept their clients, but clients must *feel* accepted. Clinicians can listen carefully to their clients, but clients must be willing and able to express their emotions so they can be heard (Zaki, Bolger, & Ochsner, 2008). Moreover, although clinicians' personality style and listening behaviors predict the strength of the alliance, clients' motivation to change and their ability to be open and cooperative rather than resistant and defensive are better predictors of positive therapeutic outcomes (Taft, Murphy, Musser, & Remington, 2004).

Problems in joining do occur. When treatment gets off-track and clients are not compliant with treatment plans, many clinicians attribute problems to clients (Bohart, 2001). Labeling clients as "treatment resistant" will, in and of itself, interfere with treatment, as will other critical and judging interventions (Serran et al., 2003). Bohart (2001) argued that joining should be more than just obtaining compliance with the treatment plan, but, instead, should involve building a true collaboration between client and clinician. When clinicians recognize that they are having a difficult time hearing and empathizing with their clients or seeing strengths as well as symptoms and problems, they should step back and focus on the therapeutic alliance.

Joining should be a continuous and ongoing process, with clinicians frequently checking in on and assessing the quality of the therapeutic alliance. Joining takes place within each session: at the beginning, when clinicians ask about the weather or the drive; in the middle, as clinicians listen sensitively to their clients' point of view; and at the end, when clinicians summarize a session or set homework that is consistent with their clients' skills, needs, and individual treatment goals. Joining occurs in the first session, but clinicians must also assess and foster the therapeutic alliance in later sessions.

Introducing New Clients to the Therapeutic Setting and Process

Even if you're improvising, the fact that beforehand you know certain things will work helps you make those improvisations successful.

—John Cale

For many people, developing a safe structure also strengthens the therapeutic alliance (Fraser & Solovey, 2007). Clinicians can develop a safe structure with new clients by introducing them to the therapeutic setting and process. This involves creating a safe setting for treatment, engaging clients in the informed consent process, and collaborating on goals and methods. When these processes are performed well, the increased clarity they provide helps clients feel respected and more able to take the risks inherent in treatment.

Creating a Safe Setting for Treatment

Change is a risky venture, and clinicians must help clients feel safe enough to take the necessary steps to change (Friedlander, Escudero, & Heatherington, 2006). When clinicians are genuine and sincere and believe in the efficacy of the interventions they offer, when they make a serious effort to understand their clients—and their clients feel that their clinicians are trying to understand them from their own point of view—clients believe that clinicians can help them change (Fraser & Solovey, 2007). Safety is further developed by creating a physical environment that promotes safety, fosters client perceptions of clinician **competence** (i.e., ability), and makes the counseling environment comfortable and free of judgment and criticism.

Clinicians create a safe physical setting by using noise screens, having client entrances that protect client confidentiality, creating client flow patterns within an office that reduce the probability that clients will run into each other, and lighting parking areas well (Friedlander et al., 2006). Starting and ending sessions on time and avoiding multiple relationships with clients set safe emotional boundaries. Furthermore, limits on self-disclosures, accepting gifts, and hugging clients can reinforce effective boundaries (Knapp, VandeCreek, & Fingerhut, 2017).

Clients draw conclusions about a practice from the way that the office is set up and decorated. Some of these conclusions concern the clinician's competence. Obtaining informed consent for treatment, displaying licenses and diplomas (as required by U.S. law), having books relevant to the nature of the practice, using appropriate assessment measures, and following accepted clinical practices communicate that the clinician is competent and that clients will be safe in treatment. Although concrete objects and practices can signal safety, safety is also reinforced at the level of client disclosures. Consider the following scene from the *Clumsy Counsellor*, paying attention to your reactions:

Client: There is something that has really been troubling me. I've been under such pressure recently. I'm just afraid that something is going to snap and that I'm going to harm the children.

Counselor: I can understand that you're under such pressure, but you know as well as I do that you mustn't do anything like that. (M. Walker, Jacobs, & Crisp, 1992, Scene 5)

This client might have felt judged and believed that her counselor saw her as incompetent and stupid. As a result, she would probably have a difficult time disclosing other potentially embarrassing or shameful thoughts or emotions. Note that she did not indicate that she was planning to hurt her children, only that she was afraid she might. People have many thoughts and emotions that they would never act on but that they nonetheless worry about.

Clinical Applications	After she came out as a lesbian, Jo's parents sent her to see Tony, largely against her will. After their second session, Jo walked back into the waiting room, where she saw her mother's best friend. Jo visibly froze. She returned to her next appointment but talked only about superficial things. What might Tony do?

Engaging Clients Through the Informed Consent Process

In an episode of the TV show *House*, an agoraphobic man with an intestinal blockage refused to leave his home (Blake & Yaitanes, 2008). To save his life, the medical team finally decided to anesthetize him for surgery, then, without his consent, take him to the hospital. This intervention ultimately saved his life, but imagine how he might feel having agreed to one intervention but awaking after receiving another, unacceptable intervention.

In general, in counseling and psychotherapy, it is advisable to obtain informed consent as early as possible in treatment. **Informed consent** is a voluntary agreement to participate in a procedure on the basis of understanding of its nature, its potential benefits and possible risks, and available alternatives. Clients have the right to know what treatment they will receive as well as the benefits and risks they can reasonably expect. They have the right to know what other treatments are available and to receive a referral to these alternative treatments when appropriate. Other issues that might be addressed—such as the clinician's fees, training, cancellation policy, and decision-making process about medications—are described in Exhibit 4.2. Acting without a client's consent is acceptable only in extreme situations, such as involuntarily hospitalizing homicidal or suicidal clients. In fact, such a situation is arguably the case in the previously described *House* episode, where, without intervention, the man with the intestinal blockage would have died. Even under such extreme circumstances, clinicians should attempt to obtain consent and intervene in the least coercive manner possible (Knapp et al., 2017).

The informed consent process assists clients in becoming true partners in treatment, encourages collaboration, enhances client autonomy, and can lead to more trusting relationships between clinicians and clients (Knapp et al., 2017). Informed consent helps clients make thoughtful and knowledgeable choices about their mental health care and forestalls lawsuits. Providing informed consent should not be thought of as occurring at a single point in time; instead, multiple informing and consenting cycles might occur over the course of treatment as decisions about alternative treatments, medication, or psychiatric hospitalizations arise (Knapp et al., 2017). However, some of these decisions are true choices (e.g., "Do you want this treatment or that one?"), whereas others simply allow clients to acknowledge that they have been informed about the clinical process (e.g., "If you report child abuse, I am mandated to report this to Child Protective Services"; Pipes, Blevins, & Kluck, 2008). Their choices in the latter situation are few: either accept these rules or refuse treatment. Nonetheless, although a client might not choose to initiate a mandated report, being informed beforehand that this is a possibility can reduce feelings of betrayal in the event that a report is made.

Exhibit 4.2 Information That Might Be Covered in an Initial Informed Consent Form or in Ongoing Informed Consent Processes

Therapy

❏ What type of therapy is used? How was it learned? Where? How does it compare with other kinds of treatment? How does it work? What are the possible risks?

❏ What percentage of clients improve with this treatment? What percentage gets worse? What percentage of clients improves without therapy?

❏ How long does therapy generally take? What should be done if therapy does not seem to be working?

❏ Will assessments be used? What kind? Why?

❏ Is a therapy manual with predetermined steps used? Why or why not?

❏ Is therapy done over the phone or Internet?

Alternatives to therapy

❏ What other types of treatment are available? What are the risks and benefits of these other approaches? What are the risks and benefits of no therapy?

❏ How is this type of therapy different from other options?

❏ Is medication prescribed? Do you work with people who do prescribe? If clients are already taking medication, do you work with the prescribing doctor? Are you knowledgeable about medications?

Appointments

❏ How are appointments scheduled? How long are they? Are fees higher for longer sessions?

❏ How can you be reached in an emergency? If you are not available, who should be called?

❏ What happens in the case of bad weather or illness? What happens when an appointment is forgotten or intentionally missed?

Confidentiality

❏ What kinds of records are kept? Who has access to them? How is confidentiality maintained?

❏ Under what conditions can confidential information be disclosed? Do family members have access to information about treatment?

Money

❏ What are your fees? How are they paid? Must missed sessions be paid for? What about telephone calls, letters, and emails?

❏ What are your policies about raising fees? Can fees be lowered if a job or insurance coverage is lost? What happens if fees are not paid as agreed?

❏ How much and what kind of information about sessions are shared with insurance companies? How much influence do insurance companies have on therapy? How are disagreements about treatment with insurance companies resolved?

❏ How would therapy be different if paid directly rather than by the insurance company?

Exhibit 4.2 Information That Might Be Covered in an Initial Informed Consent Form or in Ongoing Informed Consent Processes *(Continued)*

General

❑ What is your training and experience? Are you licensed? Are you supervised? Board certified?

❑ What is your professional background? What are the advantages and disadvantages of your credentials?

❑ Who should clients talk to if they have a complaint that cannot be resolved?

Note. Adapted from "Informed Consent Revisited: An Updated Written Question Format," by A. M. Pomerantz and M. M. Handelsman, 2004, *Professional Psychology: Research and Practice, 35*, pp. 204–205. Copyright 2004 by the American Psychological Association.

By informing clients about the treatment process, sharing expectations, and addressing common concerns from the beginning, the informed consent process can also forestall another serious problem for many clinical practices, that of cancellations and premature termination (Swift & Greenberg, 2015). About 21% of clients drop out of treatment prematurely (Swift, Greenberg, Tompkins, & Parkin, 2017). As we discuss at greater length in Chapter 10, this problem has been attributed to a number of factors, including confusion about the process, poorly developed intentions about treatment, and stigma surrounding mental health diagnoses and treatment. Unattractive and crowded waiting rooms; inaccessible offices; and culturally insensitive assessment, joining, and treatment can reduce return rates. Educating people about the process of psychotherapy—what they can expect and what is expected of them—can strengthen the therapeutic alliance and reduce cancellations and premature terminations as well as increase motivation and decrease perceived barriers to treatment (Swift & Greenberg, 2015). Client families who felt their clinician genuinely wanted to help them and felt that things might get better were most likely to return to a second session (McAdams et al., 2015).

Clinical Applications Leena decided to see a therapist, Lawrence, to resolve triggers raised by her work with her own clients. At their first meeting, Leena was given an informed consent form to sign in the waiting room. She considered walking out. Why might she have been upset? What might Lawrence do at this point when he notices her concern?

Collaborating on Goals and Methods

Setting goals and collaborating on treatment plans can be another strategy for building the therapeutic alliance. The process of being listened to and developing treatment goals consistent with their own values and goals is different from what most clients experience in other parts of their lives. This process can be a **corrective emotional experience** in which one comes to understand an event or relationship in a different or unexpected way that results in an emotional coming to terms with it. Collaborating on goals can also increase the client's investment in and commitment to the treatment process. In contrast, failing to develop cooperative goals with clients can undermine treatment and even cause serious harm.

Cases in Empathy

Conflicting Beliefs, Conflicting Treatment Goals ▮ Lia Lee

The importance of collaborative goal-setting is illustrated in the heartbreaking biographical book *The Spirit Catches You and You Fall Down*, which tells the story of a Hmong refugee family—the Lee family—and their interactions with the health care and child welfare system in the United States (Fadiman, 2012).

Lia Lee (b. 1981) was the 14th of 15 children born to Hmong immigrants. Seven were still living when she was born; the other six had died before they came to the United States. When she was 3 months old, Lia had the first of what would be numerous, eventually uncontrollable seizures (Fadiman, 2012). In the first four and a half years of her life, for example, Lia was admitted to the hospital 17 times and made more than 100 visits to the emergency room or pediatric clinic.

While Lia's physicians focused on getting her medications and stopping her seizures, her parents had traditional Hmong views of epilepsy and its cure (that it was caused by "soul loss"), preferred more traditional treatments offered by a *txiv neeb* (a shaman), believed that Western medicines caused Lia's seizures and worsened her symptoms, and had difficulty understanding and following the medication regimen prescribed. That medication regimen was, in fact, quite complex. Her prescriptions were changed 23 times

during the first 4 and a half years, with new combinations of medications, doses, and frequencies of administration. Some medications were given daily regardless of how she was feeling (e.g., vitamins, anticonvulsants), others when she was symptomatic and were to be taken until the prescription was completed (e.g., antibiotics), and still others only when she ran a fever.

Lia's parents did not speak English, were illiterate in English and Hmong, and were innumerate, which compounded problems. Because neither her parents nor her physicians spoke each other's language and did not have a translator available, they had difficulty identifying problems and preferences for treatments, gathering additional necessary information, and developing a shared understanding of the causes of her symptoms and why treatments would be helpful. Lia's doctors saw the Lees as noncompliant with her medications and treatment and as seriously endangering her life. Therefore, when Lia was almost 3 years old, she was placed in a foster home where her medication could be administered as prescribed.

Lia's parents, like most Hmong, were loving parents who took a child-centered approach to parenting. They especially loved Lia. Anne Fadiman, a journalist who listened carefully

(LIA LEE continued)

to the Lees over a 9-year period, said that it was clear "Lia was her parents' favorite, the child they considered the most beautiful, the one who was most extravagantly hugged and kissed, the one who was dressed in the most exquisite garments" (Fadiman, 2012, p. 23). They carried her all day and picked her up whenever she cried, as Hmong parents do for all of their children.

But Lia's parents had very different world-views from her physicians and social workers. They wanted Lia to be healthy, but they also believed that her epilepsy was a kind of spiritual gift, at one point stating "we are not sure we want her to stop shaking forever because it makes her noble in our culture, and when she grows up she might become a shaman" (Fadiman, 2012, pp. 260–261).

These cultural mismatches in worldview were matched by differences in communication style. In the United States, physicians expect their patients to comply with medical recom-mendations. The Lees nodded and appeared to agree with recommendations, although they may not have understood them or agreed with proposed treatments, some of which they believed made their daughter worse. As one nurse observed, the Lees "were courteous and they were obstinate. They told us what we wanted to hear. What we really knew about them wouldn't fill the bottom of a cup" (Fadiman, 2012, pp. 48–49). Perhaps because

of language and cultural differences between the Lees and their doctors, perhaps because they only saw Lia when she was ill, her doctors underestimated both the Lees' parenting ability and Lia's intellectual ability.

Some of the clinicians in the child welfare system were unable to work collaboratively with the Lees, but others worked to understand Lia's parents from their unique perspective, which allowed these clinicians to recognize and address barriers to treatment. Two of the more effective clinicians were Sukey Waller and Jeanine Hilt.

Waller, like the Lees, believed "that the long way around is often the shortest way from point A to point B." In other words, taking the time to listen to the Lee parents and understand their point of view was ultimately the quickest, most efficient way to set treatment goals consistent with their meaning system (Fadiman, 2012, p. 94). And although Hilt removed Lia Lee from her home and placed her in foster care, she also treated the family respectfully, collaborated on treatment, and helped them address other goals important to them (such as connecting the family with community resources). Effective clinicians, like Waller and Hilt, did not necessarily give the Lees everything they wanted but were respectful and more collaborative in their goal-setting and overall approach.

What Do You Think?

1. In what ways were Lia's parents' and physicians' goals, values, and beliefs about illness similar and different? How did these differences influence identification of problems?

2. What seemed to characterize those people who were more successful or less successful in working with the Lee family?

3. One kind of competence is multicultural competence. What could Lia's physicians and other workers have done to build this competence? Why might you expect that building this competence would have increased their success in working with this family?

4. Why might the setting where Lia's physicians saw her (the hospital, generally during a severe seizure) have influenced their conclusions about the Lee family?

Summary

Clients often enter treatment with some feelings of ambivalence about the process and about change. Listening to and validating clients' concerns, although not necessarily agreeing with their perceptions and conclusions, strengthens the therapeutic alliance, whereas criticism, confrontation, and judging undermine it (Moeseneder, Ribeiro, Muran, & Caspar, 2019). Clients tend to respond to the latter approaches by discrediting their clinician, devaluing the issues raised, or only superficially agreeing to change. In addition to being genuine and empathic with their clients, clinicians strengthen the therapeutic alliance by creating a safe physical and emotional space to change and providing explanations for the problem that are plausible from the client's meaning system.

Nonverbal listening strategies (a) help clinicians focus and listen well; (b) communicate interest, respect, and empathy; and (c) build and strengthen the therapeutic alliance. In Western cultures, effective listeners maintain a relaxed and open posture, with a slight forward lean and few nervous habits. They maintain good eye contact and a warm and responsive expression. Effective clinicians pay attention to the overt content in clients' statements to build understanding but also observe the process reflected in the clients' word use and juxtaposition of topics and nonverbal behaviors as well as changes in affect, mood, and relational style.

Informed consent contributes to the joining process by helping clients make thoughtful and knowledgeable choices. It encourages collaboration, enhances client autonomy, and can forestall lawsuits. Informed consent should not be thought of as occurring at a single time; instead, multiple informing and consenting cycles often occur over the course of treatment. By informing clients about the treatment process, sharing expectations, and addressing common concerns from the start, the informed consent process can also decrease cancellations and premature termination.

Finally, developing a treatment plan together and implementing it in a way that is responsive to a client's needs strengthen the therapeutic alliance. Fine-tuning the treatment plan to reflect the client's goals can also strengthen the alliance. Keeping the treatment goals in mind can help clinicians maintain a consistent and more effective course in treatment even when responding to individual crises.

For Review

Applying Concepts to Your Life

1. Describe a change you have made in your own life. How did it feel to make that change? What made it easier or more difficult to change? Compare your experience with that of your friends or fellow students. What do you conclude in comparing your story with theirs?

2. If someone—a parent, friend, minister, teacher, or therapist—helped you change, what did he or she do that seemed helpful? What characteristics and behaviors seemed particularly helpful? Compare your experience with that of your friends or fellow students. Which of these characteristics would you like to further develop to become a better helper? What steps could you take to make these changes?

3. How do you recognize that you are being treated respectfully? Would being treated respectfully be different in therapy than in other parts of your life? If so, how? If you would like to be more respectful of others, especially in the counseling and psychotherapy process, what changes would you need to make?

What steps could you take to make these changes?

4. Observe people talking to each other. What do you notice? Can you identify good listeners and poor listeners based on their nonverbal listening skills? How do others react to them?

5. Tape yourself while talking to someone else. Turn off the sound and only watch your nonverbal behavior. What do you observe? Watch your partner's responses to your nonverbal behaviors. What do you see?

6. Practice your mirroring skills by paying attention to other people's breathing patterns and making postural shifts that match theirs. What do you learn about them? How do they respond? Make your changes both subtle and respectful.

7. Speak quickly and loudly with someone who is speaking quietly and slowly. Sit up straight with someone who slouches. How connected do you feel? How does the other person react? Make sure to debrief them afterward.

Key Terms

competence, 82
content, 77
corrective emotional
    experience, 86

expectancy
    confirmation, 79
informed consent, 83
joining, 73

meta-analysis, 72
mirroring, 75
process, 78

therapeutic alliance, 72
therapeutic
    relationship, 72

Learn More

For more information about the concepts in this chapter, visit the *Empathic Counseling* companion website at http://pubs.apa.org/books/supp/slattery/.

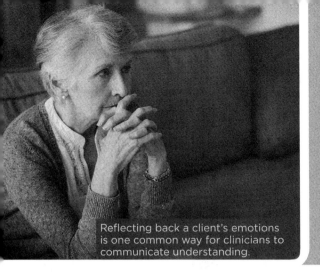

Reflecting back a client's emotions is one common way for clinicians to communicate understanding.

5 Communicating Empathy Verbally

Looking Ahead III➡

After reading this chapter you will be able to answer these questions:

1. Identify some barriers to successfully communicating empathy.

2. In what ways can clinicians express empathy verbally?

3. How can clinicians recognize when their understanding is on track?

4. How can clinicians develop their empathic understanding when clients have a difficult time expressing their thoughts and feelings verbally?

5. How do validation and hope contribute to empathy?

Cases in Empathy

"You Must Have Had a Very Good Reason" ❙ Annie G. Rogers

Annie Rogers is a gifted therapist in her own right, but she was hospitalized after a psychotic break. When releasing her from the hospital, her doctor made her promise to stay on her medication and away from psychotherapy: "What's wrong with you can be changed only with medication and time" (A. G. Rogers, 1995, p. 121). In less than a week, she broke her promise—"the need to understand what is happening to me overrode my promise" (A. G. Rogers, 1995, p. 122)—and made an appointment to see Dr. Blumenfeld, who would become her new therapist. Annie describes her first session with Dr. Blumenfeld:

Dr. Blumenfeld lean[s] in a little to listen, as if he is hearing what I have not said, what are not, in all honesty, even my thoughts. I don't look directly at him. On the periphery of my horizon of awareness, I pick up every gesture and every shift of breath. I have learned that this way I know far better what someone is thinking and feeling. (p. 123)

Annie then stated, "I took a gun and a knife to my therapist and I threatened to kill her."

Dr. Blumenfeld responded calmly, "You must have had a very good reason for wanting to do that."

(ANNIE G. ROGERS continued)

Annie responded, "I didn't want to. There were voices that told me to do that, and I, I felt compelled to follow them."

Although Annie found her own words frightening, Dr. Blumenfeld accepted them, laughing lightly: "Ah, they must have had a very good reason." His willingness to accept the meaningfulness of her voices helped her accept their meaningfulness, too. She felt understood, which allowed her to better hear and understand Dr. Blumenfeld. She exclaimed to him,

> "I can hear you in whole sentences! . . . My hearing has been messed up. Sometimes I can't hear people in whole sentences. In my journal, there are a few lines like that, whole sentences. But they are surrounded by—words that make no sense to me—gibberish! . . . And no one in the hospital could understand me when I spoke."

"No one there knew that gibberish is a language too?" (A. G. Rogers, 1995, pp. 123–124)

Annie began to cry and looked for a tissue to wipe away her tears. Instead of giving her a tissue, Dr. Blumenfeld said, "I don't want you to wipe them away. Let the tears be."

When Annie was again able to continue, she told her story from a different angle.

> "The woman who was my therapist, she won't see me, not ever again."
> "She has abandoned you," he says simply.
> "No, she loved me," I argue, swallowing hard.
> "Love? What is love then?" he asks.
> The room tilts, as if a huge wave hit us. "I don't know. I don't know what love is, or what is real anymore."
> "How could you possibly know?"
> (A. G. Rogers, 1995, pp. 123–124)

What Do You Think?

1. What do you think about Dr. Blumenfeld's work? Why?

2. If you had to briefly summarize Dr. Blumenfeld's message to Annie Rogers at this, their first meeting, what would it be? Does she accept it? How do you know?

3. What did you think about his interpretations (e.g., "No one there knew that gibberish is a language too?" or "[The voices] must have had a good reason")? What information informed his interpretations? Did they seem to be effective? How do you know?

Barriers to Communicating Empathy

Giving connects two people, the giver and the receiver, and this connection gives birth to a new sense of belonging.

—Deepak Chopra

Understanding someone, although helpful, is not enough; that understanding must be shared. Regardless of how accurate Dr. Blumenfeld's insights were, if he had maintained a poker face and kept his insights to himself, Annie would not have recognized that he understood her.

Clinicians face multiple barriers to listening empathically and sharing that understanding. Hearing someone well requires setting aside one's biases and life stressors to listen carefully and recognize that another person's perspective may be different from one's own (Pedersen et al., 2008). Listening empathically can feel intimate and be disconcerting, as becoming open enough to hear someone carefully and sensitively can leave both parties feeling more visible and vulnerable. Some men may see this intimacy as inconsistent with their gender role. For some people, intimacy can also create feelings that can feel sexual (Sherby, 2009).

Cultural norms in the United States often discourage openly acknowledging problems and people may avoid talking about difficult emotions to protect relationships: "Nice people" do not see bad things and do not talk about them. Seeing and discussing problems can feel intrusive and like an invasion of another person's "emotional space." Discussing problems can feel like creating rather than resolving problems. Similarly, clients may be reluctant to express their feelings and to risk being open about their inner experience elsewhere in their lives, especially during periods of crisis.

Genuinely listening to and hearing someone can create connections, foster feelings of belonging and understanding, and in and of itself be healing. This chapter describes basic and more advanced empathy skills, including recognizing and responding to client ambivalence and unrecognized feelings.

Clinical Applications	Isabelle, a first-year counseling student, cares about people and is insightful about them, but she has difficulty expressing her empathy because sharing her understanding of others often feels awkward, unnecessary, and not part of her cultural background (she was raised in England). Still, she wants to be successful in this profession and recognizes that better expressing her empathy would contribute to her success. What might she do at this point?

Verbal Strategies for Sharing Understanding

You only listen and say back the other person's thing, step by step, just as that person seems to have it at that moment. You never mix into it any of your own things or ideas, never lay on the other person anything that person didn't express.

—Gendlin & Hendricks (n.d.)

A variety of verbal strategies can be used to communicate understanding of someone else's experience. These strategies are types of **microskills**, the nonverbal and verbal skills that help clinicians join with clients, develop case conceptualizations, identify problems and change strategies, and help clients change. Important verbal microskills for listening and communicating understanding include paraphrases, reflections of feeling, closed questions, open questions, encouragers (including minimal encouragers), and summarizations (summarized in Table 5.1).

Paraphrases

Paraphrases are brief summaries of the content in a client's message. They promote empathy by sharing the clinician's understanding of the client's experience and are often followed by a checkout, which further clarifies the clinician's understanding. Paraphrases often take the form of (a) a sentence stem where the clinician takes ownership for what he or she heard ("It sounds like . . ." or "It seems like . . ."); (b) the essence of the content of the client's communication; followed by (c) a checkout, which clarifies the clinician's understanding ("Is that right?" "Am I following you?" "Am I on track?"). Generally, paraphrases are in the clinician's own words; however, occasionally using clients' words and metaphors strengthens the paraphrase and increases the probability that it will be useful. Because clients may discuss several ideas, paraphrases can focus on different aspects of the client's message or underlying meaning. Choosing among these different aspects depends, in part, on what best furthers the client's treatment goals.

After Sherman discloses his concerns about their fertility treatments, consider how two different clinicians might respond:

Sherman: We just found out that we can never have a child. They've done all the hormones and in vitro fertilizations that they can do. That's it. (silence) How do you go on after your whole world has been centered around making a baby for 4 years?

Clinician A: It sounds like you've focused on trying to have a baby, but now you know you can't and don't know how you can go on. Am I on track? [paraphrase, checkout]

Clinician B: It seems like trying to conceive has been the center of your world for the past 4 years, and now that you can't have a child, you're searching for a sense of purpose and meaning. Am I hearing you okay? [paraphrase, checkout]

Clinician A's response could be helpful in getting the facts out clearly to develop a strong, shared understanding of Sherman's story. Clinician B's focus on the underlying meaning would be especially helpful once she had developed a good understanding of the facts. This response would refocus the ongoing discussion on purpose and meaning.

Table 5.1 Verbal Microskills for Listening and Communicating Understanding

Skill	Characteristics	Example
Paraphrases	Promote discussion by summarizing the essence of a client's message over a short period of time, both to demonstrate the clinician's understanding and to check out that understanding.	"You said that you began the semester smoking only three cigarettes a day but smoked more and more as the semester went along, especially when you were stressed."
Reflections of feeling	Promote focus on and further discussion of emotions.	"You sound very confused and frightened as you talk about this."
	Communicate understanding by selectively focusing on the client's feelings.	"You sound pretty overwhelmed."
Closed questions	Quickly obtain specific data and discourage lengthy discussion.	"Are you almost finished?"
	Are often answered in a few words.	
	Often begin with *do, does, is, could,* and *are*.	
Open questions	Elicit major information and facilitate discussion.	"How did you come to choose psychology as a major?"
	Generally begin with *who, what, how, why,* or *could*. (But try to avoid *why* questions, which clients may experience as blaming.)	
Encouragers	Encourage elaboration of ideas and emotions by repeating one or a few of the client's main words to focus attention on the ideas contained in those words.	"Suddenly?"
Minimal encouragers	Simple sounds that help people feel heard or understood with few or no words.	"Uh-huh."
		"Awww."
		"Oooh."
		"Yes."
		"Ah."
Summarizations	Quickly organize information from a relatively longer part of a session or treatment to communicate and check out understanding.	"Last time we discussed the ways that you push people away, especially when you value your relationship with them, but also considered the ways that you are trying to approach relationships differently."
	Often used at a session's beginning or end and during changes in focus.	

The sentence stem and checkout frame the paraphrase and communicate understanding. Once comfortable with paraphrases, clinicians can use simpler paraphrases (e.g., "Your world has been centered around making a baby, and you're wondering how you can go on").

Reflections of Feeling

Reflections of feeling facilitate discussion and communicate understanding by selectively focusing on feelings. Like paraphrases, they often begin with a sentence stem (e.g., "It sounds like . . ." or "It feels like . . .") and are often followed by a checkout (e.g., "Am I understanding you?"). In between, the clinician identifies the emotion or emotions that the client is describing, implying, or expressing nonverbally, often followed by a brief statement describing the related context ("You're feeling pretty angry" + "since losing your job"). The basic form of a reflection of feeling is, "It sounds like" + "you're feeling _____." The reflection of feeling is often followed by a checkout.

Sherman: It's just been so crazy. (pause) We focused so much of our time and energy on making a baby, and it's like I don't know what to feel or do now. Sometimes I'm angry at what we've lost. Sometimes I'm depressed. Sometimes I'm almost relieved—then I feel guilty.

Clinician A: It seems like you've been feeling a lot of different things—anger, frustration, depression, relief and guilt—since you found out that the two of you can't have a baby. Am I understanding you okay? [reflection of feeling, checkout]

The feeling is the essential aspect of a reflection of feeling; the other three parts ("sounds like," the context, and the checkout) can be dropped after clinicians have developed greater therapeutic skill, especially when the therapeutic alliance between clinician and client is strong. For example, a clinician might occasionally say, "You're really feeling blue today," while making observations to determine whether she is on track. Clients signal that a clinician is on track by nodding and smiling, leaning forward, saying "Yes" or expanding on the discussion; clients signal an error by correcting the misunderstanding, leaning back, hesitating or stuttering, changing the subject, laughing nervously, discussing more superficial topics, or breaking eye contact (Thomas, 2005).

Sherman: (breaking eye contact) I guess. Um, I'm thinking about getting a new job.

Following paraphrases, clients tend to discuss content rather than feelings, whereas after effective reflection of feelings, clients tend to feel and explore their emotions more intensely. Therefore, reflections of feeling are more appropriate when trying to encourage clients to discuss their feelings and experience them more deeply, and paraphrases are more useful for gaining additional understanding of facts and ideas (Ivey & Ivey, 2014).

Closed and Open Questions

A fool may ask more questions in an hour than a wise man can answer in seven years.
—English Proverb

Questions are an important way of gathering a lot of information quickly and take one of two general forms: closed and open. **Closed questions** (e.g., "Are you tired?" "How old are you?") call for short, definitive answers. These are often answered with yes or no, and frequently start with *is, are, do, does, would, could,* or *have.* Closed questions are helpful in structured situations where a large amount of information must be gathered quickly and with very talkative clients who might talk too much in response to an open question.

Open questions encourage respondents to answer freely in their own words, providing as much or as little detail as desired. Open questions generally start with *what, how,* or *why* and are used to encourage discussion. Each question type pulls a different response (Ivey & Ivey, 2014). *What* questions lead to discussions of content (e.g., "What would you like to do after college?"). *How* questions lead to further discussion of feelings or processes (e.g., "How do you handle it when you start to get overwhelmed?"). *Why* questions focus on underlying motives (e.g., "Why did you take this course rather than the other one?"). *Why* questions should be used infrequently because clients can perceive them as blaming and may become defensive in response to them (Ivey & Ivey, 2014). *How* questions can meet the same purpose and feel less blaming (e.g., "How did you come to take this course rather than the other one?").

Here are several examples of open and closed questions. Paying attention to one's own emotional and cognitive responses to these questions can help clarify their function.

Sherman: I'm all over the place today. I'm tired of this. I just want to stop feeling.

Clinician A: What might happen if you remained open to your feelings? [open question]

Clinician B: Could you try sitting with your feelings for a while and see what happens? [closed question functioning as a directive]

Clinician C: Why do you think you should stop feeling? [open question]

Clinician D: Are you feeling like you just cannot go on any longer? [closed question]

Open questions are often useful because they encourage people to talk, but they may not be useful with people who talk at length. With such clients, closed questions may slow the therapeutic process enough that both clinician and client have more opportunity to work together productively. Teenagers often respond especially poorly to closed questions and may reply very briefly even to open questions (e.g., "How have you been doing this last week?" "Good."). Teenagers are not the only ones who respond poorly to questions, though. Consider Andrea Yates' responses to Sgt. Mehl's style of questioning in the next box.

Cases in Empathy

Transcript of Confession ▌ Andrea Yates

This is about 5% of the interview between Andrea Yates and Houston Police Sgt. Eric Mehl. The rest is available online (Associated Press, 2002). Although the murders are not described in this portion of the interview, the rest of the interview takes much the same form, with Andrea Yates responding briefly to Sgt. Mehl's questions.

Sgt. Eric Mehl: Um, after you drew the bath water, what was your intent? What were you about to do?

Andrea Yates: Drown the children.

Mehl: OK. Why were you going to drown your children? (15 seconds of silence) Was it, was it in reference to, or was it because the children had done something?

Yates: No.

Mehl: You were not mad at the children?

Yates: No.

Mehl: OK, um, you had thought of this prior to this day?

Yates: Yes.

Mehl: Um, how long have you been having thoughts about wanting, or not wanting to, but drowning your children?

Yates: Probably since I realized I have not been a good mother to them.

Mehl: What makes you say that?

Yates: They weren't developing correctly.

Mehl: Behavioral problems?

Yates: Yes.

Mehl: Learning problems?

Yates: Yes. (Associated Press, 2002, para. 107–124)

What Do You Think?

1. What did Sgt. Mehl do well? Not so well? How do you know?

2. What microskills did Mehl use during the interview? What percentage of time did he use open questions? Closed questions? Paraphrases? Reflections of feeling? Encouragers?

3. What did you think of Mehl's use of silence in his second response? Why?

4. How is this interview similar to and different from Resnick's interview of Andrea Yates in Chapter 1?

5. If this had been a clinical interview, what if anything would you have done differently?

6. What did Andrea Yates "say" about herself and, parenthetically, her relationship with Sgt. Mehl in this interview segment?

Effective clinicians resist the tendency to follow one question with another when they receive a poor response to their first question. Reflections of feeling or paraphrases of the session process may be more helpful (e.g., "It sounds like you're not ready to talk yet," "It was very difficult for you to come here today"). Of course, reflecting the difficulty of talking is only appropriate when that appears to be the problem (e.g., she is looking downward, sitting in a closed posture, struggling for words, or holding back strong emotions). When a client is not talking because he thinks therapy is boring and a waste of time—that is, leaning back in his chair, not paying attention, and making flip or off-track comments—that should be the core of the reflection (e.g., "It seems like you're angry that your mother brought you here today").

Certain types of questions may be problematic in some types of settings, especially during forensic interviews (Gilstrap, 2004). Closed questions can be leading and suggest that the correct choice is one of two options, even though neither is correct (e.g., "Did he touch you in the bedroom or in the living room?"). The clinician's preferences can be further signaled by tag questions (e.g., "He was in the living room, wasn't he?"). Asking children to imagine certain events can also be leading and distort memory (e.g., "Could you imagine what he would say?").

Asking closed questions can also encourage inappropriately dichotomous responding (e.g., "Are you feeling suicidal today?"). What degree of suicidality is enough to report? This sort of question could lead to either overestimates or underestimates of a client's suicidality. It might be more useful to ask, "On a scale from 1 to 10, how suicidal are you today?"

Finally, some statements take the form of one microskill but perform a different function. "Could" is generally a closed question but also serves as a directive (e.g., "Could you go to your 'safe place'?"). Using a closed question as a directive can be a useful way to give clients a sense of control, which is often important in the course of treatment.

Clinical Applications	Frank shares a clinical practice with his business partner, Eli. To strengthen his ability to communicate empathy and to better recognize the impact of each type of microskill, Frank practices his use of microskills with Eli. When Eli says, "It's been a long, rough winter and I don't know how I will go on," how might Frank reply if he were to use a paraphrase, a reflection of feeling, an open question, and a closed question by turn? How would you predict that his partner would respond to each of these responses?

Encouragers

Encouragers are generally several words taken directly from the client's response and used to focus further discussion. **Minimal encouragers**—"Uh huh," "Mmm," "Yup," a head nod, or an empathically appropriate facial expression—can also be used to quickly communicate understanding and encourage further discussion.

Sherman:	I just don't know what to do anymore. People keep coming up to me, to Dion, and asking about the baby-making process. I don't want to have to answer any more questions. I don't want to feel any more.
Clinician A:	More questions . . . [encourager]
Clinician B:	Feel any more? [encourager]
Clinician C:	Uh huh. [minimal encourager]

Notice how encouragers can get people talking about either content or feelings, depending on the particular encourager used. Think about what Sherman might say to the responses "more questions" and "feel any more." Minimal encouragers like "Uh huh" facilitate the discussion and influence its direction. When used well, encouragers and minimal encouragers can quickly and elegantly get clients talking, gently nudging them in a particular direction without focusing the attention on the clinician in the way that long, involved paraphrases, questions, or interpretations might.

Like any other microskill we've discussed, minimal encouragers and encouragers can be overused. Clients can perceive clinicians who repeatedly nod their head while saying "Uh huh" as stiff. Some clients may initially find encouragers awkward and be confused.

Summarizations

Summarizations are like paraphrases, but they cover a longer time period. They organize a large amount of information and help clients see the forest rather than only trees. Like paraphrases, summarizations generally take a specific form: (a) a succinct summary of a longer segment of the session, followed by (b) a checkout or question to check the client's understanding and to make sure that clinician and client are on the same page. Summarizations can be used at any point in a session, as in these two examples. They provide an effective bridge between two parts of a session or between two sessions or parts of treatment:

Clinician A:	Last session we were talking about the difficulties you've been having since learning that Dion couldn't get pregnant. We were challenging your irrational thoughts about this. How have you been feeling since then? [summarization, open question; at the beginning of the session]
Clinician B:	We've been talking about the ways that irrational thoughts cause our feelings. You've given examples of how your thinking patterns are directly related to your anger, frustration, and sadness about having to stop the infertility treatments. (nods) If you can cause these feelings, you can also control them. We discussed some ways that you could do this—and you did a great job! (pause) Is there anything else you'd want to add? [summarization, feedback, closed question; during the middle or at the end of the session]

Rather than the clinician telling clients what they got out of the session, clients can be asked to describe their own experience (e.g., "What was most important *to you* in what we did today?"). These client-generated summarizations can help them organize the session and can be empowering for the client, who then "owns" what was taken from a session. Like a checkout, a client-generated summarization can ensure that the clinician and client have the same understanding of what has happened in the session. Clinicians can also start sessions by asking, "What did you think about as you walked out of last week's session?" They can also ask, "What homework would you give yourself based on today's session?" Of course, when clients' homework assignments are too ambitious, clinicians can scale back assignments to something more manageable.

Cases in Empathy

It's Under *Your* Control ┃ D'Ja Jones

D'Ja Jones[1] (age 32) is an African American college student and mother of three. Her mother and grandmother both died when she was 16, the family who took her in stole her inheritance, and her boyfriend cheated on her and was violent toward her. Since then, she spent 3 years in therapy working on her feelings of trauma and loss. The following dialogue is from the instructional video *Trauma and Meaning*, which features Jeanne Slattery illustrating a variety of microskills with D'Ja Jones to encourage her to explore her experience more deeply.[2]

D'Ja Jones: I lost my mom suddenly when I was 16 years old.

Jeanne Slattery: Okay.

Jones: I'm an only child. My mother and grandmother raised me. My grandmother at the time was sick. We found out that she had cancer. After losing my mom, I had to sit around for 7 months and watch my grandmother die from cancer. Um . . .

Slattery: When you were 16.

Jones: When I was 16. So, my mother loved, loved, loved Luther Vandross. And she literally went to every concert that he had in Chicago. She even went to ones in Milwaukee, because I have family there. Her youngest sister. She bought every VHS back then, every LP album, cassette tape, and she literally, on her Walkman, listened to him every night. He serenaded her to sleep.

Slattery: Hm mmm.

Jones: So, I have a whole playlist. And so, sometimes when I am missing my mom a lot or am feeling really sad for her not being here for some moment, I play the whole Luther Vandross playlist, all her favorite songs. And again, it is just allowing me to *feel* how I need to feel and let it go. People always are saying, "Aw, you shouldn't be sad. Cheer up. You shouldn't feel that way. I don't want you to be sad." No, I need to feel this. Trying to *not* feel it, it just prolongs it.

[1]D'Ja is a pseudonym. We have also changed some identifying details to protect her confidentiality in this book, which is intended for a broader audience than the video.
[2]This video is available on DVD through the American Psychological Association. See https://www.apa.org/pubs/videos/4310015

(D'JA JONES continued)

Slattery: Right.

Jones: At least that's what I found for me.

Slattery: (gesturing toward self, then away) Rather than staying away from it you're going—

Jones: (gestures toward self)

Slattery: —toward it and you're *choosing* to go toward it.

Jones: Exactly. So, I have control.

Slattery: So, you have control.

Jones: Right.

Slattery: And that makes, that makes it very different.

Jones: Yes, it makes it extremely different because when you don't have control (laughs), you *become* out of control. You know, and you find yourself in *horrible* situations and you don't know how you got there. And then it's just a domino effect, a repeating of the cycle because now you have to feel upset because of whatever situation you've put yourself in. (laughs) It is, it's a vicious . . .

Slattery: Vicious cycle.

Jones: So, it's kind of like, well if I just let myself feel this way, and I keep to myself, I sit in my house, and I feel how I need to feel, then I can go on with my day and be productive and not put myself in situations that are going to cause me more harm than good.

Slattery: Mm mmm. (using hands for emphasis) And, it's under *your* control. You've *chosen* to do this. You're doing it not to bring yourself down, but to get yourself through it.

Jones: Right, it's a way to get through, instead of having it bury you. Because it will. (APA, 2020, minutes 18:54–21:38)

What Do You Think?

1. What do you think of Dr. Slattery's ability to hear and understand D'Ja Jones? What did D'Ja think? How do you know?

2. What microskills does Dr. Slattery use in this dialogue? How does D'Ja respond to these different microskills?

Accurate Empathy

> *He who does not understand your silence will probably not understand your words.*
> —Elbert Hubbard

Empathy is only effective in facilitating change if expressed. Words can communicate **accurate empathy**, reflecting what the client has said without adding any additional meaning, as Carl Rogers (1957/1992) described. However, they can also distort or lose the client's understanding (**subtractive empathy**). They can also capture the client's full meaning, both stated and not directly stated, helping a client gain insight that may not have been recognized or understood previously (**additive empathy**; Carkhuff, 1969).

Suppose a client, Sherman, states in therapy, "We worked so hard to have a child. What's next? Should we accept that we'll never have a child of our own? Should we look into adoption?" The following responses illustrate different levels of empathy:

- **Clinician A**: "It sounds like you're feeling pretty hopeless about the future right now." [subtractive empathy]
- **Clinician B**: "It sounds like this has been a difficult process and that you're feeling pretty confused about what you should do next." [accurate empathy]
- **Clinician C**: "It sounds like this has been a difficult process and that you're feeling pretty confused about what's next, but that you are also beginning to think about the future and recognize that life will go on, that you will go on." [additive empathy]

Clinician A missed the mark. After hearing Clinician A's statement, Sherman would likely respond in confusion, perhaps feeling alienated, perhaps needing to help his clinician understand him. If his clinician was lucky, Sherman would have responded by clarifying, "No, not really *hopeless*, but I am pretty confused about what we should do next." All clinicians make occasional missteps. If these mistakes are relatively infrequent and small, they might not damage the therapeutic alliance (Strupp, 1996).

Clinician B was on track, which would probably cause Sherman to expand on what he had been saying: "Yes, it has been difficult, and I'm really confused about where to go and what to do. What do I do next?" Clinician C, however, gave the most powerful response, recognizing how Sherman had been lost, but also how he and his wife were beginning to think differently about the future. Empathic clinicians do more than just parrot their clients' words; "they understand overall goals as well as moment-to-moment experiences, both explicit and implicit. Empathy in part entails capturing the nuances and implications of what people say, . . . reflecting this back to them for their consideration" (L. S. Greenberg, Elliot, Watson, & Bohart, 2001, p. 383). As seen in this and other examples, clients' statements are multifaceted, with meanings extending beyond their words. Recognizing these nuances can help clients feel heard and understood. Because Sherman felt understood by Clinician C, he responded,

> Yes, that's it! Over the past several years, we've been tossed back and forth between doctors, blindly doing whatever each doctor recommended. I didn't like it, but never recognized it at the time. Now I'm starting to feel that we have a choice and can take charge of our lives again. I feel like we can go on again.

His thoughtful expansion of Clinician C's statement suggests he felt he deeply understood.

While words communicate empathy, nonverbal and verbal empathy should be genuine and congruent because people are confused by conflicting verbal and nonverbal messages (Kolden, Klein, Wang, & Austin, 2011). Saying, "It sounds like you are having a hard time" while yawning and failing to make eye contact will probably signal a lack of interest. Saying the same thing while fully attending signals an active commitment to the person and relationship.

Lying may be common in therapy, with most clients reporting some degree of concealing their thoughts, feelings, or behavior. In one study, clients reported telling therapy-related lies because they wanted to be polite, avoid upsetting their therapist, or avoid their therapist's disapproval or because they were uncomfortable with the topic (Blanchard & Farber, 2016). Clients communicate that they feel misunderstood by blushing, fidgeting, or restlessly shifting position, avoiding eye contact or becoming silent, or making more speech disruptions, including hesitations, stammers, and rapid speech. Clinicians may do the same things when they feel bored, impatient, or inadequate, disrupting the empathic connection without being aware of doing so.

What Do You Think?

1. Return to Dr. Blumenfeld's responses to Annie Rogers from the beginning of the chapter. At what level of empathy—additive, subtractive, or accurate—would you describe his responses? How do you know? What about Dr. Slattery's work with D'Ja Jones?

Strategies for Understanding Others Deeply

I tell you everything that is really nothing, and nothing of what is everything, do not be fooled by what I am saying. Please listen carefully and try to hear what I am not saying.

—*Charles C. Finn*

Some people may be able to clearly and directly describe how they feel. Many people, however, have difficulty putting difficult thoughts and feelings directly into words. Some people (e.g., women, trauma survivors, people with borderline personality disorder) have silenced themselves, even making self-reports that are directly contradictory to their inner experiences (Blanchard & Farber, 2016). Even these groups, however, "leak" clues about how they think and feel (e.g., saying, "That's a great idea," while frowning, looking away, and quickly changing the subject).

Listening to a client's words builds empathy, but paying attention to bodily feedback can help clinicians identify their emotions and those of their clients.

Mirroring a client's breathing and following his or her movements can build understanding, rapport, and prosocial behaviors; failing to mirror can interfere with these processes (Lakin & Chartrand, 2003; van Baaren, Holland, Kawakami, & van Knippenberg, 2004). For example, speaking quickly and loudly with someone who is speaking quietly and slowly can interfere with rapport.

A client's behavior and a clinician's feelings can be misleading, however. Clients may breathe rapidly due to anxiety, but also to asthma. A clinician's anxiety during a client's discussion of her mother's illness may be related to events in his life rather than his client's anxiety. When gathering information, clinicians are generating and testing hypotheses; confidence about conclusions increases with additional consistent information.

A. G. Rogers (2001) described four strategies for deepening empathy beyond clients' choices of words. She offered the following suggestions to clinicians:

- **Approach the story from different viewpoints.** Any new interpretation— the roles of race, gender, age, ability, religion, and the like—broadens and deepens the picture. Consider things that are hinted at but never fully described. Pay attention to weaknesses as well as strengths. When and how, for example, is a client compliant with staff, and in which ways does he resist authorities? As described in Chapter 6, it is helpful to use multiple strategies during the assessment process (e.g., genograms, psychosocial histories, and timelines). The same principle applies here—multiple sources and perspectives will help with the accuracy of understanding.

- **Listen for language cues and metaphors.** Pay attention to word and metaphor choice and what they say about the speaker. When clients use active voice (e.g., "I am . . .," "I did . . ."), they may see themselves as direct and active participants with an internal locus of control, while the use of passive voice (e.g., ". . . was done to me," "It happened to me . . .") suggests an external locus of responsibility. Past tense suggests that the client sees the problem as being in the past, whereas present tense suggests it is perceived as ongoing. Metaphors can directly or indirectly describe things that may otherwise be unclear (e.g., "I sludged through an evening of work"), in this case suggesting that work was tedious, dirty, and perhaps even toxic.

  People use words for all sorts of different reasons. An unusual word choice (e.g., "I *sludged*") could indicate having (mis)heard an idiom rather than seeing it spelled out, enjoying playing with words, or even having brain damage. People's stories are influenced by various contextual factors, including cultural and temporal factors, audience, mood, environment, and chance events. Caution is necessary when drawing conclusions about people from other cultures. Language and nonverbal behaviors take different forms because of regional, ethnic, or age cohort differences that may not have the same meanings as in the clinician's culture. As suggested previously, conclusions should be drawn only after exploring other hypotheses.

Often what clients talk about can be read on several levels. For example, in saying that today is a nice day (which is true), one is also saying that the weather is not always nice. When a client says, "I really trust you," she may also be saying that she did not expect to trust her therapist, that her sense of trust is increasing, or perhaps that this trust is still wobbly. People rarely notice or talk about the things that are stable or known in their lives, often focusing instead on and talking about those things that are changeable or uncertain.

- **Pay attention to what gets omitted or muddied.** Sensitive information gets distorted or omitted in many ways. Clients may directly *deny* a problem: "I haven't cut this week" (when they did). They may change the subject to *evade* a problem: "You know, that's an important issue, but I really need to tell you about first . . .," hoping that they never get back to the problem subject. They may *revise* their story: "Well, yes, I told you that I didn't want to talk about that, but I really do." They may become *vague*, providing poorer descriptions than usual: "Yes, school is going well." Their story can be characterized by *silence*, thus actively or passively avoiding discussing a problem.

  Even when not talking about a problem (by denying, evading, revising, becoming vague, or remaining silent), clients tell a story about both the problem and themselves. For example, the client who denied cutting may be saying that she is afraid of the consequences of sharing this knowledge with someone else (or, perhaps, of admitting it to herself).

- **Track changes in the relationship.** Relationships shift and change with time. As the relationship changes, what can be told and how, as well as what is not disclosed, is altered. These changes both reflect and cause changes in the relationship. A client may disclose an intimate part of her past because she feels safe and understood, and the disclosure may in turn cause the clinician to behave in ways that draw out more disclosures.

  These dynamics should be examined in the course of the relationship, however. Some people find it easier to disclose vulnerabilities to strangers, and others can only disclose in close relationships. For example, as the therapeutic alliance develops, it may become easier to disclose some feelings, but if the client believes her clinician sees her as strong and competent, it may become more difficult to disclose vulnerabilities. Consider these ideas while listening to Anna Michener's story.

Understanding Anna ❙ Anna Michener

When Tiffany (b. 1977) was 13, she was sent to a psychiatric hospital because her grandmother said she was "disobedient" and out of control. Over the next several years, she was moved from institution to institution, then finally placed into a foster home shortly before she turned 16. There she took her foster parents' last name, Michener, to honor the people "who have been more of a family to me than any of my biological relations ever were." She also took a new first name, Anna, to make a clear separation from her past life and "to symbolize the fact that I am my own person" (Michener, 1998, p. 253). She describes her race as "mixed."

Anna's memoir was written during the period between her 16th and 17th birthdays, when she was in transition about how she saw herself and her world. In her younger years, she saw herself through her grandmother's eyes:

> My grandmother says I destroyed my mother before I was even born. A little flame of hate burns behind her ordinarily cold gray eyes when she says that. . . . [According to her] I had no conscience. I had no self-discipline. I cared for no one but myself. Apparently I was sociopathic. I was a pathological liar. I was a viciously manipulative pervert who could never love. (And thus "did not deserve to be loved," was the obvious conclusion.)
>
> My grandmother claimed to love me, however. She used to say that if she did not love me she would not have bothered to try to "save" me. She would not have pointed out everything I did wrong and explained how everything I did well could have been done better. (Michener, 1998, pp. 1–3)

In her memoir, Anna describes her grandmother putting an inordinate amount of responsibility on Anna. From the age of 6, Anna was responsible for keeping the house clean and making dinner, completing household chores, taking care of her younger brother, and making perfect grades in school. Anna was expected to put her mother's needs above her own, although her grandmother did not do so. Anna had to "earn" every good thing she received—cookies, going to the park, playing with toys. When incentives weren't enough to make Anna do as she was told, she was whipped, and when whippings no longer made Anna cry out, her grandmother whipped her little brother instead: "She knew I would rather die than see him hurt" (Michener, 1998, p. 3). Her grandmother also manipulated her with crocodile tears and spoke of "loving me so and hating to see me on the road of a person with bad character" (Michener, 1998, p. 4).

Anna's parents reinforced her grandmother's harsh view of her, demonstrating neither physical nor emotional closeness with her. For example, while her grandmother discouraged physical affection, even suggesting to Anna that touching her mother was "unnecessary stress," Anna saw her parents touch only once and did not remember being touched by her father except when he spanked her. He handled normal sibling fights with "shouting and cursing and mocking and ordering and hitting" (Michener, 1998, p. 5). When Anna was 9, she was even moved to a "small, cold room" at the back of the garage that smelled of gasoline. "In the garage I was set apart from the rest of the family, from the rest of the world" (Michener, 1998, p. 5).

This harsh view of herself and her world contrasts with Anna's current views, where she is more clearly able to identify what children deserve. Although Anna has received accolades for her criticism of the mental health system, she has also been criticized.

> I have been accused of saying in my book that I and other children institutionalized with me are perfectly innocent and everyone who worked with us was evil. But it is this interpretation, and not I who is so black and white. I do not believe anyone is perfectly innocent and I do not believe anyone is evil. I believe children become what they live and the only

(ANNA MICHENER continued)

way to combat the violent, depressed, and anti-social behavior of abuse victims is with understanding, acceptance, and love. However, I also see how this is hard to do. Mental health and social workers who do not understand the roots of certain aberrant behaviors will naturally react with fear, ignorance, and cruelty even if they are not cruel people.

I did not write this book for revenge, to point fingers, or to start fights. I hope simply that everyone who reads it puts him/herself in my place for a moment and asks—how would I feel if I had grown up this way? How would I have reacted? What would I have become? (Contemporary Authors Online, 2003, para. 2)

What Do You Think?

1. Reread this passage, paying attention to what she says without directly saying it (e.g., "My grandmother claimed to love me," *but didn't*). What else *doesn't* she say that conveys meaning?

2. As A. G. Rogers (2001) suggested, listen to Anna more closely by approaching the story from different viewpoints, attending to language cues and metaphors, paying attention to what gets omitted or muddied, and tracking changes in her relationships. What do you learn about her? What is she saying about what she needs and wants?

3. Return to Annie Rogers's story at the beginning of the chapter and listen for the thoughts and feelings embedded in her statements. How does Dr. Blumenfeld respond to these thoughts and feelings? How effective are his responses? How do you know?

The Need for Validation and Hope

This is why unpleasant events are "news"; compassionate activities are so much a part of daily life that they are taken for granted and, therefore, largely ignored.

—The Dalai Lama

Pinel and Constantino (2003) argued that people have two needs in relationships. People need to receive **validation** of their viewpoint (i.e., confirmation that their viewpoint is true or worthwhile), but they also need to hear positive things about themselves. Rather than glibly saying that everything will be better in the morning, many people prefer feedback that both validates their experience of the problem and that also suggests there is hope. Notice how Clinician C's last response was validating while also being hopeful (i.e., "It sounds like this has been a difficult process . . ., but you are *also* beginning to think about the future and recognize that life will go on, that *you* will go on").

| Clinical Applications | Frank has found himself responding to Eli with statements that include "Yeah but . . ." He has noticed that Eli now talks more slowly and more frequently breaks eye contact, but Frank isn't sure what is happening. What do you think is happening? What might Frank do at this point? |

Because the need for validation is so strong, some writers argue that clinicians should address this need very early in treatment (Ivey & Ivey, 2014; Pinel & Constantino, 2003). In sharing their understanding of clients—from the client's own viewpoint—clinicians both confirm their clients' ability to be understood and demonstrate their own clinical competence. Only when the client feels understood (validated) can a clinician hope to help a client change.

What Do You Think?

1. Did Anna Michener feel validated by the people working with her? How did she respond to this perception? What about Annie Rogers and D'Ja Jones? How did they respond?

Summary

Different microskills can be used to meet different clinical goals. Paraphrases describe the content from the client's last statement and encourage discussions of facts. Reflections of feeling focus on and encourage continued discussion of emotions. Encouragers, generally no more than a few words in length, get clients to focus on a particular aspect of their discussion and expand those ideas. Questions solicit information. Closed questions ask about specific information and are often answered with yes or no; open questions are often used to start a discussion and are less likely to be answered in a few words. The nature of the question (who, what, when, where, why, how) pulls different types of client responses focusing on different information. Summarizations succinctly pull together themes from a large part or all of a session.

Nonverbal and verbal responses, even when formed well, are not always on track. Those paraphrasing a client, without either diverting or adding to the client's understanding, reflect accurate empathy; most empathic responses used by effective clinicians are in this category. Off-track responses (subtractive empathy) interfere with the relationship when they occur too frequently or are handled poorly. Additive empathy accurately identifies both the overt message and the underlying subtext of a client's statements, thus encouraging deeper thinking and experiencing.

Developing empathic understanding can be developed in multiple ways. For example, A. G. Rogers (2001) suggested (a) approaching the client's story several times from different viewpoints, (b) listening closely to cues in the client's language and metaphors, (c) paying attention to what gets omitted or muddied in a discussion, and (d) tracking the changing emotions and relational dynamics in a session.

Generally, people respond best to messages that are both positive and validating of their self-concept. These messages must also be realistic and understandable from within the client's meaning system. Positive and validating statements reflect clinicians' deep understanding of their clients, engage clients more effectively, and build the therapeutic relationship.

For Review

Applying Concepts to Your Life

1. Pay attention to what good listeners and poor listeners do verbally. How do they demonstrate that they are listening well (or not so well)? How do others respond to them?

2. Practice using the basic verbal listening skills (e.g., paraphrases, reflections of feeling, summarization) without using questions, self-disclosures or verbal influencing skills. How does the other person respond? How do you feel in practicing these skills? If you feel awkward, remember that awkwardness is normal when learning a new skill.

3. Continue practicing verbal listening skills. What happens when you use them well? When you are intentionally poor at empathy (e.g., if someone is bouncing off the wall with joy, say, "It sounds like you had a really bad day!")? Tell your "research participant" what you were doing and why.

Key Terms

accurate empathy, 102
additive empathy, 102
closed questions, 97

encouragers, 99
microskills, 93
minimal encouragers, 99

open questions, 97
paraphrases, 94
reflections of feeling, 96

subtractive empathy, 102
summarizations, 100
validation, 108

Learn More

For more information about the concepts in this chapter, visit the *Empathic Counseling* companion website at http://pubs.apa.org/books/supp/slattery/.

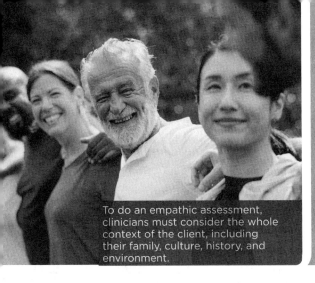

To do an empathic assessment, clinicians must consider the whole context of the client, including their family, culture, history, and environment.

6 Assessing People in Context

Looking Ahead IIII➡

After reading this chapter you will be able to answer these questions:

1. Why should clinicians attend to context during assessments and treatment?

2. How can psychosocial histories, family genograms, timelines, and mental status evaluations be used to understand and empathize with clients?

3. How does one's sources influence the information collected?

4. What can clinicians do to create a less biased assessment process?

5. What can clinicians do to create a strong case conceptualization?

Cases in Empathy

Stupid and Crazy? ▌ Raymond J. Corsini

Before leaving prison, one man made an appointment with Dr. Raymond Corsini to thank him. Dr. Corsini described this as the "most successful and elegant" therapy he had ever done. The man said to Dr. Corsini:[1]

> When I left your office about two years ago, I felt like I was walking on air. When I went into the prison yard, everything looked different, even the air smelled different. I was a new person. Instead of going over to the group I usually hung out with—they were a bunch of thieves—I went over to another group of square Johns [prison jargon for noncriminal types]. I changed from a cushy job in the kitchen to the machine shop, where I could learn a trade. I started going to the prison high school and I now have a high school diploma. I took a correspondence course in drafting and I have a drafting job when I leave Thursday. I started back to church even though I had given up my religion many years ago. I started writing to my family and they have come up to see me and they remember you in their prayers. I now have hope. I know who and what I am. I know I will succeed in

[1]Excerpts are from "Introduction to 21st-Century Psychotherapies," by F. Dumont, 2014, in D. Wedding and R. J. Corsini (Eds.), *Current Psychotherapies* (10th ed., pp. 1–17). Belmont, CA: Cengage. Copyright 2014 by Cengage. Reprinted with permission.

(RAYMOND J. CORSINI continued)

life. I plan to go to college. You have freed me. I used to think you bug doctors [prison slang for psychologists and psychiatrists] were for the birds, but now I know better. Thanks for changing my life. (Dumont, 2014, pp. 11–12)

Dr. Corsini was puzzled. How had he changed this man's life? He did not remember this man and had only given him an intelligence test. This man continued to tell him,

He had always thought of himself as "stupid" and "crazy"—terms that had been applied to him many times by his family, his teachers, and his friends. In school,

he had always received poor grades, which confirmed his belief in his mental subnormality. His friends did not approve of the way he thought and called him crazy. . . . But when I said, "You have a high IQ," he had an "aha!" experience that explained everything. In a flash, he understood why he could solve crossword puzzles better than any of his friends. He now knew why he read long novels rather than comic books, why he preferred to play chess rather than checkers, why he liked symphonies as well as jazz. With great and sudden intensity he realized . . . that he was really normal and bright and not crazy or stupid. (Dumont, 2014, pp. 11–12)

What Do You Think?

1. How did Dr. Corsini's assessment contribute to this man's changed view of himself? What about it was important?

2. Could just anyone say this so effectively? What made Dr. Corsini's statement so effective?

Recognizing Context

There's never a figure without ground.

—Kay King

Clinical assessment is the systematic evaluation and measurement of psychological, biological, and social factors in people presenting with a possible psychological disorder. Effective interventions depend on a strong clinical assessment of clients, empathically recognizing them in the context of their lives (Gutierrez, Fox, Jones, & Fallon, 2018). This chapter outlines assessment strategies that are easily implemented during initial sessions and throughout treatment. Assessing people in a three-dimensional manner is an essential part of treatment, without which clinicians may fail to be empathic, make inaccurate clinical assessments, or be outright judgmental.

Context influences and even distorts perceptions. A hard day at work might be challenging and invigorating to someone who feels well, but frustrating to someone who is ill. A woman who received sexually suggestive comments on the job might be overwhelmed while working on sexual assault issues in treatment, although a year earlier she might have felt validated by the same comments—and 3 years later, she might be able to make attributions that help her handle trauma-related triggers well.

People are embedded in an overlapping and complex set of contexts and are not necessarily aware of many of these. They may consistently recognize and identify with some contexts (e.g., religion, culture, trauma) yet be unaware of other highly influential contextual influences. For example, a woman may recognize the impact of being a lesbian from an evangelical Christian family that rejects her but fail to identify how her mother's chronic illness influences her sense of urgency about resolving family issues.

This chapter outlines four strategies for assessing people and their contexts; there are, of course, many other approaches. Yalom (2003), for example, suggested asking clients to describe the course of a "typical day" in detail to assess the pace and nature of life, as well as other details that may be so mundane that they would otherwise go unreported. Narrative exposure therapists create a visual lifeline with clients to identify important positive and negative life events, situating trauma in the person's social, cultural, historical, and political context (Schauer, Neuner, & Elbert, 2011). As Corsini's case material demonstrates, good assessments help clients to perceive themselves and their world differently and to change.

Developing Three-Dimensional Assessments

All assessment is a perpetual work in progress.

—Linda Suske

Clients are referred to treatment or for an evaluation as a result of a question, such as "Why do I feel so depressed?" This question is known as the **referral question**. In the Corsini case, the prison system asked about Corsini's client's level of intellectual functioning, which led to Corsini's decision to administer an intelligence test.

Different sources may have different questions because of their different goals. For example, each of these referral questions might have been appropriate for clinicians working with Andrea Yates in different settings:

- Court: "Is Andrea Yates competent and able to assist in her defense?"
- Attorney: "Was Andrea Yates legally sane at the time of the murders?"
- Prison: "Can Andrea Yates be safely maintained in this prison, or should she be moved to a more secure setting?"

Once clinicians understand their referral question, they can begin gathering information addressing it. While they may gather information in a focused way in the course of an interview or through focused psychological assessments (like Corsini's use of an intelligence test), often clinicians use broad and less focused strategies to help them develop a strong case conceptualization of a client. The four strategies discussed in this chapter are psychosocial history (Park & Slattery, 2009; Slattery & Park, 2012), family genogram (McGoldrick, Gerson, & Petry, 2008), timeline, and mental status evaluation. All of these strategies gather clusters of events—or their absence—to identify factors contributing to or ameliorating presenting problems, serving as obstacles, or facilitating change.

Clinical Applications	Angelika received a phone call asking her to "do an assessment" of T.R., who is being held in jail. As the phone call was from his attorney's secretary, Angelika is unclear about the purpose of this evaluation. Is she being asked to do a competency evaluation, an assessment of sanity at the time of the crime, or an assessment of treatment issues? As she thought about this, she considered the kinds of information she would need to respond to each of these referral questions. What would you suggest she consider? How would the information needed differ for each question? Why? What might she want if she were to see T.R. as a therapy client?

Psychosocial History

A **psychosocial history** is a collection of current and historical information about client behavior and functioning in a wide range of realms. Psychosocial histories gather information with a high potential to affect treatment, including relative strengths and weaknesses, obstacles to change, available resources and social supports, and client meanings. This information-gathering process helps clinicians understand their clients as three-dimensional beings, move beyond their biases and typical ways of looking at people, and develop empathy for them. Psychosocial histories can help clinicians draw a differential diagnosis, identify treatment goals and possible interventions, and assess prognosis. They help identify hypotheses about how these factors might contribute to the presenting problem and symptoms.

Rather than asking questions in a rote manner (e.g., "What is your current use of drugs and alcohol?"), most clinicians gather information for a psychosocial history in the course of an interview. They typically start with more general prompts (e.g., "Tell me why you're here today"), then move to specific questions addressing areas not spontaneously addressed earlier in the interview (e.g., "What do you do when you're stressed?"). Exhibit 6.1 identifies topics that are common to many agencies (e.g., symptoms, family background and functioning, familial history of psychiatric problems, drug and alcohol use, trauma history) and those that are more particular to our model (e.g., client's attributions about a life stressor, sense of life meaning and purpose,

Exhibit 6.1 Questions to Assess During the Assessment Phase and Throughout Therapy

<u>The problem</u>

Presenting problem or symptoms

What symptoms does the client report? How severe and chronic are they? When did they begin? To what degree do they interfere with functioning? Do they occur only in certain situations or do they occur across situations? What are the client's beliefs about what is wrong? About the appropriate treatment for his or her symptoms? Does he or she expect to get better?

   Be careful to assess major concerns, especially about suicide, rather than expecting clients to freely disclose them. Ask, *What else?*

Precipitating event and other recent events

Why is the client having problems now? Why is he or she entering treatment now? What negative or positive events have occurred recently at home, work, and school, and in important relationships? What ongoing stressors? Are reactions proportional to the stressor?

Personal and family history of psychological disorders

Has the client or family experienced either similar symptoms or different ones at some time in the past? How were problems handled? What was helpful? Specifically assess whether suicide was considered as a way to cope with problems.

   If either the client or family received formal treatment in the past, how might this affect current treatments? Were previous therapists respectful? hopeful? effective? empowering? Is current therapy an extension of previous work or, from the client's viewpoint, working on the same issues or totally new and unrelated ones?

<u>Current context</u>

Physical condition and medication use

How is the client's physical health? Can any medical conditions or medications account for the symptoms reported? Have these potential explanations been ruled out? Has the client been adherent with medications and treatment in the past? In what health-promoting (or -interfering) practices is the person currently engaging?

Drug and alcohol use

What is the client's personal and familial history of substance use and abuse? Could substance use cause symptoms? Could substances interact with prescribed medications?

Intellectual and cognitive functioning

What are the client's intellectual strengths and deficits? Could symptoms be caused by deficits?

Coping style

Does the client engage in generally adaptive or maladaptive coping strategies? What works? Are coping strategies generally short-term or long-term solutions? How do these coping strategies fit with his or her spiritual goals and values?

Exhibit 6.1 Questions to Assess During the Assessment Phase and Throughout Therapy *(Continued)*

Self-concept

What beliefs does the client hold about himself or herself? What beliefs about self or past problems are particularly helpful? Describe the client's mindset (fixed or growth) and self-efficacy.

Sociocultural background

In what culture was the client raised? If an immigrant, how long has the client been in this country? What led to the immigration? What are the client's connections to homeland and level of acculturation? What other group identifications (e.g., race, affectional orientation, gender, age, physical abilities) are most important? How do the client's cultural background and group identifications influence symptoms and reactions to symptoms? Could the behavior be "normal" in the client's culture and not in the clinician's (or vice versa)?

Spirituality and religion

What (if any) religious affiliation does he or she report? How important are the client's religious and spiritual views? In what ways are they important? How do spiritual and religious beliefs, values, goals, behaviors, and resources influence current functioning? Do they provide a supportive network? Are beliefs culture-typical or -atypical? Does the client perceive support and acceptance in the religious community (e.g., minister, congregation, God)?

Trauma history

Does the client report a history of trauma in the home, community, school, or work settings? What meanings did the client draw about it? What reactions did others have to it?

Resources and barriers

Individual resources

What does the client do particularly well or feel good about? How can these attributes (e.g., persistence, loyalty, optimism, intelligence) be resources for or undermine treatment?

Relational style

How are the client's relationships? Open? Trusting? Suspicious? Manipulative? What are the client's general views of others? What is the therapeutic relationship like? Can the client be honest about symptoms, behavior, side effects, and concerns? Honestly disclose treatment nonadherence? Correct the clinician's misassumptions?

Mentors and models

What real, historical, or metaphorical figures serve as pillars of support or spiritual guides? How have these models handled similar problems? Note: Some models may be primarily negative in tone. What are the positive aspects of these "negative" models?

Sense—and sources—of meaning

What senses of meaning does the client have and from where? Is life meaningful? Chaotic? Unpredictable? What are his or her core beliefs, values, and goals? From where is meaning drawn? Does the client have a strong sense of purpose or mission in life? How "on track" does the client perceive his or life to be regarding ultimate sources of meaning and purpose?

Exhibit 6.1 Questions to Assess During the Assessment Phase and Throughout Therapy *(Continued)*

Social resources (friends, family and school/work)

How supportive are the client's family, friends, and work relationships? Are they sufficient in both quantity and quality to meet the client's needs? Do they increase or decrease the client's stress levels? Do they empower or undermine the client?

Community resources

What agencies (if any) are involved? How supportive are they of the client and client's values and goals? How well do these agencies work with each other?

Community contributions

How does the client contribute to the community? Do contributions feel useful and meaningful to the client? Are contributions acknowledged by important people in his or her support system? Are they related to and do they feed spiritual goals?

Obstacles and opportunities to change process

What might serve as potential obstacles or aids to the change process? These can be financial, educational, social, intellectual, or spiritual. What does the client believe will (or might) happen when change occurs—both positively and negatively?

Note. From *Counseling Diverse Clients: Bringing Context Into Therapy* (pp. 14–15), by J. M. Slattery, 2004, Belmont, CA: Cengage. Copyright 2004 by South-Western, a part of Cengage, Inc. Reprinted with permission.

obstacles to change, therapeutic alliance). While learning how to write a psychosocial history, clinicians should focus less on the categories, which may change across settings, and more on developing a general strategy for gathering broad, yet detailed, information about a client.

Organizing interview and historical data into a psychosocial history can identify hypotheses that have been overlooked and make the case conceptualization process more productive and thorough (Gutierrez et al., 2018). Gathering a psychosocial history can challenge biases and prevent clinicians from missing information that does not readily fit their initial biases. Kottler (2004) described the importance of careful assessments:

> It's not that you are procrastinating when you hesitate to answer her query about how you will help her; it is just that you would be foolish to attempt any intervention without fully understanding what you are attempting to accomplish. It would be as if you went to see a doctor complaining of a stomachache and she immediately scheduled you for surgery without running appropriate tests to determine what might be wrong. (p. 198)

To illustrate the development of a psychosocial history, consider Malcolm X, a famous civil rights leader and prominent figure in the Nation of Islam in the

1960s. Malcolm X advocated for Black pride and Black nationalism. Unlike his contemporary, Martin Luther King Jr., Malcolm X supported a more militant approach to achieving civil rights, urging Blacks to acquire freedom, justice, and equality "by any means necessary" (Malcolm X, 2015). As you read his story, imagine that Malcolm Little (as he was named before he joined the Nation of Islam) had been referred to you by his caseworker at age 14, when he began running into problems at school and in his community. The caseworker's referral might include questions about why Malcolm was running into problems and whether an out-of-home placement was appropriate.

The following case material is incomplete—as it will always be, as we can never know the whole situation—but provides useful ideas to pursue further. This case material may also provide some ideas that may help you understand Malcolm X's position as a Black nationalist.

Cases in Empathy

Malcolm Little | Malcolm X

Malcolm Little was born into a society full of problems and into a family that expected him to do something about whatever problems he faced. Numerous threads contributed to his later activism: the violence that surrounded his childhood, color and race consciousness, and poverty, in particular, but also the family's mobility and search for self-sufficiency.

Born in 1925, Malcolm was Rev. Earl and Louise Little's fourth of their seven children together and his father's seventh. Malcolm was born in Omaha, Nebraska. While his mother was pregnant with him, the Ku Klux Klan threatened the family's home. His parents waited until Malcolm was born, then moved to Milwaukee, Wisconsin. Shortly after his younger brother's birth, they moved to Lansing, Michigan, a place where his parents hoped for greater financial independence. His remaining four siblings were born there. His youngest half-brother was born 7 years after Malcolm's father's death.

In 1929, his family was threatened again, this time by the Black Legion. The previous attack had broken their windows; this time their home was burned to the ground. The police and fire departments that were called to the fire just stood and watched the devastation. The Little family moved outside of East Lansing, Michigan, where they could be largely self-sufficient. Four of Malcolm's uncles were killed by White men, one in a lynching, and Malcolm blamed his father's death—ruled as a streetcar accident by local officials—on the Black Legion. He believed that he, too, would die as a result of this systemic violence targeted at Blacks: "I have done all I can to be prepared" (Malcolm X & Haley, 1964/1999, p. 2).

Race and the racism permeating his environment were formative factors in Malcolm's development. Malcolm's father, a Baptist minister, was a follower of Marcus Garvey, a Black separatist, who believed that Blacks must return to Africa because Black freedom, autonomy, and self-respect could never happen in the United States. Malcolm and his father traveled to meetings of Garvey's followers. He admired the people he met there, whom he saw as forceful and intelligent, yet down to earth. Being surrounded by others who saw themselves as capable and confident inspired him to feel that way too, and he looked for this same naturalness and intensity in others, even as an adult.

Malcolm received mixed messages about race, however. He suspected his father favored him because he was light-skinned, as was typical for many Black parents. His mother, whose mother had been raped and impregnated by a White man, was born in Grenada and looked White. Malcolm believed that his mother favored her darker children as a result and worked to prevent him from developing color-superiority.

Mrs. Little was a force to be reckoned with, holding high standards for her children and making sure they were well educated. Her oldest son, Wilfred, described their childhood like this:

> When we were doing our homework, there was always a dictionary on the table, and when we mispronounced a word my mother made us look it up and learn both to spell and to pronounce it correctly. By reading that Marryshow paper day after day, we developed reading and writing skills superior to those of our white classmates. By reading Garvey's paper and Marryshow's paper, we got an education in international affairs and learned what Black people were doing for their own betterment all over the world. (Carew, 1994, p. 117)

Although much of the violence that Malcolm saw was overt—including violence between his parents and toward their children—other violence was more subtle and pervasive. Police and firefighters did not respond when their family home was attacked. The insurance companies paid off the smaller, but not the larger, of his father's life insurance policies after his murder. The welfare system undermined, then split up, Malcolm's family after his father's death. He saw this as unnecessarily destructive and reflective of society's failures. "I have no mercy or compassion in me for a society that will crush people, and then penalize them for not being able to stand up under the weight" (Malcolm X & Haley, 1964/1999, p. 22). He recognized that systemic racism and violence takes many forms.

In Malcolm's childhood, Whites were at best a benign presence, generally helpful when he excelled by their rules—as he did in school—and when he did not rock the boat. When he spoke out, when he tried to take more than they thought he should have, they quickly backed off or moved him to a safer distance. For example, as he described in his autobiography, when he was 13, a teacher asked what he wanted to be when he grew up. He responded that he wanted to be a lawyer. His teacher responded both with surprise and condescension.

> "Malcolm, one of life's first needs is for us to be realistic. Don't misunderstand me, now. We all here like you, you know that. But you've got to be realistic about being a nigger. A lawyer—that's no realistic goal for a nigger. You need to think about something you *can* be. You're good with your hands— making things. Everybody admires your carpentry shop work. Why don't you plan on carpentry? People like you as a person—you'd get all kinds of work."
> The more I thought afterwards about what he said, the more uneasy it made me. It just kept treading around in my mind. (Malcolm X & Haley, 1964/1999, p. 38)

As he considered this incident, Malcolm became more and more uneasy. Mr. Ostrowski had encouraged his classmates to be whatever they wanted, "yet nearly none of them had earned marks equal to mine. . . . But apparently I was still not intelligent enough, in their eyes, to become whatever *I* wanted to be. It was then that I started to change—inside" (Malcolm X & Haley, 1964/1999, p. 38, italics in original).

Malcolm's native skills in many areas— academics, interpersonal, dancing, carpentry, hunting—gave him a leg up. But several other things also influenced him. His father was

(MALCOLM X continued)

a Baptist preacher, his mother a Seventh Day Adventist. However, he struggled with Christian views and with many Christians: "I had very little respect for most people who represented religion" (Malcolm X & Haley, 1964/1999, p. 5). He had two powerful and assertive role models: his father and his half-sister Ella. His father believed that things could be different for Blacks and worked to make it happen. Ella, a "really proud black woman," showed him that one could aim high, be successful, and reach out to help other Blacks (Malcolm X & Haley, 1964/1999, p. 34). From his quiet brother, Wilfred, who often went hungry as a result of his lack of assertiveness, he learned that "if you want something, you had better make some noise" (p. 8). He watched and learned from others' successes, as he recognized that their successes could tell him something important.

What Do You Think?

1. What questions would you want to ask to further flesh out your understanding of Malcolm? How would you go about asking them?

2. If you tended to focus on problems as you read his story, go back and identify strengths. Why might identifying strengths be useful in your work with him?

3. Why might it be important to attend to the systemic violence affecting other Blacks when working with Malcolm? Would attending to this systemic violence and racism be as important for someone less politically active?

As seen in the case material and the psychosocial history in Table 6.1, Malcolm's story is complicated, including considerable violence and family stressors (e.g., parental arguments and domestic violence, murders, poverty, early fighting and thieving) but also numerous strengths (e.g., good health, academic success, an assertive and gregarious nature, strong work ethic, and strong spiritual background). One could assess either the weaknesses or strengths; systematically gathering them encourages a more complete clinical assessment. Other issues of note:

- Malcolm has considerable supports, but many of these supports seem conflictual in nature. The conflictual nature of his supports may affect how he sees and interacts with others and influence his expectations for treatment.

- Malcolm reports numerous racist experiences (e.g., his family members' murders, his family home being burned, his family's color bias) that influence how he sees the world. Failing to pay attention to race in treatment would probably undermine the therapeutic relationship.

Table 6.1 A Psychosocial History for Malcolm Little in 1940, Age 15

	Objective description	Client's global and situational meanings	Hypotheses about treatment
The problem			
Presenting problem or symptoms	Caught stealing food and other items, engaging in small mischief (e.g., tipping outhouses), and fighting with his brother and other teens.	Feels justified in these actions, both supporting family and opposing a system he sees as racist.	Does not see himself as source of problems and may be unmotivated to change.
Precipitating event and other recent events	In the past 4 years, his siblings were split up and put into foster care. His mother was placed in a psychiatric hospital 2 years ago. The family has not had enough food to eat following his father's alleged murder.	Sees life as unfair and frequently racist.	Joining may necessitate recognizing and naming racism in his life.
Personal and family history of psychological problems	Denies a history of psychological symptoms, attributing problems to the racist society he lives in. His mother has been recently hospitalized as a result of a "nervous breakdown."	Angry at the system that forced his mother's hospitalization, which he attributed to psychosocial stressors, especially pervasive racism.	Aligning with his meaning of these events, at least initially, may be necessary to join.
Current context			
Physical condition and medication use	Is strong and in good health. Good basketball player. No medications reported.	Values his health, which he sees as outward manifestation of his personal vitality.	His physical health influences his self-concept, an asset that can be harnessed in treatment.
Drug and alcohol use	None reported for client or family.	No problem.	
Intellectual and cognitive functioning	Reports being one of the top students in his class. He thinks abstractly, recognizing both what is but also what could be.	Feels smart and competent and sees this as a means for meeting personal goals.	More strengths to harness in treatment.
Coping style	Reports identifying problems, recognizing their societal causes, and protesting these loudly.	He sees this coping style as healthy and adaptive.	Treatment should be active and consider societal injustices.

Table 6.1 A Psychosocial History for Malcolm Little in 1940, Age 15 *(Continued)*

	Objective description	Client's global and situational meanings	Hypotheses about treatment
Self-concept	Sees self as smart, "intuitive" like his mother, and capable of addressing or circumventing problems.	Values his style of approaching the world.	His growth mindset and self-efficacy can foster change. Treatment should be active and both rational and intuitive.
Sociocultural background	Is African American in a racist society. His parents have had two houses threatened, one burned to the ground. Five of his uncles and his father were murdered in race-related violence. He attended Marcus Garvey's group as a young child with his father and felt that the members of this Black separatist group were "more intense, more intelligent and down to earth" than other Blacks.	Sees world as racist and unfair, with normal means to success being blocked. He sees the activist and separatist approach of Marcus Garvey as offering an avenue for success.	Race and issues of social justice must be addressed in treatment. He describes several positive African American models. White workers, especially those failing to acknowledge and challenge racism, will have difficulty creating an effective therapeutic alliance.
Spirituality and religion	Was raised in a family with strong religious beliefs. His father was a Baptist minister. His mother is a Seventh Day Adventist and has been criticized for refusing "unclean foods," given their obvious poverty. He reports not respecting most religious leaders or doctrines.	Feels disillusioned with much organized religion.	Although he feels disillusioned with organized religion, religion has been both a family strength and a unique part of their family identity. This may be a resource to access in treatment.
Trauma history	His father was reportedly murdered when he was 5; his uncles were also murdered. Insurance company denied payout, and community was perceived as unsupportive. Parents were violent toward each other and their children.	This history of race-related violence has alienated him from mainstream (White) community and created an expectation that he will die young as the result of violence.	This sense of alienation and hopelessness might undermine the therapeutic relationship and may be a significant barrier to change. What does he see himself as able to change?

Table 6.1 A Psychosocial History for Malcolm Little in 1940, Age 15 *(Continued)*

	Objective description	Client's global and situational meanings	Hypotheses about treatment
Resources and barriers			
Individual resources	Has strong reading and writing skills, and is a good problem-solver. He debates well; is hardworking and assertive; and a good carpenter, gardener, and hunter. Recognizes that he can learn from anyone, including people who are more successful than he is.	Sees these individual strengths as attributes that will make him successful in almost any situation.	Has considerable self-efficacy and high aspirations that can be helpful in treatment. These may counterbalance his feelings of hopelessness about racial injustice.
Relational style	Dominant, gregarious and argumentative. He is intuitive and able to read others well. He is able to get people to like and help him.	Appreciates his social skills. Believes that reading others is a way of meeting his individual goals.	He may initially say what he believes is expected, but his social skills could be a significant strength.
Mentors and models	Sees both his father and oldest sister as proud and capable and had strong, positive relationships with both. His mother emphasized the importance of learning and hard work. On the other hand, he saw his brother Wilfred going hungry because he was quiet and unassertive. He learned that you've got to "make some noise" to get what you want.	He sees people as getting ahead by being strong, proud, capable, assertive, and smart. His family valued these qualities, although they were not valued within the racist society in which he lives—at least when others perceived him as "uppity."	These mentors and models indicate social resources, but also attributes that he wants to develop. They can be accessed when he looks for positive ways to resolve problems.
Sense—and sources—of meaning in life	He is both acutely aware that the world is racist, color-conscious and unfair, but also believes that if one makes "some noise," things can be changed. Although surrounded by violence throughout his childhood, he believes his mind was a more important agent of change than violence alone. He believes that he will die a violent death.	Recognizes the importance of being smart, but also of "making noise" to make a difference. Does not see a positive personal outcome to his struggles.	His focus is individual, familial, and societal. Framing treatment goals only individually would miss an important part of his picture.

Table 6.1 A Psychosocial History for Malcolm Little in 1940, Age 15 *(Continued)*

	Objective description	Client's global and situational meanings	Hypotheses about treatment
Social resources (family and friends)	Client is the seventh of 11 children (fourth in his father's second marriage). Despite numerous stressors, his family has considerable strengths. His parents were strong role models who worked hard to create a sustainable life in a racist society. His father strongly supported him, while his mother challenged him. He and his siblings fight with each other but are also loyal and supportive. Since his father's alleged murder, the family has been poor and without food, leading to some children being placed in foster care.	Values his family's social support and attributes recent problems to racism and ways that the system has undermined his family.	He wants the welfare system and treatment to support rather than undermine family.
Work/school	He is near the top of his class in school; however, when he announced wanting to be a lawyer when he grew up, a favorite teacher instead encouraged him to be "realistic" and become a carpenter.	Sees teacher's evaluation of his future as unfair and as a major impetus to his recognition of racism.	He needs to find some way of resolving this discrepancy between his abilities and his treatment by society.
Community resources	Families in the community have been buying food for client and his siblings, as well as sharing food with the family. The welfare system is actively monitoring the family since his mother was hospitalized; they are considering placing her younger children in foster care.	Is ambivalent about his neighbors' support and very negative about the welfare system's involvement in his family.	Wants supportive relationships, not those that he sees as undermining his family or himself.
Community contributions	Is actively supportive of family and neighbors.	Feels strong and capable.	A strength to harness in treatment.

Table 6.1 A Psychosocial History for Malcolm Little in 1940, Age 15 *(Continued)*			
	Objective description	Client's global and situational meanings	Hypotheses about treatment
Obstacles and opportunities in change process	Is bright, capable, with strong sense of self-efficacy. Has been undermined or treated as a "pet" by authority figures.	Distrusts most Whites and authority figures. Does not see himself as having a problem, attributing problems to societal factors.	Should consider racial identity in assigning clinician. Choose goals that he is willing to work towards, while acknowledging societal contributions to problems. Acknowledge and access considerable strengths in treatment.

- Despite numerous stressors, Malcolm was resilient. He recognized injustice and believed he could do something about rectifying it. He had considerable self-efficacy and an internal locus of control and admired assertive action in others. Taking a passive or neutral stance in treatment would likely be ineffective. Perhaps treatment should focus on helping him identify positive ways of responding to stressors and oppression.

- Although there are considerable stressors and conflict within his family, Malcolm also reported considerable support and numerous positive role models. As a result, perhaps treatment should identify ways of making these supports more effective for him.

Often the write-up of a psychosocial history follows a standard format that includes the first two columns from Table 6.1, although generally using headings and brief paragraphs. We include two additional columns: the meanings clients draw in response to factors described in the psychosocial history and hypotheses about the impact of these events on treatment (Slattery & Park, 2012). Although these last two columns are not normally included in psychosocial histories, they illustrate the kind of thinking in which a reflective clinician might engage while gathering or reading a psychosocial history, the sort of thinking that builds empathy.

Clinical Applications

During a psychosocial history, Terrell noted that he was the first member of his family to attend college. He struggled to explain what it meant for him to be "the first" because this felt normal for him, although he noted that his family was simultaneously putting a lot of pressure on him to succeed and also saying things like "Terrell wouldn't understand." What positive and negative meanings might you hypothesize that being "the first" has for him?

Family Genogram

The **family genogram** (McGoldrick et al., 2008) is a visual means of generating hypotheses about familial factors that may contribute to the problem or serve as resources for treatment. Genograms generally include genealogical material but also show relationships, patterns of mental health diagnoses or substance abuse, and major events in a family history. They include basic information about number of marriages and children, birth order, and deaths. See Figure 6.1. Genograms can also include information on disorders running in the family (e.g., alcoholism and depression), alliances, the nature of relational interactions (e.g., cutoffs and enmeshments), and living situations. Slattery (2004) described using genograms also to track family strengths. Their use is only limited by the imagination.

Genograms can be useful in keeping track of complicated family information, which would certainly be helpful when working with Malcolm Little. See Figure 6.2. Another, more important use of genograms, however, is to generate hypotheses about family relationships. For example, family events can have either unique or common meanings across family members; these familial patterns may be carried forward to impact future generations (either repeated or reacted to). **Enmeshed** families have permeable and unclear boundaries; members of such families often have difficulties with privacy and may be unable to separate their emotional experiences from each other's. Some questions and hypotheses that could be drawn based on the patterns in Malcolm Little's genogram include the following:

- How might being his father's fourth child in his second marriage, seventh of 11 children total, have influenced Malcolm? What about the relatively close spacing of children in his parents' marriage—seven children in 9 years?

- Malcolm reported that his skin color created and, perhaps, undermined alliances in his family. How might these influences be affected by his grandmother's rape? How did people's reactions to his skin color influence how he saw himself and his relationships with others?

- How did his father's and uncles' murders by White men—and his grandmother's rape—influence Malcolm's self-concept, activism, and attitudes about race?

- In genograms, a **triangle** indicates when there is an unstable relationship between two people. That relationship is stabilized by bringing in a third either for comfort or to redirect tension. In this case, there appears to be an important triangle between Malcolm's parents, which was stabilized by his parents diverting their positive and negative emotions toward Malcolm. What was the impact of this triangle on his family status? How might that triangle influence his later relationships?

- How can family alliances be accessed in treatment to support Malcolm during this vulnerable period?

FIGURE 6.1 A Brief List of Standard Symbols for Genograms

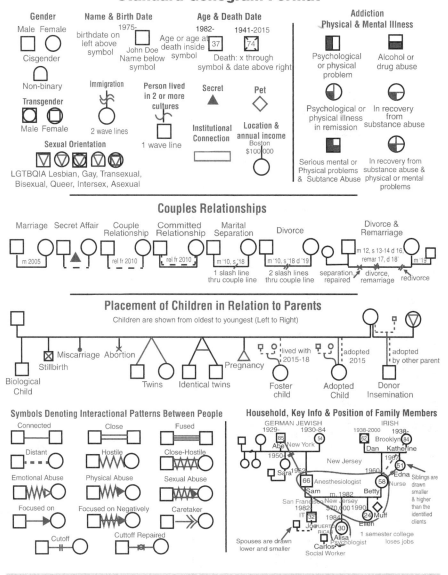

From *Genograms: Assessment and Intervention* (4th ed., Inside book cover), by M. McGoldrick, R. Gerson, and S. Petry, 2020, New York, NY: W. W. Norton. Copyright 2020 by M. McGoldrick, R. Gerson, and S. Petry. Adapted with permission.

FIGURE 6.2 Family Genogram for the Young Malcolm X in 1939, at the Age of 14

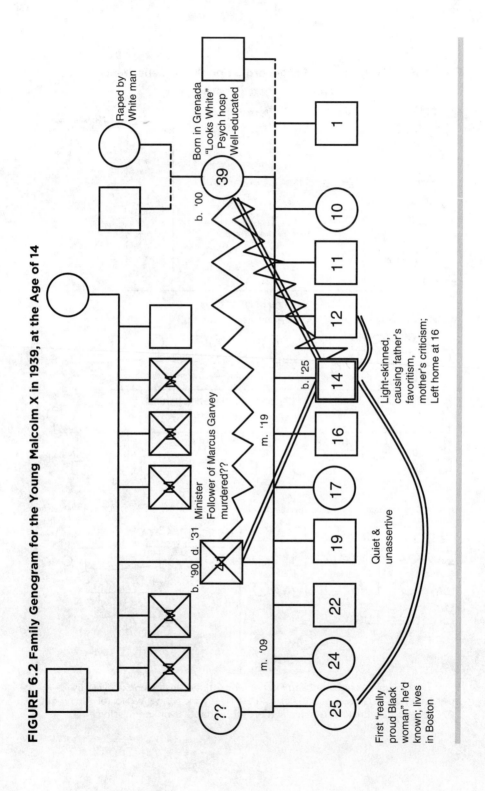

Timeline

People exist in a family and systemic context; however, they also exist in a temporal context. One useful strategy for describing clients' temporal and historical contexts is a timeline. A **timeline** is a record from birth to the present describing major events for clients and their immediate family. It organizes information and highlights the temporal contiguity of events. Timelines generally include information gathered during a family genogram, including dates of births, deaths, marriages, divorces, and so on in the immediate family. Timelines record both the mundane (e.g., a voluntary job change) and the unusual (e.g., being charged with statutory rape). Timelines can be especially useful with people who have complicated histories or for whom the relationships among events are unclear.

A timeline contains stressors and major events *from the client's idiosyncratic point of view* over his or her life span. That is, although flying may not be a stressor for most people, being told that one has to fly across country as a regular and ongoing part of one's job could be a major stressor for someone who has a flying phobia. Furthermore, timelines afford the opportunity to look at clustering of stressors as well as reactions to them. Losing a job is almost always a stressor, but its meaning may be amplified during a year when a child has been diagnosed with cancer, one's partner has asked for a divorce, and the mortgage has gone into default. In addition, the person who experiences four major stressors in a relatively quiet life may perceive these stressors differently from a person who has had major stressors throughout life.

Generally, the assessment process also notes reactions to these stressors, including depression, suicide attempts, ulcers, and increased drinking. How does the person respond to stressors? Do relatively trivial stressors overwhelm the client, or can clusters of stressors be handled well? Has this pattern of reactions changed across time, with the person seeming to become either more easily overwhelmed or hardier and more stress-resistant? What sorts of stressors seem to overwhelm the client (e.g., job-related, interpersonal, familial)? Is there any sort of theme to these stressors (e.g., personal threat, loss of control, perceived abandonment)?

A number of the themes raised in the timeline echo those seen in Malcolm Little's psychosocial history and genogram. See Exhibit 6.2.

- Malcolm reports his parents had a number of children in rapid succession, echoing the questions raised in the genogram about physical and emotional resources in the family.

- He had numerous significant traumas throughout his life, including five murders, two house fires, his mother's psychological decline, and his placement in foster care. To what extent are concerns raised by the referring agency related to trauma rather than to poor parenting?

- The family's level of functioning appeared to decline in the years after his father's murder. To what extent was this decline related to grief and to what extent poverty?

Exhibit 6.2 A Timeline of Malcolm Little's Early Life[a]

1924—Family and home threatened by the KKK while Mrs. Little was pregnant with Malcolm.

1925—Malcolm was born.

1926—Moved to Milwaukee, WI.

1927—Reginald was born.

1928—Moved to Lansing, MI, hoping for financial independence. Wesley was born.

1929—Yvonne was born. Home was threatened and burned to the ground while fire department watched. Moved outside of East Lansing, MI.

1931—Earl Little was run over by a streetcar and died; he was rumored to have been murdered by a White supremacist group. Two of their three insurance policies refused to pay, claiming Mr. Little had committed suicide. Family had difficulty putting food on the table.

1936—Mrs. Little was courted by a "large, dark man from Lansing"

1937—Mrs. Little's relationship ended—perhaps because of the number of mouths to feed. Mrs. Little began to decline: "the beginning of the end of reality for my mother." Family was "destroyed" by state, which began placing children in foster care.

1938—Robert was born. Malcolm was expelled from school. Mrs. Little was declared legally insane and committed to a state hospital.

Note. Data from Malcolm X and Haley (1964/1999) and Twenty-First Century Books (2008).

[a]Information included here is not presented for its historical accuracy (although we have done the best we can) but to describe how one might use biographical information to understand a person. Official sources provide inconsistent dates for Malcolm X's life.

Note that each hypothesis suggests the problem is treatable, although in different ways.

This timeline is useful in organizing information from Malcolm's life, but it provides an incomplete picture of his experience. Rather than being a defeated and traumatized child, Malcolm is bright, astute, and assertive. How did he get that way? Although his psychosocial history begins to answer this question, his timeline should also incorporate these strengths to provide a three-dimensional clinical assessment that will engage him in therapy. Adding the information in Exhibit 6.3 begins to round out this story.

Clinical Applications

During his intake interview, Terrell outlined a number of events on his timeline: being raised by a single mother, being African American at a White-majority high school, being diagnosed with exercise-induced asthma, coming out as gay at 15, and being the first in his family to attend college. His therapist, Ruby Dee, considered both a negative story he might tell about his life based on this information alone, but also a more positive story. What stories might she tell? What might the implications be for each story?

> **Exhibit 6.3** **Strength-Based Additions to Malcolm Little's Timeline**
>
> 1929—Family moved outside of East Lansing, MI, hoping to become self-sufficient, and built home.
>
> 1929–1931—Traveled with father to the meetings of Garvey's followers. Described believing that Blacks at these meetings were "more intense, more intelligent and down to earth."
>
> 1931–1938—Attended school and was recognized as one of the smartest and most talented children by both adults and children, Whites and Blacks.
>
> *Note.* Data from Malcolm X and Haley (1964/1999) and Twenty-First Century Books (2008).

Mental Status Evaluation

An important part of most assessments is a description of mental status. The client's mental status in numerous areas, including mood, affect, cognition, and impulsivity is normally assessed in the course of other assessments or during treatment. Along with other assessments, a mental status evaluation creates a three-dimensional description of the client's psychological status during the assessment. A **mental status evaluation** is an assessment of the client's functioning in a number of realms (e.g., appearance, relationship with interviewer, affect and mood, speech and language use, cognition, and memory, disorders in thinking, and insight and judgment). This tool is helpful to the process of differential diagnosis and can help a clinician conclude whether social isolation, for example, is related to depression, psychosis, an autistic spectrum disorder, or dementia.

Mental status evaluations include both client strengths and weaknesses. The specific content of the mental status evaluation varies considerably depending on the evaluation setting and population assessed (e.g., an adult in an Alzheimer's wing of a nursing home, a preschooler suspected to have autism) but generally includes the following:

- **Appearance.** The client's age, race, sex, relational status, dress, grooming, gait, posture, level of activity, and coordination.
- **Interviewer–client relationship.** The client's interpersonal skills, the rapport between client and interviewer, and the perceived validity of the interview. **Validity** is the extent to which an observation or assessment measures what it is supposed to measure. A weak relationship between interviewer and client can cause the client to withhold or disguise information, which introduces bias in interpreting other indicators.
- **Affect and mood. Mood** refers to the client's "emotional atmosphere," which is internal, subjective, and relatively more sustained, although may vary across time. Mood is often inferred from the client's verbal tone and subjective report. **Affect** refers to the client's observable

emotion. Descriptions of affect usually include level of reactivity (i.e., flat, blunted, constricted, normal, labile) and congruence between affective expression and verbal content. Indicators of anxiety or affective disorders are noted (e.g., eye contact, posture, nervous mannerisms).

- **Speech and language use.** The exam assesses volume, speed, fluency, length, and articulation quality of responses, their situational appropriateness, clarity of answers, and unusual speech components (e.g., echolalia, overgeneralization, poor word choices).

- **Cognition and memory.** Includes alertness, attention, concentration, and orientation (to person, place, time, and purpose of interview), long and short-term memory, general intellectual level and fund of knowledge, abstract thought, and ability to perform simple tasks (e.g., arithmetic, reading and repeating sentences, ability to understand and perform tasks, and ability to copy or generate figures).

- **Disorders in thinking.** Disease processes may be observed in reports or behavioral indications of hallucinations, delusions, obsessions, dissociative processes, derealization, depersonalization, and confusion about one's identity. Thought processes may be marred by irrelevant detail, unnecessarily repeated words and phrases, interrupted thinking (thought blocking), and loose, illogical connections. The assessment should include thoughts of suicide or homicide as well as indicators of level of dangerousness.

- **Insight and judgment.** The former refers to an awareness of the presenting problem and its nature, severity, and need for treatment, whereas the latter refers to the ability to identify reasonable and appropriate responses to commonsense problems. Judgment is often identified by considering a client's pattern of coping with problems, including whether coping efforts tend to increase or decrease problems.

Do Malcolm's actions reflect sociopathy? Mental retardation? Depression? Poor social skills and social awareness? Cultural alienation? Notice how the write-up of a mental status evaluation for Malcolm provides a new perspective on his behaviors that, with previously gathered information, helps to draw a differential diagnosis. See Exhibit 6.4.

Although a mental status evaluation can be useful in identifying the presence of problems and pinpointing their nature, it can be subjective and biased by the meaning systems of client and clinician. Being aware of this subjectivity and its impact on the validity of the interview is important, especially for assessments of clients raised in an ethnic community, another country, or those for whom the interview language was not their first language. Even when clinicians and clients share a language and country of origin, nonverbal

Exhibit 6.4 Mental Status for Malcolm Little in 1940, When He Was 15[a]

Malcolm Little is a tall, thin, 15-year-old, African American boy, who appears older than his stated age. He was well groomed and neatly dressed in a dapper green suit, of which he appeared proud. His gait was athletic and exuberant, his gestures loose. He was charming and affable and responded openly to questions, suggesting that the observations made would be valid. He is currently in the eighth grade, where he reports he is excelling. His mother has recently been placed in Kalamazoo State Mental Hospital after a nervous breakdown; his father was reportedly murdered in racial violence when he was 5. Michigan Department of Human Services is considering placing Malcolm in foster care after a series of small thefts and petty mischief in school and the community.

Malcolm's affect was broad and generally matched the content of the interview. He appeared neither depressed nor anxious, reporting no symptoms of either. He leaned forward and maintained good eye contact and a relaxed open posture throughout the interview. He displayed no nervous habits except tossing a ball that he had brought to the interview and playing with small objects on the desk. Despite his apparent relaxation, at several points he seemed to become vigilant and less disclosing verbally and nonverbally, especially in response to questions about the welfare system's involvements with his family.

Malcolm reported no hallucinations or delusions; no evidence of these or any sort of dissociative or other disease process was observed. He reported no history of suicidal or homicidal ideation and, although he had a number of visible scratches, scrapes, and bruises, reported no history of self-injurious behavior, instead attributing injuries to a recent hunting expedition through underbrush.

Malcolm is a bright, abstract thinker who responded nimbly to questions. Rather than responding only to the direct questions asked, he was able to respond cogently to the underlying question and identify patterns in his life. His speech was within normal limits in rate, tone, and modulation, varying in volume to verbally underline his points. He used an unusually large vocabulary with well-developed sentences, carefully chosen words, and a sophisticated use of alliteration and puns, evincing a history of wide and thoughtful reading. He was assertive and outspoken, his speech clearly and forcefully articulated with few stutters or interruptions.

Malcolm was observant and socially curious, noticing small details and drawing good insights into his and others' behaviors. He appeared self-confident and interacted comfortably with adults. However, his recent thievery and petty mischief is impulsive and demonstrates poor judgment. He admitted to having committed the thefts with which he was accused, justifying his acts based both on his family's current poverty and the ways that his family has been mistreated.

Note. The information included here is consistent with Malcolm X and Haley (1964/1999); however, because Malcolm X's accounts are retrospective, selective, and incomplete, this material is included for its educational rather than its historical value.

behaviors and colloquial language can have very different meanings for each party. As a result, written reports of mental status evaluations include both inferences and the observations leading to them. These observations allow the reader to evaluate the data used to draw conclusions and determine whether other interpretations of the interview data might be more valid.

Case Conceptualizations

If we are facing in the right direction, all we have to do is keep on walking.
—*Buddhist Proverb*

Assessment tools such as psychosocial histories, genograms, timelines, and mental status evaluations all help clinicians put together case conceptualizations for their clients. A **case conceptualization** is an integrated set of hypotheses about the causes and treatment of the presenting problem, which are based on the assessments of, interviews with, and observations of the client and on reports from outside parties. Case conceptualizations help identify problems, goals, and interventions.

Not everyone will draw the same conclusions about the nature of the problems to be addressed and appropriate goals for treatment because of the theoretical frame that they use to approach the case. For example, the National Organization of Women provided a radically different viewpoint of Andrea Yates than that generally given:

> The National Organization for Women is troubled by the March 12 guilty verdict in the Andrea Yates trial and its implications for the one in 1,000 new mothers who will suffer from postpartum psychosis. Our society cannot wash its hands of this tragedy by locking up Yates for life, or putting her to death.
>
> Who shares in the responsibility for these five deaths and possibly another? What about the hospital that sent a dangerously psychotic woman home? What about the doctor who inexplicably stopped Yates' anti-psychotic medication 13 days before this tragedy? What about the weak support system that left Andrea Yates, delusional and suicidal, alone with five young children? The health care system and the medical establishment failed all of them. (Gandy, 2002, para. 1–2)

This statement makes an argument about the cause of problems (societal; inadequate support for a woman who was "dangerously psychotic") and treatment (a more responsive and supportive "health care system and the medical establishment"). Just as NOW's statement proposes a plan for action (in this case, political action), clinical case conceptualizations lead to some sort of an action plan—specifically, a plan for treating the individual or family.

Different theoretical viewpoints lead to different useful pictures of the person and symptoms. For example, rational emotive behavior therapists emphasize the role of irrational beliefs; cognitive behavior therapists emphasize thought patterns and skill deficits. Structural family therapists emphasize hierarchies and boundaries in the family system, while feminist therapists emphasize issues of power and oppression and the social and political contexts in which they occur. Case conceptualizations are also influenced by the available research and client and clinician preferences. Finally, clients and clinicians may choose among possible interventions on the basis of time, costs, and possible side effects.

As seen in Exhibit 6.5, there is no single "correct" way of conceptualizing a person's problems because most people can be well understood and effectively worked with from several theoretical perspectives, as long as the case conceptualization engages both the client and clinician (Wampold & Imel, 2015). That there is no single correct case conceptualization can be frustrating for beginning clinicians, who may be more comfortable with knowing the "right" answer. Developing multiple conceptualizations of clients, however, strengthens a clinician's understanding of the role of research and theory and allows flexible and multimodal interventions.

Exhibit 6.5 Explanations for Andrea Yates's Depressive Symptoms From Diverse Theoretical Perspectives and Corresponding Treatments

Biological model. Ms. Yates had a genetic vulnerability to depression, exacerbated by postpartum hormonal changes. Depression can be countered through a variety of treatments including antidepressant and antipsychotic medications and electroconvulsive therapy.

Psychoanalytic model. Ms. Yates's childhood encouraged development of a strict, overly rigid superego, leading her to ignore her needs. Her marriage reinforced this pattern. Her ego was unable to negotiate between a demanding superego and often-ignored and "unacceptable" impulses. Treatment should develop more reasonable expectations and strengthen her ability to negotiate between id impulses and her rigid and demanding superego.

Cognitive model. Ms. Yates held rigid and unreasonable expectations and beliefs about herself and her children that were dichotomous and unrealistic (good vs. evil). Treatment should help her recognize her beliefs, resulting interpretations of situations, challenge irrational beliefs, and identify healthier ways of thinking.

Behavioral model. Ms. Yates was rewarded for parenting godly children but received social sanctions when her behavior—as a woman and as a mother—deviated from the social norms of the religious group with which she was associated. She had few interactions with people outside her family and other followers of Michael Woroniecki, and few social reinforcers. Treatment would encourage Ms. Yates to become more active and broaden the number and sources of positive reinforcement.

Person-centered model. Ms. Yates was raised in a demanding household that did not accept her for who she was. As a result, she believed she had to be someone other than who she truly was to be accepted. Listening to her empathically and genuinely, accepting her for who she is, allows her to accept herself as she is and begin to actualize her self-concept.

Multicultural model. Ms. Yates can be understood in terms of her race, gender, class, and religion, and other contexts. These cultural influences caused her to set unrealistic standards for herself, repress anger, avoid discussions of concerns, care for others while making her own needs a low priority, and ultimately murder her children. Treatment should help her identify more flexible ways of perceiving herself and responding to these pressures.

Taking Multiple Perspectives

It does not do to leave a live dragon out of your calculations.

—J. R. R. Tolkien

Strong case conceptualizations take advantage of several sources in order to gain multiple perspectives on clients and avoid rigid cognitive sets. With an oppositional child, a behavioral observation of the child, interview with parents, parental reports on standardized assessments, and consults with teachers are often standard protocol. Empathic, effective clinicians listen to clients but also observe their behavior—in their offices, waiting rooms, and other settings. They talk to family members and contact other agencies involved in the case (e.g., Juvenile Probation, Child Protective Services, psychiatrists, and physicians). Clinicians can also have their clients make observations of the frequency, severity, antecedents, and consequences of their behavior.

To produce fair and unbiased clinical assessments when gathering material from multiple sources, clinicians should consider the following questions: What other perspectives of behaviors, problems, and symptoms can be taken? Which respondents report more problems and which fewer? What is different about those settings or respondents? What things do some sources omit? Are these differences related to differences in the observer's meaning system and context? Are they related to differences in the settings in which the observer sees the client?

What Do You Think?

For Andrea Yates (see also Chapter 1), numerous original source materials are available on the Internet. Although these sources have influenced descriptions in this book, draw your own conclusions by reading the original sources. Pay attention to the writer's viewpoint and biases.

CNN.com. (2006). *Yates' confession*. Retrieved from http://transcripts.cnn.com/TRANSCRIPTS/0608/01/ng.01.html

Denno, D. W. (2003). Appendix 1. Time line of Andrea Yates' life and trial. *Duke Journal of Gender Law and Policy, 10,* 61–84.

Yates, R. (n.d.). Welcome. Retrieved from http://www.yateskids.org/

1. What do you conclude after reviewing these materials? If your viewpoint shifted as you read additional sources, how did it shift? What influenced you?

2. Given that everyone has biases, how can you listen to or read sources so as to reduce bias in your clinical assessments?

Research Informs Treatment

You certainly usually find something, if you look, but it is not always quite the something you were after.

—J. R. R. Tolkien

When developing a case conceptualization, clinicians frequently draw on scientific research on an issue, problem, or group. This research helps clinicians develop their case conceptualization. What **comorbid**, or co-occurring, disorders can be expected? What kinds of typical obstacles can be anticipated in the course of treatment? What treatment strategies are most effective? What ancillary treatments increase the effectiveness of treatment? What makes treatment less effective? What risk factors should be considered? What role, if any, does medication have in treatment?

Clinicians should also consider research on the client's culture(s). What challenges or stressors do people of the client's cultural backgrounds typically face? What values are commonly shared? What messages do people of this culture generally receive about self, family, sex, parenting, and their bodies? What resources and supports are commonly available? What are unavailable? Many people identify with multiple groups. For example, Malcom Little identified as a young Black man, as a follower of Marcus Garvey, as agnostic, and as a son in a strong but traumatized family. Andrea Yates identified as a Christian and a follower of Michael Woroniecki, a wife, and a mother. These multiple identities and associated meaning systems should be considered in the course of the case conceptualization process.

Most clinical practices see a number of clients who present with similar problems or issues (e.g., depression, anxiety, substance abuse, or cognitive impairments). Knowledge gained by doing research for one client develops an expertise helpful to others. Even when working with a relatively homogeneous population, clinicians will begin working with clients with new presenting issues. For example, at an in-home family therapy program, many children and teens may be depressed or oppositional and have school or legal problems; however, occasional clients may be enuretic or diagnosed with obsessive compulsive disorder. A clinician may generally work with an African American population, but sometimes work with Latinx. As new issues and populations present, wise clinicians do additional research.

Research alone, however, should not drive treatment, but be one driver, along with clinical judgments about the client's conditions and needs and the client's preferences, values and context (American Psychological Association Presidential Task Force on Evidence-Based Practice, 2006; Morales & Norcross, 2010). This process is analogous to a three-legged stool—research, clinical judgment, and client preferences—each leg in balance with the others. Without each of these legs, we will be unable to offer strong treatment tailored to the individual client.

What Do You Think?

1. Consider the research on postpartum depression. See Exhibit 6.6. Given this research, how would you approach treating Andrea Yates if you had worked with her before her hospitalization? How does this research fit with your earlier case conceptualization?

Exhibit 6.6 Summary of Research Findings on Postpartum Depression and Postpartum Psychosis

Although often a positive experience, childbirth can also be characterized by increased psychosocial stressors, sleep disruption, weight gain, decreased physical activity, and first depressive episodes (Saxbe, Rossin-Slater, & Goldenberg, 2018).

Poor perceived social support is related to greater rates of postpartum depression (Tambag, Turan, Tolun, & Can, 2018).

Women whose partners were involved in caregiving did better after their child's birth. This was most marked for mothers who wanted more involvement from their partners (Powell & Karraker, 2019).

Attributions that a woman's postpartum depression are temporary rather than stable and not her fault increased sympathy and decreased stigma, thus increasing willingness to provide social support and relationship closeness (Ruybal & Siegel, 2017, 2019).

Pulling Assessment Strategies Together

For every complex question there is a simple answer—and it's wrong.

—H. L. Mencken

As discussed in this chapter, the process of assessing clients and generating hypotheses builds a careful and contextualized understanding of a client. We have described systematically gathering behavioral observations and information obtained during formal assessment strategies, drawing inferences and hypotheses from these strategies and then organizing these various types of information into an overall clinical assessment to guide treatment. When conducted well, this integrated assessment process creates a three-dimensional picture that moves the clinician beyond symptoms and problems to an empathic and contextualized understanding of a client. This empathy and contextualized understanding is essential for engaging clients, developing treatment goals and interventions, recognizing factors that increase or diminish problems, motivating change, anticipating barriers and obstacles to change, and harnessing strengths for treatment.

As the examples throughout this book demonstrate, a web of interrelated factors often influences a person's behavior and current status. For example, abuse does not necessarily cause current deficits in a client's functioning; its effects are moderated by the meanings drawn about the abuse, subsequent changes in social support, and a client's trauma history (Park, Currier, Harris, & Slattery, 2017). A strong assessment attends to these factors, identifies strengths and vulnerabilities, and generates treatment strategies. Exhibit 6.7 demonstrates how assessment materials and a case conceptualization could be used in a report addressing the referral questions that might have brought Malcolm into treatment.

Exhibit 6.7 Sections of an Evaluation Report for Malcolm Little[a]

Reason for Referral: Malcolm Little was referred by Michigan Department of Human Services as a result of a series of small thefts and petty mischief in the community. The department requested an assessment to identify why he is running into problems and a recommendation as to whether out-of-home placement is appropriate.

Ms. Little was made aware of the nature and purpose of this examination. First, that it was being performed at the request of Michigan Department of Human Services to identify what services would be necessary to stabilize her son and determine whether an out-of-home placement would be appropriate and necessary. Second, that a report based on this interview, third-party consultations, and completed assessments would be compiled for Michigan Department of Human Services and that this report would be used for the purpose of making recommendations regarding treatment. Given this, Ms. Little agreed to participate in this assessment.

Evaluation Procedures:

Interview with Malcolm Little (1.0 hr)

Interview with Mrs. Louise Little at Kalamazoo State Mental Hospital, gathering family genogram, psychosocial history, and timeline (2.0 hrs)

Teacher Consult, Mr. Ostrowski (.25 hr)

Review of summary of client records, Michigan Department of Human Services

. . .

Summary and Recommendations: Malcolm Little is a 15-year-old African American male with significant intellectual, physical, and social strengths. He has recently been acting out in school and engaging in petty thievery and mischief in the community.

Malcolm is the fourth of Mrs. Little's seven children. Both Malcolm and Mrs. Little report a significant history of violence and trauma, with at least five family members, including Malcolm's father, being reportedly murdered in racial violence. They also report that their home was threatened on two separate occasions, once being burned to the ground, and that Mrs. Little's mother was raped, leading to Mrs. Little's birth. Malcolm also described a positive history of domestic violence between Mr. and Mrs. Little, as well as physical abuse of most of their children, including Malcolm.

Exhibit 6.7 Sections of an Evaluation Report for Malcolm Little[a] *(Continued)*

Malcolm admits that this pattern of violence has caused significant problems in the family but reports as much or more concern about how he and his family have been mistreated within the community, especially by his White teachers, neighbors, and social workers. He believes their actions are often racist and have undermined his family. Both he and Mrs. Little report that she has been increasingly depressed since Mr. Little's murder 8 years ago and with their increasing poverty. He is especially concerned that his siblings have been placed in foster care and about the low expectations that a previously favorite teacher holds for him.

Malcolm has high self-efficacy and an internal locus of control but an external locus of responsibility; he does not attribute the family's problems to himself or his mother. He sees his current actions as appropriate responses to a racist society that is systematically undermining his family. Malcolm has significant strong leadership skills, is assertive and believes in active responses to stressors, engages adults easily, and responds well to their mentoring when their behavior is racially sensitive.

Given these concerns, barriers to treatment, and individual and familial strengths, the following recommendations are made:

1. The Little family possesses significant strengths and appears to have been functioning well until Mr. Little's death, which led to a significant loss in family income and social supports. Rather than removing the children to meet their physical and emotional needs, they would probably respond best to referrals to programs that provide financial support and access to food. Foods previously provided have not been sensitive to Mrs. Little's religious beliefs, which should be considered in future referrals.

2. Although Malcolm's current problems may be related to trauma and grief, he is unlikely to be receptive to traditional forms of psychotherapy, especially if he saw himself or his family as blamed. He may accept more active treatments, however, especially treatments that would mentor him and help him identify positive ways of responding to stressors. He has had positive experiences with Marcus Garvey's church and might be open to a mentor there.

3. Because Malcolm has felt that Whites have acted in oppressive and condescending ways, whoever works with him should be responsive to perceptions of racism and oppression in both the stressors that he reports and the services that he receives.

4. Some of the family's instability stems from Mrs. Little's current depression and recent hospitalization. Although she is open to treatment currently offered at Kalamazoo State Mental Hospital, many of her symptoms seem to be reactive to the poverty and severe stressors that her family faces. Initial sessions should help her family stabilize, meet their basic physical needs, and develop natural supports in the community.

Note. Although this information is consistent with historical data, it is not based on an original evaluation. Information included here is not presented for its historical accuracy but to describe how one might perform an assessment and write about its products. Information leading to the summary and recommendations are omitted in this example but are presented in rough form in earlier exhibits and the table.

Summary

People are three-dimensional beings, although they may come to therapy describing only one part of their lives, usually their symptoms and problems. We enrich the picture of a client by using a range of informants (e.g., client, parents, teachers) and types of information. Such a process generates additional hypotheses to explain the client's behavior and identifies opportunities and potential barriers to change.

Four kinds of assessment strategies were discussed in this chapter: (a) psychosocial histories organize diverse information about clients' functioning in a variety of settings, (b) genograms illustrate family relationships and family patterns, (c) timelines list major events in clients' lives in chronological order, and (d) mental status evaluations carefully describe a client's psychological functioning in a number of realms. Each of these assessment strategies gathers information that might otherwise be overlooked and leads to a case conceptualization supported by theory and research.

For Review

Applying Concepts to Your Life

1. Consider the Summary and Recommendations for Malcolm Little. See Exhibit 6.7. What theoretical perspective was taken in this report? Try writing from another perspective.

2. Choose a problem in your own life and describe the factors influencing and maintaining it. Next, create a psychosocial history, family genogram, and timeline for yourself. What new meanings and understandings emerge as you complete these assessments? How do these strategies change your view of this problem? What psychological resources, social supports, and barriers to the change process do you identify? What factors would you need to consider if you were to decide to make changes?

Key Terms

affect, 131
case conceptualization, 134
clinical assessment, 112
comorbid, 137
enmeshed, 126
family genogram, 126
mental status evaluation, 131
mood, 131
psychosocial history, 114
referral question, 113
timeline, 129
triangle, 126
validity, 131

Learn More

For more information about the concepts in this chapter, visit the *Empathic Counseling* companion website at http://pubs.apa.org/books/supp/slattery/.

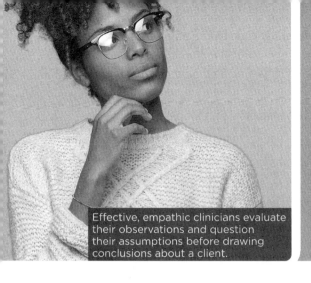

Effective, empathic clinicians evaluate their observations and question their assumptions before drawing conclusions about a client.

7 Thinking Critically to Ensure Empathic Assessments

Looking Ahead III➡

After reading this chapter you will be able to answer these questions:

1. How do observations and inferences differ?

2. How does meaning influence perceptions and assessments?

3. What social psychological processes can bias assessment?

4. How can critical thinking be seen in clinical work?

5. How does context influence assessments?

6. Why is recognizing strengths important to developing a strong assessment?

7. Why should assessments recognize both strengths and weaknesses?

Cases in Empathy

I Call It Being Honest I Eminem

Eminem (b. 1972), a White rap musician, has said and done things that offend people, especially women and gays and lesbians. In "Fall," for example, Eminem rapped, "Tyler create nothin', I see why you called yourself a faggot, bitch" (the word *faggot* is partially obscured by a sound effect).

When asked why he says such things, Eminem's answer has changed across time. In 2001, he explained, "I come from Detroit, where it's rough, and I'm not a smooth talker" (Gabriella, 2001, para. 15). He also said that words like "faggot" don't have the same

meaning to him: "It just means you're being a fag. You're being an asshole or whatever. . . . Battling with somebody, you do anything you can to strip their manhood away" (Gabriella, 2001, para. 13).

More recently, Eminem has attributed his "missteps," as attempts to get a reaction:

All the bullshit around that—I'm not making an excuse, but the mentality that I've had since I was rapping at open mics was that you better have shit that's going to get a reaction or you will not be accepted when you're on the mic. Your first, second, third,

(EMINEM continued)

and fourth line better grab attention or you're done. That attitude morphed into my music. A lot of times I'm saying stuff just to get that reaction. Maybe I took it too far sometimes. (Marchese, 2017, para. 61)

At other times his lyrics seem to be offensive for more impulsive reasons:

I've grown and sometimes I want to reflect that—but when I'm writing, a line will pop in my head that's so fucking ridiculous that it's funny, and depending on the punch lines I need and the rhyme schemes in the song maybe I'll use it. (Marchese, 2017, para. 6)

Eminem has also claimed to be misinterpreted: "You know, I call it being honest, but some sick asshole who does sick things on the sly and doesn't talk about it is cool?" (Gabriella, 2001, para. 17).

What Do You Think?

1. How did you feel about Eminem as you read this? How might these feelings influence your work with him? What might help you work more effectively with him?

2. What do you know about Eminem and his meaning systems based on his interviews? What evidence supports your conclusions?

3. People sometimes say things that are not true. Eminem says that he is being honest when he uses homophobic slurs. How else could you explain the things he says? How would you know whether he is being honest?

4. Eminem was raised in inner-city Detroit, in a working class family. How do his statements and actions reflect that upbringing and his social class? See Table 7.1.

Assumptions and Values in Clinical Practice

We don't see things as they are, we see them as we are.

—*Anaïs Nin*

Most people believe that they can understand others, yet the social psychological literature clearly demonstrates that people tend to make consistent and predictable errors. This chapter provides tools for effectively using the frameworks developed in the previous chapters. In particular, we emphasize looking for other explanations for observations, recognizing the role of context, and seeing strengths as well as weaknesses.

Accurately and carefully observing behavior before drawing inferences is an important first step to being a good observer and effective clinician. However, strong work depends on being aware of and testing **assumptions**—underlying beliefs about others and the world, which are often invisible and outside of awareness. Clinicians may believe that clients behave with others the way they behave during a counseling session, that their behavior is reflective

Table 7.1 Social Class Differences in Parenting Among European Americans

Lower socioeconomic status	Upper-middle socioeconomic status
Parenting—method and goals	
Parents raise children with a "hard" individualism. Children must be "toughened up" to maintain their identity and values in an uncertain world. Children are teased, contradicted, and exposed to negative events and emotions.	Raise children with a "soft" individualism. Children are "delicate flowers" who must be allowed to discover themselves and blossom in a welcoming world.
Children are encouraged to become self-reliant, self-disciplined, honest, fair, and reliable.	Children are encouraged to self-actualize and express themselves, and are given choices.
Parents are less likely to request help for poor achieving children.	Parents are somewhat more likely to monitor poor achieving children and more likely to request help.
Values	
Value honesty, fairness, reliability, adjusting to contingencies, and resisting social influence.	Especially value growth, control, and productivity.
Economic and political opportunities	
Generally earn less money, have fewer and more dangerous housing options, less geographic mobility, poorer health, and less leisure time.	Often earn more money, have more housing options, safer living conditions, more geographic mobility, better health, and more leisure time.
Have more feelings of powerlessness, greater sense of constraint and external locus of control, and lower self-efficacy. Emphasize self-control and are more accepting when they do not get what they want.	Expect greater ability to control their world and become more frustrated when they cannot do so. Expect that getting what they want should be possible and easy.
Nature of work	
Work is often more physical. Intellectual work and education are less valued.	Work often depends on intellectual skills and may be invisible to the casual observer. Intellectual skills, per se, are valued.
Communication	
All communication, including anger, is expected to be direct and forthright.	Talking directly about conflict and problems creates problems and disrupts the social fabric. Anger should be disguised, repressed, or indirect.

Note. Data from Nelson, Englar-Carlson, Tierney, and Hau (2006); Robinson and Harris (2013); and Snibbe and Markus (2005).

of underlying personality traits, or that they cannot be trusted to tell the truth. They may believe that children of divorcing parents are best placed with their mothers, that men are not insightful or interpersonally interested, or that change is always happening, both in and out of therapy. These assumptions may or may not be true. And clinicians should consider both evidence supporting their assumptions and evidence that might disconfirm it (Taleb, 2010).

Recognizing assumptions and their consequences is important to the therapy process. Some assumptions have positive consequences. For example, the belief that people have strengths that can be used to resolve problems can help a clinician identify intervention strategies. Other assumptions—for example, that court-referred clients do not want to change—although sometimes accurate, may interfere with the therapeutic alliance and the change process.

Clinicians' values vary widely and influence their perceptions and goals (Cummings, Ivan, Carson, Stanley, & Pargament, 2014). Their values appear to have a direct impact on choice of therapeutic approach, problem definition and goals, and even clients' ability to change (Cummings et al., 2014; Mohr, Weiner, Chopp, & Wong, 2009). Concluding that a child is oppositional has different treatment implications than believing that her parents engage in power struggles with her. Rather than painting a client's behavior with a broad brush, it is helpful to wonder when a child is oppositional and with whom, when parents set up power struggles and when they can bypass them. Unfortunately, clinicians often underestimate these influences (Zapf, Kukucka, Kassin, & Dror, 2018), and this bias especially affects experienced clinicians.

What Do You Think?

1. Consider your assumptions about people who talk the way that Eminem did. How would your assumptions help or interfere with treatment?

Social Psychological Processes Influencing Clinical Judgments

What happens when good people are put into an evil place? Do they triumph or does the situation dominate their past history and morality?

—*Philip Zimbardo*

Errors made during decision-making have been well described in nonclinical settings and, increasingly, in assessment and treatment (cf. Autin, Batruch, & Butera, 2019; Schwartz, Docherty, Najolia, & Cohen, 2019). In fact, unless clinicians recognize and challenge factors biasing their judgment, these factors will interfere with their assessments.

One of the most common errors in thinking is **confirmation bias**, the tendency to gather evidence that confirms preexisting expectations, typically by emphasizing or pursuing supporting evidence while dismissing or failing to seek contradictory evidence. This bias can be illustrated in a short example. When Ryan, a man with a history of significant heroin abuse, shows for his first appointment, confirmation biases may already be operating: The clinician may look for characteristics consistent with her already-existing schema about heroin addicts and overlook behaviors that are inconsistent with it, including his commitment to family, his love of animals and the outdoors, and his desire to help others (Taleb, 2010). Further, traits consistent with stereotypes are more likely to be recalled and reported (e.g., he is currently unemployed and significantly ambivalent about treatment) while disconfirming information is ignored (e.g., that he has not missed a session and completed six of seven homework assignments). Divergent opinions tend to disappear during **case conferences**—group discussions about a client's treatment that are often multidisciplinary—due to **groupthink**, the tendency for each person to conform his or her opinion to the group consensus (Kassin, Fein, & Markus, 2017).

The case conceptualization of Ryan is also influenced by **trait negativity bias**, which causes clinicians and other observers to weigh mistakes, symptoms, and problems more heavily than positive coping strategies, successes, and effective functioning (Bebbington, MacLeod, Ellison, & Fay, 2017). In practice, this bias may mean that Ryan overlooks the fact that for much of the week he handled his cravings well, instead reporting that he had a bad week because he used heroin once.

When clinicians see Ryan's heroin use as reflective of his "addictive personality," rather than as a coping mechanism to handle stress or as something that he does around friends who also use drugs, they have engaged in the **fundamental attribution error**, the tendency to see others' behavior as due to internal traits while overlooking or minimizing the contribution of external and situational factors (Kassin et al., 2017). What is striking about this process is that although people underestimate the role of context for others' behavior, they tend to make situational attributions for their own problematic behavior (e.g., "I am not a big drinker. I only drank too much last night because everyone else was getting hammered too"). However, when clinicians overestimate the role of traits in clients' behavior and fail to see the roles of situations and context, they miss opportunities for change.

What Do You Think?

1. Return to the opening description of Eminem. Do any of these problems factor into your reactions to him? In what ways?

Critical Thinking

The first step toward success is taken when you refuse to be a captive of the environment in which you first find yourself.

—Mark Caine

Banaji and her colleagues have repeatedly demonstrated that people may behave in a biased way, even when they believe they are not prejudiced (Banaji & Greenwald, 2013). Good intentions are not enough; one must be vigilant to counter **implicit biases,** unconscious beliefs about a social group. In short, making strong assessments depends on vigilant awareness of, and critical thinking about, the factors biasing perceptions. **Critical thinking** is the purposeful and reflective process of evaluating observations and drawing conclusions about them. It includes identifying assertions, evaluating evidence supporting and contradicting these assertions, identifying other explanations of this evidence, and choosing the most reasonable explanation.

Most people fail to question their expectations and biases, accepting initial perceptions as reality. They often seek simple, black-and-white explanations of complex and difficult problems. Rather than testing their expectations and beliefs, they often seek confirmation of them. Perhaps when many bad things seem to happen in the same day (e.g., a flat tire, a forgotten appointment), we are just noticing those things fitting that expectation that it is a bad day (confirmation bias). Further, the causal nature among the setbacks may not be recognized (e.g., being stressed after the flat tire caused distraction, leading to the forgotten appointment).

Critical thinking involves making strong and systematic **observations,** or sensory data (things that are seen, heard, felt, tasted, or smelled). It means recognizing alternative explanations for why people behave as they do and looking for data that help discriminate among these explanations. It requires becoming aware of biases and challenging them. It also demands becoming aware of the role of context and culture in observations.

Good and careful observations are important tools for developing a strong, empathic understanding of others. Observations are sensory-based bits of information that can be seen, heard, felt, smelled, or tasted. Each of the following is an observation:

> Danny slowly said, "She doesn't want me anymore," his statement marked by two hesitations and one stutter. His cheeks were flushed, his hands cold. His posture was closed and his head down. He made little eye contact while talking.

In contrast to observations, **inferences** are the meaningful interpretations of observations and are influenced by one's biases and global beliefs. Although people generally agree about sensory observations, even reasonable people can disagree about the inferences drawn from a set of observations because multiple inferences can be used to explain any single observation. For example, why are Danny's cheeks flushed? They could be flushed because he is embarrassed, angry, hot, recently sunburned, having an allergic reaction to some food, or hypertensive. Alternately, his face could be red because that is his normal coloration.

In fact, people are poor in making at least some sorts of assessments. Although most people believe they can identify liars, for example, their ability to do so is little better than chance (Costanzo & Krauss, 2017). In fact, in a survey of people from 75 countries, most reported inaccurate cues of lying (i.e., avoidance of eye contact, squirming, touching and scratching themselves, and telling longer stories than usual; The Global Deception Research Team, 2006). Bond and DePaulo (2008) concluded that people differ little in their abilities to recognize lies and more in their abilities to believe they can recognize lies. Meissner and Kassin (2004) concluded that

> When cognitive resources are limited (possibly due to time constraints or various social pressures) or when a theory is held in great confidence, individuals may neglect to gather evidence altogether and instead rely upon prior beliefs or expectancies in reaching a decision. (p. 94)

Well-collected observations and well-drawn inferences lead to clinical assessments about the causes, maintenance, and treatment of problems and symptoms. Clients—and their family members, friends, and referral sources—will offer explanations of their behavior; some explanations will be accurate, others inaccurate. While considering these explanations, think about the motives and assumptions of the source. Is the explanation extreme? Is it reasonable? Is it supported by evidence? Good assessments require being open to such explanations, without excluding others prematurely. Good assessments also require being open to alternative explanations. Are there mitigating factors? Exceptions to the behavior? What is the positive intent in the behavior?

Clinical Applications	Brett has worked for years with people with substance abuse problems and is beginning to wonder whether he is getting burned out because he finds himself assuming that his new clients do not want to change even before he meets them. What cognitive biases might have contributed to this change in attitude? What would you suggest he do to perform more effective assessments?

Choosing Among Alternative Explanations

Consider the T-shirts in Figure 7.1. What would you guess about the person wearing each T-shirt? What other explanations are there? How could you choose among these hypotheses?

FIGURE 7.1 What Hypotheses Do You Draw About the People Wearing These T-Shirts?

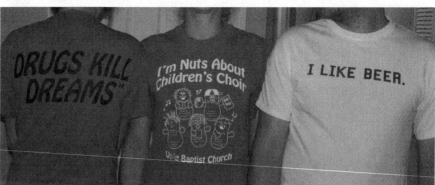

Several behavioral strategies lead to stronger clinical assessments. As we have discussed, effective clinicians make observations in multiple situations and recognize the factors potentially biasing their perceptions. Effective clinicians recognize the tentative nature of their inferences and test their hypotheses rather than jumping to conclusions (Kassin et al., 2017). They do more than simply read the words on these T-shirts to gain an empathic understanding of their clients but also pay attention to grooming, other clothing, and speech patterns to identify whether the T-shirts directly reflect their wearers' values, are an ironic statement about cultural mores, or were the only clean clothing in their roommate's closet.

Some inferences initially look like observations. Many people, upon meeting Danny, might say that he was depressed, believing this to be a simple observation. Although he might be depressed, when clinicians draw this inference without identifying and excluding other explanations for his behavior, their assessment could misdirect treatment and bypass other more accurate explanations of his behavior.

The validity of assessments is increased when a broad range of observations is obtained: from different days, situations, or kinds of measures. The clinician's confidence in the validity of Danny's diagnosis is increased when he is interviewed on several days, observed both in the office and in his second-grade classroom, and understood through his mother's responses to a questionnaire about his sleep, eating habits, friendships, and behavior in the home. His lethargy during an assessment could stem from the fight he had with his mother earlier in the day or a poor night's sleep. It could be a side effect of the medicine that he was recently placed on or a signal of his perception of the clinician's goals for the interview (e.g., out-of-home placement).

Clinical Applications	Brett has begun working with Lawrence, who was referred for treatment with a history of substance abuse. Lawrence is currently unemployed but had been a social studies teacher at a local high school. Lawrence showed up late for his second and third appointments, and Brett found himself angry and assuming that Lawrence doesn't want to change. What other explanations might there be? How could Brett choose among these alternatives?

Countering Observer Biases

Taken out of context I must seem so strange.

—Ani DiFranco

One of the paradoxes of making observations is that simply paying attention to people or groups changes their behavior (Dale & Vinson, 2013). The **observer's paradox** is a particular case of the systemic nature of all interactions, which are both affected by and affect observers and their contexts. Clinicians' contexts influence what they observe and how they interpret it. For example, if Danny's social worker had an argument immediately before their session, she might have difficulty paying attention to his statements or perceive innocent remarks as threats. Because she is part of Danny's context, her size, appearance, dress, grooming, and interpersonal style may cause Danny to respond differently toward her than he would to someone else.

Children with attention-deficit/hyperactivity disorder (ADHD) may behave differently in two settings, and observers may perceive the same behavior very differently. Because clinical observations can introduce bias, Pitts and Wallace (2003) suggested viewing children's behavior in a culture- and context-sensitive manner. Their process, although developed for African American children who might have ADHD, is appropriate for any population and behavior:

1. **Description.** Identify and carefully describe the problem.
2. **Frequency.** Compare problem frequency with baselines for the general population and the client's specific population (e.g., 9-year-old African American boys).
3. **Intensity.** Compare problem intensity with cultural norms and established baselines.
4. **Environmental setting.** Note the environment in which the behavior was observed or in which it was reported to have occurred. Then determine whether the behavior could be better explained by environmental or biological factors including hunger, stress, or abuse.

5. **Bias.** Recognize, minimize, and account for reporter values, judgment, and biases. What are the costs and benefits of the "problem behavior" for all parties?

What Do You Think?

1. Consider Malcolm Little (Chapter 6). How might the preceding five factors influence your perception of Malcolm's behavior?

Recognizing Strengths and Exceptions to Problems

Strength does not come from winning. Your struggles develop your strengths.
When you go through hardships and decide not to surrender, that is strength.
—Arnold Schwarzenegger

Clinicians and clients tend to focus on problems in their efforts to resolve them, while overlooking strengths. However, no person is totally good or bad. Focusing on problems and weaknesses to the exclusion of strengths interferes with empathy; creates a poorer assessment of the person, devoid of clients' strengths and natural success strategies; and interferes with the therapeutic alliance. It forms a one-sided clinical assessment that creates distance rather than understanding and connection. Challenging derogatory descriptions of clients and recognizing their strengths as well as their weaknesses can strengthen the therapeutic alliance.

Pejorative attributions about behavior have negative consequences. A review of the literature concluded that being diagnosed with a significant mental illness interferes with equal access to jobs and housing. Further, people with a significant mental illness are more likely to lose custody of their children, even when the diagnosis is unrelated to ability to parent, ability to profit from parenting interventions, or even the presence of ongoing problems (Benjet, Azar, & Kuersten-Hogan, 2003).

Clinical assessments and diagnosis can also create a **self-fulfilling prophecy**, which is a belief or expectation that helps to bring about its own fulfillment (cf. Wurm, Warner, Ziegelmann, Wolff, & Schüz, 2013; Zwebner, Sellier, Rosenfeld, Goldenberg, & Mayo, 2017). This process can work in negative ways, as when a man is diagnosed with bipolar disorder and concludes that he cannot do anything to control his moods ("It's biological and I can't do anything about it"). This phenomenon has been observed in a variety of settings, including classrooms, courtrooms, and physicians' offices (Kassin et al., 2017).

Problems are important to recognize, describe, count, and contextualize, but strengths and exceptions to problems are equally important. Exceptions to problems can reframe a situation and provide a foundation for change. For example, the Lees' social worker might ask, when do the Lees give Lia her medicine (Chapter 4)? When don't they? What's different about these two sets of circumstances? Are they more likely to give some sorts of medicines than others (e.g., those with particular side effect profiles or that are more acceptable to their cultural and spiritual beliefs)?

One way of identifying exceptions to problems is to have clients complete a **functional analysis**, an assessment procedure in which either the client or clinician observes and records a behavioral problem, including what is happening when the behavior occurs (antecedent) and the consequences of the behavior. Although clients should be asked to record when there is a problem, they should also record when there could have been a problem but it did not occur. See Table 7.2.

Recognizing real strengths builds hope and self-esteem, identifies resources for solving problems, and builds the therapeutic alliance. Clients feel heard and understood and the clinician is more likely to respond compassionately, caringly and empathically. However, good assessments and treatment require hearing people from their own point of view while also being objective about their symptoms, strengths, and weaknesses.

Table 7.2 A Hypothetical Functional Analysis for the Lees' Administration of Medicine

Antecedents	Behavior	Consequences
8 a.m. Lia woke up in a good mood.	Gave medication with breakfast.	She laughed and spat out medicine. Felt mean giving her medicine when she does not want to take it. No seizure this morning.
12 p.m. At sister's apartment. Forgot to bring medicine. Sister disapproves of Western medicines.	Did not give medicine.	Relieved that sister does not hassle me about giving medicine. No seizure this afternoon.
7 p.m. Lia's brother was tired and feverish. Everyone went to bed early.	Gave both noon and evening medicines.	Slept well and woke late. No seizure.
8:30 a.m. Lia overslept. Could not find one medicine.	Gave other medicines.	Lia laughed and spat it out. Do not have extra pills and cannot afford to refill prescription.

Note. Data from Fadiman (2012).

Cases in Empathy

Seeing Strengths *and* Weaknesses ▐ Dylan Klebold and Eric Harris

One of the most horrifying events in 1999 was a high school shooting in Littleton, Colorado, known as the Columbine Massacre. This was by no means the first recorded school shooting in the United States (there were at least 53 shootings between 1970 and 1999), and tragically there have been many shootings in the years since then. However, the Columbine massacre shocked the nation because of the scale of bloodshed. The shooters, Dylan Klebold (age 17) and Eric Harris (age 18), brought guns to school, killed 12 students and a teacher and wounded more than 20 others, and then killed themselves. This single incident accounted for almost 30% of the deaths by school shootings in the 1990s (Cai & Patel, 2019).

Is it possible to empathize with these shooters? It can be helpful to look at their history. Dylan and Eric had been arrested during their junior year for breaking into a commercial van and stealing electronics; at the time of the shooting, both were on probation. They felt lonely, alienated, and disrespected by peers, who would throw them into lockers and call them names. In 1997, Dylan wrote in his journal, "I swear—like I'm an outcast, and everyone is conspiring against me" (Abelson, Frey, & Gregg, 2004, p. 314). He repeatedly wrote about being depressed and wanting a gun so he could kill himself.

Dylan and Eric were believed to be members of a group of social outcasts, the Trenchcoat Mafia, and to have talked about getting back at the jocks and minorities who put them down. Eric had threatened a fellow student with a gun and described how to make bombs on his web page. Both were enamored of Nazi culture (they would eventually commit their infamous shooting on Adolf Hitler's birthday).

Reports written by Dylan and Eric's probation officers before the Columbine Massacre illustrate the difficulty of seeing things going against our biases. Although the reports describe the struggles and bad behavior of the two teens, the teens were also described as coming from good families. Eric's father was a recently retired Air Force officer, Dylan's father was a geologist. Both were excellent students; Dylan quoted Shakespeare easily and was in the gifted and talented program at his grade school. Eric was described as a leader, Dylan a follower. Both played Little League when younger and enjoyed the video game Doom. Dylan operated the lights and sets for high school play productions, was involved in video productions there, helped maintain his school's computer, and built his own.

What did their probation officers conclude in their reports? One wrote of Dylan, "Dylan is a bright young man who has a great deal of potential. . . . He is intelligent enough to make any dream a reality but he needs to understand hard work is part of it." Eric was described as "a very bright young man who is likely to succeed in life. . . . He is intelligent enough to achieve lofty goals as long as he stays on task and remains motivated" (Bai, 1999, para. 7). Of course, predicting violence is notoriously difficult, and these reports were written before the shooting, when important information was unavailable.

Clinicians need to recognize clients' strengths and exceptions to their problems. However, recognizing strengths does not mean overlooking weaknesses and problems. Before the shooting, Eric wrote in his journal, "It's my fault! Not my parents, not my brothers, not my friends, not my favorite bands, not computer games, not the media, it's mine."

What Do You Think?

1. What factors might have contributed to the probation officers' underestimates of Dylan's and Eric's potential for violence? Why?

2. How could you see Dylan's and Eric's strengths, while also considering the risk for violence?

3. Later reports suggest that Dylan and Eric were not part of the Trenchcoat Mafia, had not been bullied by fellow students, and had not targeted jocks and minorities (Brockell, 2019). How does this development influence your perception of them, as well as the usefulness of secondhand reports at the time of a crisis?

4. How might this persistent error in describing Dylan and Eric be related to some of the cognitive biases that we have been describing?

Summary

Making good observations is a difficult process, complicated by many factors. Many people confuse observations (sensory data), with inferences, the conclusions people draw about observations. Inferences are influenced by many factors, including the beliefs and values of one's own meaning system. Assessments are clinical judgments, based on a number of observations and the inferences drawn from them.

In many nonclinical settings, people jump to conclusions rather than thinking critically. In professional work, assessments are strengthened by questioning expectations and biases and considering other hypotheses. Being open to complex answers to difficult problems and testing hypotheses rather than only seeking confirmation of them further strengthens the assessment process.

People's judgments are biased by a series of factors that interfere with critical thinking and the development of an empathic understanding. People engage in expectancy confirmation, the tendency to look for what they believe, and operate by confirmatory biases, the tendency to recall observations that confirm beliefs, both of which compromise the accuracy and usefulness of observations. People are more likely to notice problems, particularly when observers are primed to look for symptoms and problems (trait negativity bias). Because of such processes, behaviors are seen as reflecting internal and persistent traits rather than environmental or transient factors (fundamental attribution error). Furthermore, even when people report being bias-free, they often have implicit biases against some groups that affect their inferences and behavior.

There is no such thing as pure, unadulterated observations: Observers both affect that which they observe and are affected by their observations (observer's paradox). Clients are also influenced by their own expectancies (self-fulfilling prophecy). Although working in groups can bring in new points of view, groups can engage in groupthink, with diverging opinions disappearing in favor of the group's consensus. Challenging this tendency in treatment increases critical thinking and retains openness to other viewpoints and options.

To counter these factors in treatment, clinicians can approach their observations systematically. Rather than describing behavior globally and vaguely, a practice susceptible to bias, Pitts and Wallace (2003) suggested carefully describing behavior; observing its frequency, intensity, and the setting in which it occurs; and acknowledging and challenging biases. Finally, although recognizing strengths and exceptions to problems strengthens our empathic understanding of clients, recognizing strengths should not exclude recognizing weaknesses.

For Review

Applying Concepts to Your Life

This chapter focused on the observer in the assessment and treatment process and how biases influence the conclusions drawn.

1. Pay attention to your style of observations. What do you generally pay attention to? What do you tend to overlook?

2. Pay attention to how you draw inferences about others. Are your inferences useful, respectful, and based on a range of information, or do you tend to jump to conclusions that are primarily positive or negative in tone? Do you tend to draw a single type of conclusion (e.g., that you cannot trust others)? If so, what kind? How can you increase your confidence about your interpretations?

3. Pay attention to the assumptions that underlie your perceptions and decisions. What types of assumptions do you tend to make? Do they tend to be useful and accurate? Are they likely to be helpful in therapy? When? How?

Key Terms

assumptions, 144
case conferences, 147
confirmation bias, 147
critical thinking, 148
functional analysis, 153
fundamental
    attribution error, 147
groupthink, 147
implicit bias, 148
inferences, 148
observations, 148
observer's paradox, 151
self-fulfilling
    prophecy, 152
trait negativity bias, 147

Learn More

For more information about the concepts in this chapter, visit the *Empathic Counseling* companion website at http://pubs.apa.org/books/supp/slattery/.

Part IV

Facilitating Positive Change

The chapters in this part of the book describe how to help clients make positive changes in their lives. First, the clinician needs a map to guide the change process. We describe the process for creating that map, which includes developing goals that address the client's problem and a treatment plan that specifies which interventions will be used, in which situations, to help the client progress toward the goals. Like all phases of therapy, this planning phase should be a collaboration between the clinician and client.

Next, the clinician implements the treatment plan by delivering the agreed-on interventions. We present several interventions designed to change clients' problematic thoughts, emotions, behaviors, or a combination of these. If the interventions are ineffective, or if the client changes his or her goals, then the clinician and client work together to revise the goals and treatment plan. Ideally, therapy will not only help the client meet specific treatment goals but also empower the client to continue to address life goals outside of and beyond therapy.

Ideally, treatment ends only after all or most goals are met. The therapist and client collaborate to achieve closure, often by discussing treatment successes and strategies for clients to maintain and extend treatment gains into the future. However, premature or abrupt termination can harm the client and even the clinician. We present several strategies to help clinicians minimize risk and facilitate a successful termination.

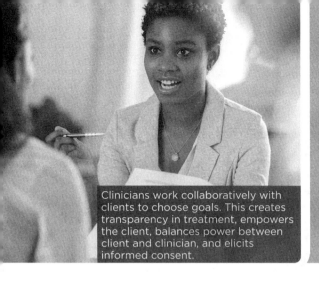

Clinicians work collaboratively with clients to choose goals. This creates transparency in treatment, empowers the client, balances power between client and clinician, and elicits informed consent.

8 Developing Goals and a Treatment Plan

Looking Ahead ||||➡

After reading this chapter you will be able to answer these questions:

1. What makes change difficult?

2. How does a client's readiness for change affect treatment?

3. How do relapses and lapses differ, and what are their implications for treatment?

4. What are the characteristics of good treatment goals?

5. What happens when clinicians' goals are incompatible with their clients'?

6. Why is recognizing strengths important to treatment?

7. How do clinicians write treatment plans?

8. How do clinicians assess treatment?

Cases in Empathy

"Jail Was My Saving Grace" | Reymundo Sanchez

In Chapter 2, Lil Loco described his involvement with gangs in Chicago. When he was 21, he was sent to prison on drug charges. He described this period as "my saving grace," a "blessing in disguise." His nightmares stopped, and he began to think differently. Reflecting on the bad things in his life, paradoxically, now made him aware of the ways that he had been lucky, rather than only cursed: He recognized that guns pointed at him never fired, that some did surprisingly little damage, that he had lived whereas others had died in similar circumstances. In thinking these things, he began "to consider my conviction [on drug charges] as a blessing. It was actually the first blessing I counted" (Sanchez, 2003, p. 73).

Two older men served as mentors: one when Reymundo was in jail, another when he was on work release. They helped him think about the directions in which he might go, although in very different ways. King Leo, a member of the Latin Kings, serving a life sentence at Shawnee Correctional Center, took Rey (as he was now called), under his wing. Reymundo had begun writing poetry, an outlet for his frequent pain and anger. Leo supported his writing and

(REYMUNDO SANCHEZ continued)

encouraged him to connect his writing and drawing with his newly emerging sense of inner peace. Leo said,

> "Look at those brothers over there," . . . looking in the direction of the weight pile. "All of them short-timers, a couple of years and they're back on the street. *Son pendejos, mi pana* (They are idiots, my partner). *En ves de enfuenzar sus mentes, enfuerzan sus cuerpeos* (Instead of strengthening their minds, they strengthen their bodies). They leave just as stupid as they came in, only stronger." Leo turned to face me. "Most of them will come back, some of them lifers like me. *No seas haci de pendejo* (Don't be an idiot like that)." (Sanchez, 2003, p. 84)

Reymundo listened, understood, and continued to think about how he could change his life for the better.

Reymundo's other mentor, Kalil, was Jamaican-born and Muslim. He was a member of another gang, the El Rukn. Reymundo met him while they were on work release. Kalil said,

> "Can you deny that the time you spent in jail was the salvation for your life? Not many brothers can say that, nor can they even begin to think it. Allah works his miracles for those who seek them faithfully."
>
> "But I don't believe in or even recognize Allah," I responded.
>
> "Call him what you will," Kalil answered. "It's faith that will lead us all to the promised land. As I sit here talking to you, all my questions regarding the path my life suddenly took are being answered. Your journey has just begun, young brother. Just be faithful, even when faith seems not to exist." (Sanchez, 2003, p. 113)

Kalil's words stuck with Reymundo and helped him consider and reconsider his life's journey. He now believed that he had a future. He wrote,

> I didn't want to do anything that would risk my losing the new freedoms I had gained. I could smell total freedom just ahead in my life, and I lived every day with the intention of gaining it and keeping it. (Sanchez, 2003, p. 112)

What Do You Think?

1. What goals would Reymundo work toward that Lil Loco (Chapter 2) would not have worked on? What goals would Lil Loco work toward that Reymundo would not? Why might they have different goals?

2. What did Kalil and Leo do that was so powerful for Reymundo? Would they have had the same impact if Reymundo had been mandated into treatment and they were his suburban-born counselors, saying these same things? Why or why not?

3. If you were working with Reymundo, how might you tailor your interventions with him in a way that was genuine for you and helpful for him?

Change

Most people readily identify what others can do to change, although they may see their own problems as difficult to change. Sue Monk Kidd (2006), who very much wanted to be less depressed, talked about the process this way:

My husband, Sandy, was as exasperated as he was bewildered. He wanted things to go back to the comfortable way they were before. He wanted me to "snap out of it." I did too, of course. I had ordered myself to do just that numerous times. But it was sort of like looking at an encroaching wave and telling it to recede. Demanding didn't make it happen. (p. 5)

Failures in empathy, such as Sandy's, can make change even more difficult.

Often the change process is emotion-laden. Some people may feel overwhelmed and stuck, unable to change. Others may believe that the problem is unchangeable or that they cannot control that change (e.g., Bandura, 1997; Dweck, 2006). They may be ambivalent about change, recognizing both its benefits and the losses they will incur (Norcross, Krebs, & Prochaska, 2011; Weaver, 2014). They may see numerous barriers to change, including a loss of freedom, financial and transportation barriers, and stigma (Hundt et al., 2018; Stecker, Shiner, Watts, Jones, & Conner, 2013; Weaver, 2014). People reporting difficulties with either a therapist or the agency were less likely to access services (Hundt et al., 2018). People perceiving multiple barriers are less likely to change. For example, one study found that cancer patients who profited from a pain intervention perceived fewer barriers to change than did those who did not (Ward et al., 2008).

Despite the real and imagined costs of change, many people are willing and able to change. One study found that people who perceived fewer structural barriers (e.g., cost of treatment or barriers to attending treatment) or attitudinal barriers to treatment (e.g., stigma, believing they should be able to handle problems on their own) were more likely to access needed mental health treatment (E. R. Walker, Cummings, Hockenberry, & Druss, 2015).

Clinical Applications	Teenie's new client, Jacob, wants to become a better father. He frequently gets home from work exhausted and sits in front of the TV. When he finally recovers, he tends to yell at his young children, who have been running and yelling around the house. Before working on a treatment plan with Jacob, Teenie discussed the advantages he expected would come from his goal of becoming a better parent. They also considered the potential barriers and costs. What are some advantages, barriers, and costs that they might have discussed with regard to this goal?

Stages of Change

Just do it!

—*Nike*

"Just do it!" is a good advertising campaign, but as Sue Monk Kidd (2006) observed, it is an ineffective way to help people change. To change, people must first recognize that they have a problem and commit to change. As we saw with Reymundo Sanchez, people vary markedly on these dimensions. Clients most committed to change are also most likely to change, although Norcross and his colleagues (2011) encouraged clinicians to tailor interventions to their clients' readiness for change. In fact, doing so improves treatment outcomes, depending on problem and treatment modality (Norcross et al., 2011). The following sections describe both the stages of change and some strategies for responding to people at each stage.

Precontemplation

At some point, most people have had what other people would identify as a "problem" but have been unaware of its negative consequences. Prochaska and his colleagues (Norcross et al., 2011; Prochaska & Norcross, 2010) called this stage **Precontemplation**. People in the substance abuse field often call this lack of insight *denial*. Clients in this stage may appear uninterested, unaware, or unwilling to change, even though friends and relatives are often very aware of the problem. When these clients end up in treatment, it is often because a third party (e.g., parents, an unhappy spouse, or a judge) has forced them. One study found that clients feeling most pressure to attend therapy were those least likely to report commitment to change (Moore, Tambling, & Anderson, 2013). Clients at this stage may say things like, "I don't know why I should change. They're the ones with the problem!"

Clients must first recognize that they have a problem. Questions such as, "How would you know that this is a problem?" could be useful at this stage (Zimmerman, Olsen, & Bosworth, 2000). Supportive and empathic responses are often helpful, whereas confrontational and conflict-laden responses can increase resistance and interfere with treatment (Serran et al., 2003).

Contemplation

Even when clients have identified a problem, they may not necessarily be willing to change. Many people acknowledge that they are having difficulty but also recognize the significant costs associated with change and are ambivalent about accepting those costs (Norcross et al., 2011; Prochaska & Norcross, 2010). A study of college students found that those who perceived fewer benefits and more costs to changing their alcohol use were less likely to do so (Carey et al., 2018), consistent with the notion that to commit to change, one must perceive more benefits to changing when perceived costs of change are also high. For example, a woman in a violent and abusive relationship may know that her relationship is unhealthy but also worry that if she leaves her husband, she will be unable to pay her bills; receive disapproval from her family, friends, and church; and lose a father for her children, along with the financial and emotional support that he offers. She may be afraid that she cannot parent their difficult children on her own, will not find a job that will support the family, does not have the skills to keep their bills paid and their car and house running smoothly, and will not find another man who will love her. She may also feel guilty that she has not done enough to make their relationship work. These high costs and low perceived benefits may reduce commitment to treatment.

Clients in **Contemplation** recognize a problem but are not yet ready to change. They need to assess barriers to change as well as identify the benefits of changing. Questions such as, "What are the benefits of changing at this point in time?" and "What might keep you from changing at this point?" are helpful for clients in this stage (Zimmerman et al., 2000). Paraphrasing change talk (e.g., "You like getting high, but you don't like that it keeps getting you in trouble") facilitates change, while paraphrasing reasons not to change (e.g., "You have fun getting high with your friends") discourages change (D'Amico et al., 2015). At this point, the goal of treatment is to heighten motivation and tip the balance toward committing to change.

Preparation

Once clients have identified obstacles as well as motivators for making change and have worked through their ambivalence about change, they often need to prepare to change. During **Preparation**, clients test the water, often by making small initial changes (Norcross et al., 2011; Prochaska & Norcross, 2010). This stage is characterized by planning, gathering information, getting support, problem-solving, and obtaining needed skills. Clinicians can help their clients identify and build needed skills and acquire the support needed to change.

Action

Prochaska and his colleagues (Norcross et al., 2011; Prochaska & Norcross, 2010) defined **Action** as the stage when the desired behavior (e.g., leaving a spouse or quitting smoking) has occurred for at least 1 day. Although the focus in Precontemplation and Contemplation was on motivating clients, in Action, clinicians need to help clients identify effective change strategies.

Although clients in Action are committed to change and are actively changing, change can be difficult. Clinicians need to be generous and genuine with positive feedback. For example, in working with a client who is quitting smoking, a clinician might remark, "Wow! It's been a week since you last smoked! What are you doing that is making this happen?" Some clients may attribute their change to luck or chance. Clinicians can empathize with their client's feeling that the change was outside their control but help their client identify his or her contribution to the change.

I know it feels like *he* changed, but I want you to think about what *you* did, so you can do it again. What changes did *you* make—no matter how little— that caused this week to be such a good one?

Notice the active, first person focus of the question. Also note that this clinician ended with an open question. If it had been a closed question, the client might have believed that an extreme and dichotomous response was acceptable: "Nothing!"

Maintenance

It is easier to make a positive change (e.g., stop drinking, lose weight, become more assertive) than to maintain that change. A **slip** is a return of the problem behavior, which can be seen as either temporary and an opportunity to learn (**lapse**) or more permanent and without eventual positive consequences (**relapse**). Clinicians can help clients frame problems as lapses rather than relapses.

Many people may cycle through the stages of change more than once despite having gained insights and skills (Norcross et al., 2011; Prochaska & Norcross, 2010). For example, relapse rates from substance abuse are high (between 40% and 60%), and relapse rates for diabetes, hypertension, and asthma are similar (National Institute on Drug Abuse, 2012). Similarly, relapse rates after antidepressant treatment for depression are high: About 80% of responders relapse in 2 years, even when maintained on an antidepressant (DeRubeis, Siegle, & Hollon, 2008).

Transferring skills to other situations, maintaining them across time, and preventing relapses are other important tasks in **Maintenance** (Norcross et al., 2011; Prochaska & Norcross, 2010). Two essential issues to consider to reduce and prevent the frequency and impact of relapses are (a) reducing **triggers** to the problem behavior (i.e., emotions, settings, and situations that increase the probability of a lapse or relapse of the problem behavior) and (b) challenging negative cognitive and emotional responses to slips. Slips do not occur at random but in predictable situations, including periods of boredom, loneliness, interpersonal stress, and exposure to triggers (Laudet, Magura, Vogel, & Knight, 2004). Some triggers can be avoided (e.g., bars, for people who are trying to quit smoking or drinking); others can be minimized or prevented (e.g., stress, fatigue). In addition, thinking about slips using a growth mind-set rather than a fixed mind-set can be useful (Dweck, 2006). A **growth mind-set** views the problem behavior as a bad habit that can be changed, while a **fixed mind-set** views it as an unchangeable trait. Fixed mindsets interfere with treatment; growth mind-sets facilitate change.

People with high self-efficacy and positive self-attributions following a lapse are less likely to have a second one (Moos & Moos, 2006). Pay attention to clients' successes to modify their attributions and bolster their self-efficacy: "It sounds like a rough situation, but you walked away without blowing up. What made the difference?"

Clinical Applications	Although Jacob initially told Teenie that he wanted to become a better father, as they talked about his parenting, it became clear that Jacob felt ambivalent about doing the work they discussed. Jacob stated that he needed to put in long hours at work, had few supports at home once he picked up his children from daycare, and did not have family to help him. What might Teenie do given this unclear motivation?

∗ ∗ ∗

One part of the difficulty that Jacob has in changing is that he is not confident that he can change: "This is how the men in my family are. We blow up and then back off." If Teenie believes Jacob has a fixed mind-set about his ability to parent, what might she do?

Good Goals

If one does not know to which port one is sailing, no wind is favorable.

—*Lucius Annaeus Seneca*

One thing that influences a client's readiness for change is the usefulness of the treatment goals. **Treatment goals** are the planned objectives for treatment, and they can be either long term or short term. A **long-term goal** is the primary treatment goal, while a **short-term goal** is an immediate goal that helps the client work toward the long-term goal.

Clients often are ready to commit to working on some goals, but not others—perhaps Reymundo Sanchez would be more willing to work on staying "free" rather than on anger management. Obviously, it is important to choose goals that clients are willing to work toward. Additionally, effective goals must be framed in a way that is useful to the clients. The acronym SMART summarizes five attributes of good goals (specific, measurable, achievable, realistic, and time-bounded). Because these attributes only partially describe effective goals, we've also added two other attributes (intrinsic, committed), making our acronym **SMART-IC**.

Specific and Measurable Goals (SM)

Good goals are simple, concrete, and specific, providing detailed descriptions of the client's problems and goals (Michalak & Grosse Holtforth, 2006). Rather than focusing on what *not* to do (**avoidance goals**), it is more useful to focus on the specific and observable changes clients want to make (**approach goals**). What will they be doing instead of yelling? What will they be doing instead of being anxious? Attending to approach goals is associated with stronger therapeutic relationship and better treatment outcomes (Grosse Holtforth & Castonguay, 2005).

These specific goals should be able to be broken down into action steps. Approach goals facilitate change by clarifying the nature of tasks and goals of treatment. For example, it is unclear what "being less angry" (an avoidance goal) would be; however, "being more assertive" (an approach goal) offers a clearer path for treatment. Being assertive can be broken down into positive and achievable steps (e.g., recognizing feelings, identifying personal and interpersonal rights, expressing feelings in ways that are respectful both to the client and others).

In addition, good goals are objective and quantifiable, which helps people to monitor the extent to which treatment is on track, identify progress in treatment, and remain motivated to continue the often-difficult work of therapy (Michalak & Grosse Holtforth, 2006). Measurable goals help client and clinician assess treatment and recognize change. One of us, for example, had a client who was frustrated during a treatment plan review, feeling like things had not changed at all in the 3 months we had seen each other. When she had begun treatment, her sleep was interrupted and unsatisfying; she was chronically suicidal and had held a gun to her head during a crisis call. As we discussed her progress, she recognized that she now slept much better, although more briefly than she would like, and although she still had passive suicidal ideation, these thoughts tended to be fleeting and had not escalated to an active attempt.

Achievable and Realistic Goals (AR)

Strong goals are under a client's control and, thus, achievable and realistic. They are actions rather than end results and often can be phrased as a verb rather than a noun. See Table 8.1. Grades and weight loss (nouns) are at least somewhat outside clients' control, although clients can study more, use different study skills, and exercise and eat differently (verbs). Each of the latter puts change under the client's control. As they develop treatment plans, clinicians might ask, "What will you be doing differently when you're on track?" or "How will you be thinking differently?"

Strong goals are achievable. Failing at a goal can be demotivating, cause negative emotions, and interfere with performance (Soman & Cheema, 2004). As a result, goals should be designed so that a person is likely to experience success rather than failure. Goals should be challenging, but realistic. For example, a student on academic probation who sets a goal of earning a 4.0 GPA may be demotivated by a C on an exam, even though that grade may be better than that earned in previous semesters. Also, that student may perceive anything less than an A as a failure. Such dichotomous goals can be problematic. It may be more helpful to choose minutes spent studying as a goal because this is a behavioral goal under the student's control, which can be set more realistically and evaluated on a gradient of change rather than a dichotomy.

Table 8.1 Bloom's Taxonomy of Learning and Goal Statements Associated With Each Level

Level	Action verbs	Possible goal
Remembering	Define, name, list, tell	"Identify three approaches to parenting."
Understanding	Explain, discuss, identify, recognize	"Discuss the role of self-talk in emotion."
Applying	Apply, practice, illustrate, use, demonstrate	"Practice assertiveness skills in settings outside the office, starting with easier situations first."
Analyzing	Distinguish, analyze, criticize, relate	"Distinguish between the emotional responses elicited by validating and invalidating responses."
Evaluating	Judge, evaluate, choose, measure	"Determine whether your approach to parenting meets your description of *effective parenting*."
Creating	Design, plan, propose, organize	"Design an approach to responding to your child's anger that uses the skills discussed today."

Note. Data from Anderson and Krathwohl (2001).

Clients often think about ways that their life would be better if others were to change. Although this may be true, it may not be realistic to expect someone else to change. Neither clinician nor client can directly change a client's family and friends. They can, however, change the person in the consulting room, which may, in turn, cause others to behave differently. Clinicians cannot make a client's husband stop his abusive tirades. A clinician can help the client change how she reacts to such tirades. She can consider her role in problems and respond to requests assertively rather than aggressively. She can hear the pain behind his tirades.

Time-Bounded Goals (T)

People often run into difficulties with tasks that are too large or that extend too far out into the future. Rather than waiting for change to happen, effective clinicians encourage clients to think about how they can begin to change right now. They might ask, "As you leave here today and you are on track, what will you be doing differently?" This focus encourages clients to recognize their role in the change process and commit to changing now.

Intrinsic Goals (I)

Clients experience more success with treatment goals that they choose rather than goals imposed by others, intrinsic rather than extrinsic goals (e.g., self-acceptance rather than money or status), and approach rather than avoidance goals (what they want to do rather than what they don't want).

When goals match the individual's motives, clients report greater change and more likelihood of meeting their treatment goals (Klug & Maier, 2015; Lindhiem, Bennett, Orimoto, & Kolko, 2016). When goals are well integrated and congruent with each another, clients report greater subjective well-being and life satisfaction (Michalak & Grosse Holtforth, 2006).

Given this association between goal type and therapeutic outcomes, Michalak and Grosse Holtforth (2006) argued that clinicians should pay attention to client goals. People who primarily pursue hedonistic and materialistic goals, for example, should be encouraged to develop more intrinsic and internal goals (e.g., self-acceptance, autonomy, relatedness), which are likely to provide a sense of meaning, purpose, and subjective well-being.

Committed to Change (C)

Finally, people change more rapidly when they are committed to a particular goal (i.e., are in Action; Norcross et al., 2011), and experience a good fit between motivations and goals (Michalak & Grosse Holtforth, 2006). Further, they should see their life circumstances as favorable for working on that goal and that it is not in conflict with other goals (Michalak, Heidenreich, & Hoyer, 2004). Barriers like lack of social support, time, and money can hinder motivation for change (Michalak et al., 2004).

One way to develop goals that clients are committed to is to ask them to imagine their preferred future. This can be done with the **miracle question**, which asks clients to imagine a miracle happened and how they would first know that the miracle had occurred (Stith et al., 2012).

> Imagine that you go home tonight, do the dishes, go about your daily life, go to sleep, and a miracle happens. The problem that brought you here has disappeared! What would be the first thing that you would notice letting you know that this miracle happened to you?

This exercise allows clients to imagine change, recognize where the miracle is already happening, and concretely visualize the steps needed to make that miracle happen more frequently. Asking clients what their family members would see might also help make the miracle more visible and tangible (Stith et al., 2012). This exercise also frames change in such a way that clients likely own the problem identified.

What Do You Think?

What goals would you want to address with Reymundo Sanchez? What do you think he would see as important to address? These goals might include developing positive coping skills for responding to stressors, building a positive support network in prison, acquiring career and life skills for after prison, and identifying a sense of direction and purpose for the future.

1. Which of these goals would you want to work on first? Would your decision be influenced by whether you expected that he would be released from prison?

2. Would it be enough that he stopped some behavior (e.g., drug use)? Would you also want him to make a positive change of some sort? Why?

3. How well do each of these goals match the SMART-IC recommendations? How could you rewrite these goals so they would be more effective?

Collaborative Goal-Setting Process

Let us never negotiate out of fear. But let us never fear to negotiate.

—John F. Kennedy

The SMART-IC model is a useful structure for developing good treatment goals; however, the goal-setting *process* is at least as important as the content. An effective process of goal setting requires listening closely to a client's values and preferences to collaboratively identify treatment goals. Notice how Leo and Kalil listened to and influenced Reymundo Sanchez in the case material at the beginning of this chapter. Such a collaborative process may be therapeutic in its own right (Grosse Holtforth & Castonguay, 2005). Further, setting goals with a client fosters the therapeutic relationship, guides treatment, focuses both client's and therapist's attention, and provides criteria for them to assess treatment outcomes (Michalak & Grosse Holtforth, 2006; Wampold & Imel, 2015). Collaborative goal-setting is also central to ethical treatment, as it creates transparency in treatment, empowers the client, balances power between client and clinician, and elicits informed consent (Knapp, VandeCreek, et al., 2017).

Good goals can be difficult to develop and depend on a strong and accurate assessment of the problem. Timelines, genograms, psychosocial histories, and behavioral observations can broaden clinicians' and clients' perspectives while helping them to look past symptoms and problems to the larger concerns (i.e., past individual trees to the larger forest). Nonetheless, goals that make sense to a clinician may not make sense to the client.

One reason why there may be a mismatch between client and clinician is that it can sometimes be difficult to identify who the client really is. Court-referred clients may not be the "real" client; instead, the court and probation or parole office may have mandated the client into treatment and chosen treatment goals; the referral source may have very different goals from the client's own goals. One partner may be more committed to change in couples therapy than the other. Children and their parents may have different—even conflicting—treatment goals, but clinicians must find a way of contracting for treatment with each (Hawley & Weisz, 2003). Feeling pressured can decrease client commitment to change (Moore et al., 2013).

Different cultural groups may have differing values and goals that influence setting treatment goals. Latinx immigrant parents are generally more collectivistic in their approach to school situations than are many European American teachers, disagreeing on the importance of individual achievement, the use of praise rather than criticism, the relative importance of academic rather than social skills, and individual expression rather than respect for authority (Greenfield et al., 2006). Hmong immigrants and their U.S. physicians often differ both in goals for treatment and in acceptable strategies for approaching it (Fadiman, 2012). Even willing clients may have goals for themselves that are different than their clinician's. Lent (2004) described one such case:

> I am reminded of a supervisee whose client admonished her for moving too quickly toward prescribing actions to help the client feel better. After a figurative tug-of-war in one session, the client announced, "I know how to get myself to feel better. And I know how to make decisions. What I could use your help with is figuring out how I get myself into messes like this to begin with." (p. 489)

Clinicians and clients must also make decisions about what to talk about during treatment, how to talk about it, and what approach to take. They may also have different and contradictory values. Liszcz and Yarhouse (2005), for example, highlighted the role of clinician values in the treatment goal identification process with clients questioning their sexuality. Religious clinicians and those specializing in work with lesbian and gay clients each tended to choose treatment goals consistent with their own values and attitudes. When there was a conflict in goals, clinicians tended to choose goals consistent with their own values over clients' goals. Failing to collaborate effectively can damage goal setting, treatment plan development, and the therapeutic alliance.

One final consideration: The problem and goal must fit each other. Sometimes clients and clinicians choose goals that fail to address the problem identified. A student with poor grades may say that she needs to study more (although she cannot concentrate when she does study). A man who is overweight may believe that he needs to eat less (although he eats a normal number of calories but rarely exercises and consumes more than 1,200 calories per day in beer). A father may conclude that he needs to be stricter with his daughter (in fact, he is strict enough but fails to tell her that he loves her). The following strategies can help clients and clinicians find common ground and work effectively together.

Work From Where the Client Is

Clients must feel understood and safe enough to change. Clinicians can create this sense of safety by listening carefully to their clients and accepting their perceptions of the world. Only when clients feel understood can clinicians begin to help them perceive their situation or problem differently (Ivey & Ivey, 2014). In this hypothetical dialogue, notice Liam's drug and alcohol counselor's approach.

Rosaria 1: Why are you here today?

Liam 1: The judge and social worker think I should be here.

Rosaria 2: I hear you saying this was their idea. I wonder why they think you need to be here.

Liam 2: They took my kids because they said I was neglecting them. (pause, clenching jaw) The judge says that if I want to get my kids back, I have to see you.

Rosaria 3: (Gently) This is hard.

Liam 3: Yes, real hard. All I have is my children. I think about them all the time—whether they are safe, what they're doing. I just want them back.

Rosaria 4: You want them back. (pause) They're saying you need to parent differently? Is this your goal too?

Liam 4: I suppose. Yes, I think so. (pause) I need to stop drinking, too. When I'm drinking, I'm not such a good parent.

In this dialogue, Rosaria listened to Liam and shared her understanding in R2 ("I hear you saying this was their idea") and Liam recognized this ("They took my kids because they said I was neglecting them"). Once Liam recognized and accepted Rosaria's understanding, Rosaria could begin to get Liam to identify and set goals ("They're saying you need to parent differently? Is this your goal too?").

Build Clients' Commitment to Change

Clients in Precontemplation do not recognize the problem that the court or their parents, spouse, or employer sees (Norcross et al., 2011; Prochaska & Norcross, 2010). Clients in Contemplation are ambivalent about change, seeing both the pros and cons for changing. Clients in any stage may have different goals than their clinician or referral source. Such goal conflict is related to poorer subjective well-being (Kelly, Mansell, & Wood, 2015)

In the exchange between Rosaria and Liam, Rosaria accepted Liam's feelings and listened seriously to him. She respected Liam's choices while holding him responsible for the consequences of his decisions. If he had been forced to enter a parenting class, Liam might have dug in his heels and refused. When it was his choice, she was willing to commit to make changes. Rosaria also helped build Liam's commitment by noting and highlighting Liam's motivation to change (in R3 and R4), "This is hard. . . .You want them back." Still, Rosaria let Liam set his own goals.

Address Obstacles to Change

From the outside, change looks straightforward and easy. From the inside, it's often hard. Liam may want to change, but in becoming a better parent, he has to develop new skills, which takes time and comes with no guarantee of success. He also has to admit that he has made mistakes and that some other approach to parenting may be better than the one he has been using. Liam might have to tell others that his drinking has been a problem and that he has made mistakes. He needs to identify triggers to his drinking and find ways of changing his behavior during those situations. He needs to find better ways of handling stress and other strong emotions that he quieted with alcohol. He might have to make new friends and find new pastimes in place of drinking. Assuming that Liam is in Contemplation about stopping drinking, Rosaria needs to recognize and address both sides of Liam's ambivalence: his desire to change and the barriers to doing so. Many clinicians are hesitant to raise and address problems, believing that doing so might undermine a client's self-efficacy. Talking about ambivalence can be done without undermining hope.

Rosaria 5: It sounds like you want to stop drinking and that getting your children back would be a real incentive for doing so. I'm wondering what things we should be prepared for. What might make stopping difficult for you at this time?

Liam 5: (putting face in hands) I hate thinking about this . . .

Rosaria 6: Thinking about this *is* difficult, but it can help prepare you to cope with problems. (pause) You've tried quitting before? What happened?

Liam 6: Uh, okay. (pause) The hardest thing last time was my friends. They all drink and I could either go out with them or sit home alone. I hate being alone.

Rosaria 7: That is important to remember. Anything else?

Respect Clients' Strengths and Contributions to Treatment

Recognizing and using client strengths builds hope, self-confidence, and self-efficacy; strengthens the therapeutic relationship; and increases the probability of recovery (Norcross & Lambert, 2011). As seen in the last exchange, clinicians can acknowledge and use client strengths in many places. Liam is committing to changing both his drinking behaviors and parenting and is willing to work on each goal, even though doing so is difficult for him. He is socially oriented and insightful, readily identifying situations that have previously put him at risk of relapsing. Rosaria recognized these strengths, normalizing the difficulty of discussing these issues in therapy (R6) and the importance of patterns Liam had already observed and described (R7). Liam is open and honest with Rosaria, and they appear to be developing a good relationship.

Build Self-Efficacy and Mastery

Clients often enter treatment with a number of previous "failures," sometimes believing they will never be able to change. Assignments with a high probability of success can increase clients' perceptions that therapy can be successful, while dichotomous goals that are too challenging increase perceptions of failure and can be demotivating (Soman & Cheema, 2004). Rosaria's request that Liam consider where he has run into problems abstaining from alcohol in the past could be framed as a homework assignment that will be successful, regardless of what happens over the next week. This assignment would allow Rosaria to normalize Liam's cravings and reframe them as useful observations rather than as a problem in motivation.

Rosaria 8:   Liam, I'm impressed with your ability to observe when and where you've run into problems abstaining from alcohol. [pause] Could you expand this and think about when and where you crave alcohol this coming week? Can you record your observations throughout the week, including as much detail as you can? [Okay.] I also want you to observe the times when you *don't* have cravings. You're probably doing something special there that we want you to develop and expand.

Focus on the "Forest" While Respecting Clients' "Trees"

Many clients bring in the crisis of the week to discuss. It is important to take clients' crises seriously while also seeing the big picture. Paying attention to the big picture addresses treatment goals; discussing the current crisis can build an understanding of the problem's context and help clients recognize their clinician's empathy and understanding.

Rosaria 9:   Liam, it sounds like you "lost it" when you couldn't find a sitter when you'd planned to go to a meeting but that you eventually pulled things together, smoothed things out with your kids, and made it to a later meeting. Right?

[Uh-huh] Have you thought about how this example relates to the issues we've been talking about for the last several weeks?

Liam 9:   Yeah. Things don't go as I plan, and I lose it. I didn't drink this time, I didn't hit my kids, but I thought about it.

Rosaria 10:   But you didn't. That's a big change from a month ago.

Notice how Rosaria first paid attention to Liam's crisis in R9 ("Liam, it sounds like you 'lost it' when you couldn't find a sitter when you'd planned to go to a meeting but that you eventually pulled things together, smoothed things out with your kids, and made it to a later meeting"), making sure that she and Liam were on the same page but then related this to the larger treatment goal ("Have you thought about how this example relates to the issues we've been talking about for the past several weeks?"). In doing so, Rosaria developed a shared understanding with Liam, which allowed her to intervene and successfully reframe Liam's behavior.

Clinical Applications	At her first four therapy sessions, Faith described problems communicating with her partner, frustrations with being "heard" at work, believing that her children walk all over her, and feeling anxious "all the time." Her therapist, Yasser, felt more and more confused and lost in their work together. Yasser's supervisor suggested that he step back to think about the big picture. What commonalities among these problem statements might Yasser observe to identify a treatment goal?

Use Client Metaphors and Work Within Their Meaning System

One way of getting on track with clients is by using their metaphors and key words. Clients' own words reflect their ways of seeing themselves and their world and describe their familiar ways of looking at the problem. As seen in the following example, using their words communicates our empathic understanding, which strengthens the therapeutic relationship.

Liam 10:   There's a wall between the two of us, like we will never get close again. She just doesn't talk to me anymore.

Rosaria 11:   You feel like there's a wall between the two of you, and you don't know what you can do to climb over it or to tear it down. (Yeah.) What can *you* do *now* to make a door through this wall?

Liam 12:   Maybe we could try to understand each other . . .

Rosaria 12:   What could you do *today* to begin to tear down that wall?

Liam 13:   I could tell her how much I've missed having fun with her.

Note that although Rosaria accepted Liam's metaphor in L10 ("There's a wall between the two of us"), she didn't accept that the wall was permanent or impenetrable. She expanded Liam's way of thinking about the problem in by referring to standard attributes of walls (e.g., that they have doors, can be climbed over, or can be torn down). Her questions also helped Liam develop a concrete and specific picture of what he wanted to change and what needed to be done to get there.

What Do You Think?

1. For some of the people we've met earlier—Andrea Yates, Tara Westover, or Reymundo Sanchez—would their wishes influence your decisions about treatment goals? Why or why not? Would you be willing to defer to some people's goals for themselves and not others? Why?

2. If your goals differed from theirs, how would you negotiate this difference in goals? Why?

Writing Treatment Plans

Without goals, and plans to reach them, you are like a ship that has set sail with no destination.

—Fitzhugh Dodson

Treatment plans are detailed plans specifying the client's long-term goals, written as **goal statements**, as well as specific **interventions**, strategies that the client and clinician plan to use to meet those goals. They are a standard part of treatment, often required by agencies and insurance companies, and they facilitate collaborative work toward the same goals. Without a treatment plan, treatment can be rudderless, going hither and yon with the weekly concerns of a client: fighting with a spouse, disrespectful children, being bypassed for a promotion. Each of these symptoms (i.e., the fighting, disrespectful children, and work problems) might be seen as problems with effective and assertive communication. Treatment plans remind clinicians to step back and see the big picture.

Focusing on the big picture can help clinicians develop a consistent course in treatment and ensure that the client's full range of concerns is addressed

(Makover, 2016). Developing short-term goals and interventions provides client and clinician with a "map" that helps them identify the steps toward meeting their goals and recognize when goals have been met. Treatment plans can increase client hopefulness and self-efficacy and can make change easier to identify. Collaboratively developed treatment plans can build an understanding of the problem and empathy for the client, ultimately strengthening the therapeutic alliance.

Although long-term goals such as we have been focusing on are useful (we've just been calling them goals), they do not provide a detailed plan for treatment. They can be like trying to travel the country without a map. Most clinicians expand client goal statements by identifying short-term goals (e.g., "Client will practice challenging irrational beliefs") that help clients progress toward long-term goals (e.g., "Client will report feeling less depressed and having a greater sense of meaning"). In general, focusing on goal *progress* rather than goal *attainment* is related to greater well-being (Klug & Maier, 2015). Thus, treatment plans include short-term goals that help the client progress to the long-term goals.

Even short-term goals are often broken into smaller steps: the actual interventions that will be used to meet these goals. These interventions may include **implementation intentions**, if–then plans outlining the specific actions the client will take to meet the goal under specific circumstances (e.g., "If rated depression is greater than 6, client will attend to situational beliefs and challenge their irrational aspects"). When plans include implementation intentions, clients are somewhat more successful in meeting their goals (Bélanger-Gravel, Godin, & Amireault, 2013; Gollwitzer & Sheeran, 2006). In fact, although the effects of using implementation intentions are often moderate in size, they are larger for people with "difficulties regulating their behavior," such as people with psychological problems (Gollwitzer & Sheeran, 2006, p. 94). Implementation intentions seem to help people recognize how to regulate their behavior more effectively.

Attending to Strengths and Resources as Well as Weaknesses

Success is achieved by developing our strengths, not by eliminating our weaknesses.
—Marilyn vos Savant

When developing a treatment plan, it is tempting to focus on weaknesses that will be targeted. But effective treatment plans also draw on the client's strengths and resources—and every client has strengths and resources. Consider a glass of water. Many of us are used to asking whether it is half-empty or half-full. Nonetheless, this question illustrates the dichotomizing tendencies of humans, as the glass is no more one than the other. Each aspect—its emptiness and its fullness—are valid ways of looking at the glass of water.

Similarly, our strengths and weaknesses, problems and exceptions to problems, successes and failures, are equally valid aspects of who we are and each important to consider in our work with clients.

When clients present for therapy, they are rarely at their best. In crisis, they focus on the things that are not working. They may rely on maladaptive coping strategies and only describe the parts of their life that are problematic, either because they believe that is what their clinician is interested in or because they want to make sure that their clinician recognizes the significant help they need. Sometimes clinicians fail to look for or ask about strengths.

Recognizing obstacles to change is helpful when creating a treatment plan (Bélanger-Gravel et al., 2013), but identifying strengths is equally helpful (D. Gutierrez, Fox, Jones, & Fallon, 2018; S. J. Lopez & Snyder, 2003). Using and developing client strengths increases school achievement; leads to meaningful, productive work; and improves mental health.

The importance of identifying strengths can be seen in an example. Char and Robin had been married for 10 years but were fighting more and more frequently, especially since their daughter was diagnosed with diabetes. Char felt taken for granted and believed that she had to take on a disproportionate amount of the health care for their daughter, and Robin believed that they needed to resolve problems and was frustrated by Char's avoidance. Char was surprised when, late in treatment, their therapist noted that they were beginning to communicate more effectively. In fact, she believed that they had communicated well before their daughter's diagnosis and continued to do so in many situations.

Failing to recognize that their relationship had been strong in the past was hurtful to them but, more important, meant that their therapist formed a weak case conceptualization that undermined her empathy for the couple. Their therapist might have asked, although Char and Robin frequently fight, do they always? Have they always? What distinguishes between the bad and better times? What do they do well? How can their strengths be used as a resource in treatment? As this example illustrates, looking for strengths and exceptions to problems has multiple benefits. In particular, it can build empathy, strengthen the therapeutic alliance, develop stronger case conceptualizations, and identify resources for treatment.

Consider what a treatment plan for Char and Robin might look like. They have each identified different problems, leading to different long-term goals. First, ensure that their long-term goals are appropriate (i.e., they meet SMART-IC criteria).

> Char's problem statement: He never talks to me. He treats me like I'm a maid and nothing more.

> Char's long-term goal: I want him to talk to me and treat me as his partner, someone whom he loves.

Robin's problem statement: We fight like cats and dogs, each wanting to be King of the Hill.

Robin's long-term goal: I want us to work together well and have a common vision for our future.

Of course, these statements are inferences and would need to be verified before going further (e.g., "What I hear you saying you want is . . . Am I on track?").

When Char and Robin's long-term goals are assessed with regard to SMART-IC criteria, we see potential problems with their goals. Char's goal, for example, is specific, measurable, and in her own language, but not under her control, so perhaps not achievable. It is unclear whether she is committed to making the changes she is asking for. Char's goal could be better phrased as "I am going to consider my values and goals in our decision-making process and ask that my partner do so too."

Furthermore, Char's long-term goal only partially matches her problem. Perhaps this was because a more complete description of her problem would be "He rarely talks to me and, when he does, he treats me like I'm a maid. I think about myself in this way too and allow others to treat me that way." This new version of her problem helps her recognize her role in the problem and identify what she can do to change. In other words, she can identify an appropriate short-term goal, such as "If he treats me like a maid, I will challenge any automatic thoughts that I don't deserve to be treated better, then respond in a positive but assertive manner."

The second half of Robin's goal (i.e., "a common vision") is not a behavioral outcome and should be described more specifically to be realistic and achievable. Furthermore, it is not clear whether Robin has control over the desired outcomes and should be more clearly under her control.

Although there are different formats for presenting a treatment plan, if Char entered individual therapy to work on problems leading to difficulties in her relationship, her treatment plan might look like that in Table 8.2. Most plans have several short-term goals, acknowledging the multidimensional causation of many problems. Some people also include dates to meet goals and outcome measures.

Realistically, will all goals be completely met in the course of treatment? Probably not. Treatment should empower clients to continue to address life goals outside of and beyond treatment. Further, treatment goals and life goals should be distinguished (Makover, 2016). Writing a novel may be an important life goal, but staying in therapy until that novel is published is probably unrealistic. Instead, a good treatment goal might be to challenge cognitive and social barriers to writing.

Table 8.2 Treatment Plan for Char, Whose Relationship Is Characterized by Frequent Fighting

Problem 1: He never talks to me and, when he does, he treats me like I'm a maid. I think about myself in this way too and allow others to treat me that way.

Long-Term Goal 1: I am going to begin taking myself more seriously and ask others to do so too.

Short-term goals	Interventions	Outcomes
If he treats me like a maid, I will challenge automatic thoughts that I don't deserve to be treated better.	Discuss relationship among beliefs, emotions, and behaviors. Monitor and analyze beliefs, emotions, and behaviors, especially during periods of strong emotion. Recognize irrational beliefs and their impact on emotions. Challenge irrational beliefs, first during therapy then in balance of life.	Decreased depression, as measured by the Beck Depression Inventory.
If he treats me like a maid, I will respond in a positive but assertive manner.	Discuss assertiveness, distinguishing it from passive, aggressive, and manipulative behaviors. Practice assertiveness in controlled settings then move up the hierarchy.	Decreased number of fights and reported severity of fighting.

Problem 2: When I get stressed or upset, I am more likely to misinterpret my partner's actions and start a fight.

Long-Term Goal 2: I want to cope with my feelings without stressing my relationship.

Short-term goals	Interventions	Outcomes
I will cope more effectively with stressors.	Discuss coping mechanisms, evaluating their impact on self and valued goals, including but not limited to relationships. Increase use of adaptive coping strategies, evaluating their success, identifying better ways of coping as necessary.	More frequent reports of coping effectively with stressors.
If I get upset by something my partner says, I will first consider other explanations of his behavior and evaluate these.	In session, practice generating alternative explanations of partner's behavior, then evaluating predicted outcomes of each interpretation.	Decreased number of fights and decreased reported severity of fighting.

Determining Services

Details create the big picture.

—Sanford I. Weill

Treatment planning includes not only developing appropriate long- and short-term goals for clients (i.e., the details of treatment) but also determining the nature and level of services needed by that specific client (i.e., the big picture; Seligman, 2004). What intensity of services is necessary to stabilize the client? What option would be least restrictive and most helpful? The following questions may be helpful in this process:

- Is counseling appropriate? If so, what modality (e.g., individual, family, group) and approach? In what setting (e.g., outpatient, day program, inpatient, residential)?

- What community services can help stabilize the client (e.g., housing, transportation, medical assistance, parenting classes)?

- What natural supports can be engaged to help stabilize the client (e.g., grandparents, babysitters, softball coaches, pastors, neighbors)?

- Is medication appropriate? Should a psychiatric consult be requested?

- Has the client had a recent physical? Could some disease (diagnosed or undiagnosed) cause or complicate the client's symptoms?

- Can drug and alcohol issues be sufficiently addressed in the primary treatment setting? Are adjunctive services necessary to do so?

- Could prescription or recreational drugs cause symptoms?

- Does the client have strong preferences for the clinician's gender, race, or religion? Is there a reason to consider these issues when assigning a clinician?

Some issues are especially complicated and may require multiple types of interventions. Because trauma and abuse affect many dimensions of a person's life, for example, treatment should focus on multiple aspects, including safety planning, grief work, and family functioning (Faust & Katchen, 2004). Treatment should address symptoms that arose in response to the trauma and behavior that puts clients at risk; challenge problematic thoughts while building skills; and assess functioning in all realms, including work and school performance.

Although adjunctive services can be helpful, more is not necessarily better. Clients can be overwhelmed when too many workers and services are offered at the same time. It can be advisable to identify and work first with issues or services that will most rapidly stabilize the client or create change. Finally, a shared, consistent picture among the treatment team and other involved professionals facilitates change and can be built in phone calls or by sharing reports.

What Do You Think?

For Reymundo Sanchez, Tara Westover, or Andrea Yates:

1. What strengths do they have? How could these be used in treatment?

2. What do they want to happen in treatment? What treatment goals would they be willing to work toward?

3. How might their goals differ from their support system's goals for them? How might their goals differ from your goals for them?

4. What supports or services might they be open to and willing to accept?

5. Write a treatment plan for one of these individuals (a) using goals that he or she would find acceptable; (b) recognizing current strengths and exceptions to the problem(s) faced as well as current symptoms; (c) breaking the goal into concrete, recognizable steps that build on each other; and (d) considering natural supports, substance use, and health issues.

Revisiting the Treatment Plan Periodically

Know what's weird? Day by day, nothing seems to change, but pretty soon . . . everything's different.

—*Calvin from* Calvin and Hobbes

A treatment plan might not be effective because the problem was poorly or incompletely assessed, the treatment plan does not really address the problem, the client and clinician do not identify shared problems and goals, the proposed plan was unacceptable to the client, or the plan was poorly implemented. As a result, after developing a treatment plan, it is important to evaluate progress on treatment goals on a regular and ongoing basis.

There are a variety of ways to determine whether treatment has been effective. The easiest way is to ask a client. This can be performed using an open question, "How are things relative to when you came in?" One could also use a **scaling question** to assess where the client is relative to the desired change, "On a scale from 1 to 10, with 1 being the day that you called to make your appointment and 10 being how it will be the day after the miracle, where the problem is resolved, where are you today?" When a client's response is different from the last assessment, ask, "What is different?" This series of questions gets people thinking about change and what they can do to make the desired change happen more frequently.

There are also short satisfaction questionnaires designed for adults and teens (e.g., Client Satisfaction Questionnaire [CSQ]: Larsen, Attkisson, Hargreaves, & Nguyen, 1979; Youth Satisfaction Questionnaire [YSQ]: Stüntzner-Gibson, Koren, & DeChillo, 1995). Unfortunately, satisfaction questionnaires such as the CSQ and the YSQ are only moderately related to either therapist perceptions of outcomes or client behaviors (Turchik, Karpenko, Ogles, Demireva, & Probst, 2010). The weak validity of these measures has been attributed to several factors. Clients, family members and therapists might each focus on different aspects of a client's behavior (e.g., subjective depression, energy levels, or sick days taken); offer positive ratings of progress because of the positive therapeutic alliance; or provide feedback designed to protect a clinician's feelings. Despite these problems, most clinicians believe that client satisfaction is necessary to effective treatment.

Change can also be assessed with paper-and-pencil measures at intake and some later point in treatment. Borckardt and his colleagues (2008), for example, recommended a daily or weekly measure of distress, as well as a standardized outcome measure such as the Beck Depression Inventory (BDI; Beck, Steer, & Carbin, 1988) or the Outcome Questionnaire—45 (OQ–45: Lambert, Gregersen, & Burlingame, 2004). Self-reports like the BDI are short and easily responded to and scored, although because their intent is fairly transparent, can be biased by the desire to look good or bad, by client denial, or lack of insight. Multidimensional scales such as the Child Behavior Checklist (CBCL; Achenbach & Rescorla, 2004) are useful because they can identify growth and strengths while also identifying relative weaknesses.

One can also monitor change using behavioral measures (e.g., number of fights, number of instances of self-injury), preferably behavioral outcomes that are under the client's control (e.g., time studying rather than grades, calories consumed rather than weight change). Char's therapist hypothesized that if treatment was effective and moving toward treatment goals, there would be both fewer and less severe fights. See Figure 8.1. She could have

FIGURE 8.1 Effects of Treatment on the Severity and Frequency of Fighting Between Char and Her Partner

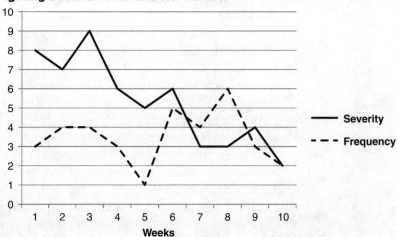

instead assessed monthly ratings of their relationship, Char's scores on the BDI, or distress scores from both Char and her partner. In this case, Char and her therapist noticed that although they did not fight less frequently, their fights were much less severe than before. When they discussed this change in treatment, Char decided that she didn't care as much about the number of fights because sometimes their fights helped them solve problems, but the severity of these fights really mattered to her. They used this information to fine-tune and further target her goals.

Clinical Applications	Autumn has a history of sexual abuse as a child, chronic depression, and frequent self-injury. She decided that her initial goal in therapy is to decrease her self-injury. When her therapist, Reyna, consulted with her clinical supervisor, the supervisor recommended that Reyna work with Autumn to identify at least three behavioral measures to track change across the course of therapy. However, Reyna and Autumn are having difficulty identifying possible outcome measures. What measures might they consider?

✳ ✳ ✳

If Reyna discovered that there was little progress in her work with Autumn at their first treatment plan review, what might she consider? Why?

Summary

Change is often difficult because people may have mixed emotions about change and identify a number of obstacles to changing successfully. Helping people change requires a strong understanding of the change process. People enter treatment at different places and with different motivations to change (Norcross et al., 2011; Prochaska & Norcross, 2010). Recognizing these different levels of commitment helps match intervention styles to individual clients.

Not all goals are useful, and not all goals are realistic. Good goals are specific, measurable, achievable, realistic, time-bounded, and intrinsic, and the client is committed to working on them (SMART-IC). Clients and clinicians may identify different goals, which may reflect differences in values or a clinician's inaccurate assessment of the client's commitment (stage of change). Wise clinicians work from where their clients are, strengthen their clients' commitment to change, address obstacles for change, respect their clients' strengths and contributions to treatment, and build their clients' self-efficacy and sense of mastery. They pay attention to their clients' individual concerns but are also able to see how weekly crises relate to the larger issues that brought clients to treatment and work at both levels.

Treatment plans guide treatment. The approach outlined in a specific treatment plan should be a function of the clinician's theoretical viewpoint, research on the problem, and the client's strengths and resources—as well as those of the clinician. In effective treatment plans, the long-term goals align with the problem, the short-term goals help clients progress toward long-term goals, and the interventions help clients meet short-term goals. When possible, clients and clinicians should collaborate on treatment plans to develop a shared map and goals for treatment; this process strengthens the therapeutic alliance.

Treatment progress and outcomes should be regularly assessed, preferably from the beginning of treatment and along several types of outcomes. Multidimensional scales and multiple measures (e.g., self-reports, paper-and-pencil measures, behavioral outcomes) can identify strengths, weaknesses, ongoing issues, and alternative interpretations of problems.

For Review

Applying Concepts to Your Life

1. Identify your stage of change for a change you made or attempted to make. How difficult was change? How was this level of difficulty influenced by your readiness to change?

2. Are there changes that others think you should make that you don't see as important? How have you handled these potential conflicts?

3. For a current "problem" in your life: What is your goal? How can your strengths be useful in approaching this goal or resolving this problem? What do exceptions to the problem tell you about how you can handle it?

4. Imagine not having a clear "treatment plan" (e.g., a course without a syllabus, a vacation without destinations or plans, medical interventions that are not clearly described). If this lack of planning sounds good under some circumstances but would be uncomfortable at other times, consider why. When and why might this work?

5. For a "problem" that is important to you, write a brief treatment plan. As you do so, pay attention to the research on the problem, exceptions to the problem, and strengths that may be useful in resolving the problem. Consider your conceptualization of the problem and develop concrete, recognizable steps toward your goals. Identify natural supports, when possible.

6. How would you assess progress towards your goals? How have you identified change on a goal you have previously set?

Key Terms

action, 163
approach goals, 165
avoidance goals, 165
contemplation, 163
fixed mind-set, 164
goal statements, 175

growth mind-set, 164
implementation
    intentions, 176
interventions, 175
lapse, 164
long-term goal, 165

maintenance, 164
miracle question, 168
precontemplation, 162
preparation, 163
relapse, 164
scaling question, 181

short-term goal, 165
slip, 164
SMART-IC, 165
treatment goals, 165
treatment plans, 175
triggers, 164

Learn More

For more information about the concepts in this chapter, visit the *Empathic Counseling* companion website at http://pubs.apa.org/books/supp/slattery/.

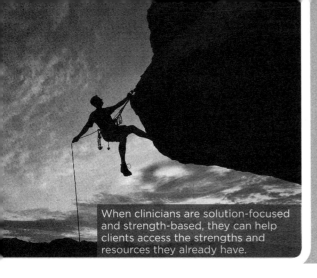

When clinicians are solution-focused and strength-based, they can help clients access the strengths and resources they already have.

9 Providing Empathic Interventions

Looking Ahead

After reading this chapter you will be able to answer these questions:

1. What intervention strategies are shared across most theoretical viewpoints?

2. Why is listening before intervening important in facilitating change?

3. What can clinicians do to help clients change behaviors, thoughts, and feelings?

4. What are common barriers to treatment, and how can these barriers be effectively addressed?

5. How can clinicians assess the success of their interventions?

Cases in Empathy

I Don't Drink Every Single Day | Beth Schneider

Beth Schneider is an attractive, middle class White woman in her 30s. She is 8 months pregnant, described as healthy, active, fun-loving, and carefree. She has become more careful about her diet since becoming pregnant, but also made a controversial decision about drinking alcohol. "I don't drink every single day. It's probably four or five days a week that I enjoy a glass of wine. A beer. (sound of a cork popping from a wine bottle) Love that sound. (laughing) You know, when you get one glass a day, you milk the hell out of it."

She continued, "I've heard of fetal alcohol syndrome, and of course, you know, every-thing scares you as a pregnant woman, and they put fear in you."

Her husband Jeff said, "There is a chance. How big of a chance? We don't know. It's not something to worry about or stress about."

Linda Murray, editor-in-chief of *BabyCenter*, admitted, "We have quite a few women . . . who've told us that for the first time in their lives [now that they're pregnant], they really want beer. They love the smell of it, they love the taste of it."

A number of women reported that they drink, but never in public. One observed, "It's not really worth risking public ridicule or scorn or all the advice I'm sure I'd get."

Beth concluded, "I don't care. I'm a firm believer that anything in moderation is OK." (Chang, Chan, & Stern, 2008)

What Do You Think?

1. Assuming Beth's obstetrician had recommended that she stop drinking, but she continued to talk about her drinking in this way, in what stage of change would she be in? How do you know? What prevents her from stopping drinking?

2. If her obstetrician asked you to help Beth stop drinking during pregnancy, how would you approach this? Why?

3. How do your feelings about drinking during pregnancy influence your reactions to Beth? How would they influence your ability to work with her?

The Process of Intervening

So when you are listening to somebody, completely, attentively, then you are listening not only to the words, but also to the feeling of what is being conveyed, to the whole of it, not part of it.
—Jiddu Krishnamurti

Once clients and clinicians have developed goals and treatment plans, they follow through with the treatment plan, providing the agreed-on interventions. How do clinicians identify what is appropriate and timely and what the client will be receptive to? How do they get clients to become "the engine" driving treatment? How we choose to do so will depend on the client's stage of change and treatment goals, as well as the quality of the therapeutic alliance. Receptivity may change across sessions and within a single one; thus, throughout treatment, clinicians should consider whether their clients are receptive to further interventions (Ivey & Ivey, 2014).

Depending on their clients' stage of change, clinicians help them recognize the problem, resolve their ambivalence about changing, or identify strategies for changing or staying on track (Norcross, Krebs, & Prochaska, 2011; Prochaska & Norcross, 2010). Simple agreement with the client ("You're right, you should leave him") can be nonproductive and nontherapeutic, whereas criticism ("You can't just sit around! Get up and do something!") may come across as invalidating the client's experience, which may lead to resistance to change (Beutler, Rocco, Moleiro, & Talebi, 2001). Such critical, judgmental, and blaming responses put people with a history of mental illness at increased risk of relapse (Hooley & Miklowitz, 2017; Masland & Hooley, 2015).

Ivey and Ivey (2014) described a more helpful approach to facilitating change. They suggested that clinicians should listen, share their understanding, and intervene only after that understanding is recognized.

Listen

As clinicians listen deeply to their clients, they assume their clients' perspective makes sense to them (Fraser & Solovey, 2007; Ivey & Ivey, 2014).

Rather than jumping in too quickly to intervene, they become curious about how their clients see the world, their place in it, the problem, and their ability to change it. With suicidal clients, for example, listening can be essential to the engagement process because family and friends may not have wanted to listen to their story (G. K. Brown et al., 2006). Listening carefully to their story can help clinicians identify risk factors and develop a strong case conceptualization.

Share Your Understanding

Once clinicians believe they understand, they must share their understanding of the client and the problem from the client's point of view. Clinicians undermine treatment when they prematurely intervene, even when their interpretations and interventions are "right." Only when clients recognize their clinician's empathic understanding can clinicians share a new perspective to motivate change. See a description of verbal influencing skills in Exhibit 9.1. In the following case, pay attention to whether Antonia feels understood and how she signals her understanding.

Exhibit 9.1 Verbal Influencing Skills

Reframe. Provides a new way of looking at behavior. Can either make the behavior more desirable or less desirable. "Your 'helping behavior' enables him to continue getting high." "Your 'enabling' is a sign of your deep compassion for the people around you."

Interpretation. Identifies a deeper, underlying meaning to client behavior. "I wonder whether your lateness to sessions might indicate your ambivalence about being here."

Self-disclosure. Discloses material that is somewhat personal to the clinician (e.g., reactions, memories, dreams, actions). "I was thinking that we have been moving very quickly today." "I had a very difficult time starting college and missed my parents something fierce."

Feedback. A special case of self-disclosure sharing the clinician's perception of or reaction to the client. "You say others see you as distant and cold, but I don't see you that way."

Information giving. Provides information to help client understand the problem, symptoms, or others. "Many people with a history of child abuse have a difficult time trusting others."

Normalization. Reframes a behavior that client has perceived negatively. "Everyone has both good days and bad. The problem occurs when the bad days are too frequent or severe."

Directives. Tells client what to do, generally in a relatively circumscribed situation to help meet a treatment goal. "Take three slow breaths and begin to center yourself." "Monitor your thoughts over the next week, especially when you're having strong feelings."

Advice. Tells client what to do, especially how to solve a problem. "I would kick her out."

Confrontation. Identifies a discrepancy within or across realms, for example, between client's behavior and goal, or between behavior and values. "You say that your children are everything to you, yet you've been out drinking each night this week."

Antonia 1:   (looking down, talking slowly) I've had a really difficult week. I keep struggling to stay on track with the things that we were talking about last week. It all seems like so much. Even getting out of bed seems like too much.

Jon 1:   It sounds like you've been having a really difficult time, that you're struggling to stay on track with what we talked about last week, even getting out of bed. [paraphrase]

Antonia 2:   (nods) Yeah. I don't want to get out of bed, but I have some important things to do. I have to decide whether to fire someone at work. I have to choose a new day care for the twins. Mostly, though, Tomas has been manicky lately and I have to decide whether I can continue living with him. (pause) It's all too much.

Jon 2:   It's all too much. (Antonia nods and looks up) And, yet, you *have* gone on and have even begun to make some very difficult decisions at work and with your family. (Yeah.) [encourager, feedback]

In her second comment (A2), Antonia felt at least partially understood: "Yeah. I don't want to get out of bed." Still, she signals that she has not felt completely understood when she continues, "but I have some important things to do" (i.e., "I cannot afford to stay in bed"). When clients are feeling ambivalent and hopeless, there's a danger of falling into a "yeah, but . . ." game. When either the client or clinician responds with a "but" (unless the clinician is paraphrasing the client's ambivalence), there is a disruption in understanding. In this case, Jon would be premature to follow up with a more action-oriented intervention and should instead focus on listening.

Sometimes, however, the "but" is only expressed nonverbally, through hesitations or breaks in eye contact (Thomas, 2005). As in the next example (A3), hesitations and breaks indicate a failure to reach agreement and should be interpreted as a signal to slow down.

Antonia 3:   Uh . . . (pause, eyes drop) You're right. I really shouldn't stay in bed. I have important things to do. (turns away slightly, posture becomes more closed)

Antonia's hesitations and changes in body language (e.g., break in eye contact and change in body posture) signal that she is not yet on board, despite language suggesting agreement. The word *should* also signals a possible problem: She believes she *ought* to agree rather than that she does.

Empathic understanding is developed when clinicians hear the **discrepancy** between where clients are and where they want to be (Slattery & Park, 2012). Clinicians must validate both poles of the client's dilemma and experience: how a client is failing to meet her goals but sees these as essential; she is symptomatic but wants to change (Fraser & Solovey, 2007; Slattery & Park, 2012). Without the former, clients may not feel understood; without the latter, clients may not feel hopeful enough to begin to change.

Jon 4: You *should* do "important things" (Uh huh), yet don't want to get out of bed. (Yeah) It sounds like you want to do these things, but are ambivalent about them. How can you solve problems when you don't know what you want to do? [paraphrase, open question]

Antonia 4: Exactly. (making eye contact, posture relaxing somewhat) How can I solve these things when I don't know what I want to do?

In this exchange, Antonia indicated both verbally and nonverbally that she believed Jon understood her. She said, "exactly," while making eye contact and relaxing, then paraphrased Jon, demonstrating she accepted they were on the same page.

What Do You Think?

1. The consequence of failing to listen well, of imposing views on clients, was seen in Beth Schneider's reaction to criticisms of her drinking in the opening case material. Using this strategy of listening and intervening only after the client feels heard, reevaluate your initial approach to helping Beth change. How did you do? What would you do differently?

* * *

2. How would you respond to the Lee family (Chapter 4), attending to traditional Hmong approaches to and values about healing; addressing Lia's specialness, as seen in the Hmong view of her epilepsy; and her parents' concerns for her physical health? How does this match what her doctors did? If the Lees said they were willing to use a medicine to stop her seizures, how would you handle their unstated ambivalence—their willingness to try something different but also the barriers that prevented them from consistently following through with medical care in the past?

* * *

3. If you were working with the young Malcolm X (Chapter 6) in the period after his father's murder, how could you acknowledge the feelings that motivated his acting out while also seeing the positive qualities characterizing this blossoming activist? If he talked about beginning to follow the school's rules, how could you address both the part of him that wants to change and the part that might be unwilling to do so? Why might this be important?

Then, Introduce Change

God grant me the serenity to accept the people I cannot change, the courage to change the one I can, and the wisdom to know it's me.

—*Anonymous*

When clients signal that they have been understood and are receptive to interventions for meeting a goal, clinicians can help them change. Interventions must be grounded in an empathic understanding of the person but be different enough from their current perception of the problem to motivate change (Fraser & Solovey, 2007). Like Goldilocks's experience with the Three Bears, reframes, interpretations, and other interventions that are too similar to the client's current viewpoint provide insufficient justification for change, whereas those that are too discrepant are often rejected as failures of empathy. Further, effective interventions must also be plausible and believable to both the client and clinician. Interventions should motivate more benign self-perceptions and adaptive change rather than maladaptive ones (Park, Edmondson, & Mills, 2010; Slattery & Park, 2012).

When Antonia says, "Tomas's moods are up and down and I never know what I'm going to walk into next. I'm feeling pretty hopeless about things ever getting better," imagine how three different clinicians might respond to Antonia and how these fit within this model.

- Clinician A: "It seems that it's pretty unlikely that you'll ever get out of this." [a weak paraphrase accepting Antonia's perception of the problem; subtractive empathy]
- Clinician B: "Oh, things will be easy, just wait and see!" [groundless feedback rejecting Antonia's perception of the problem; subtractive empathy]
- Clinician C: "You're feeling pretty hopeless right now (Yeah . . .), feeling stuck (Uh huh), but I also notice that you're saying that you're *feeling* hopeless rather than that the situation *is* hopeless. (Yes) You don't *yet* know what you can do to handle Tomas better." [reflection of feeling, reframe; additive empathy]

Clinician A made a poor paraphrase that failed to catch Antonia's hesitancy—that she *feels* hopeless rather than that her situation *is* hopeless. Clinician B's glib response may be based in the clinician's own fears, anxiety, boredom, or restlessness and is so far off the mark that Antonia is unlikely to feel heard. Clinician B's response could easily be framed as "yeah, but . . ." (e.g., "Yes, but things will be easy, just wait and see!"). Clinician C empathizes with Antonia's feelings of hopelessness, while also noticing her hesitation. The additive empathy in this intervention can help Antonia feel listened to and, in reframing the situation ("You don't *yet* know . . ."), could develop her motivation for change.

Timing is important to an intervention's effectiveness. If stated prematurely, the mild reframe in Clinician C's last sentence ("You don't *yet* know . . .") will be rejected. However, when it was withheld until after Antonia accepted the reflection of feeling, Antonia was able to relax slightly, nod, and begin to consider other ways of seeing this problem.

With the Goldilocks approach, interventions must be similar enough to a client's meaning system to allow "safe" change, yet different enough to motivate change toward treatment goals. Interventions can offer a new way of seeing things (e.g., that there are as yet undiscovered ways of handling Tomas better) or a different approach to an old problem (e.g., taking a breath before talking to Tomas). As seen in the following examples, changing clients' perceptions of themselves and the problem can lead to changes in their behavior. In a reciprocal fashion, changing their behavior can change the way they see the problem.

- When Kerin begins to see her daughter as bright and curious rather than as having attention problems, instead of attempting to refocus her daughter, she may begin to support her daughter's curiosity. Her new assumptions change her behavior, which in turn changes the ways that she sees herself and her daughter. Further, her daughter's behavior may also change in response to the new parenting style. (Beliefs → Behavior → Beliefs → Behavior)

- Gib began taking a breath before talking to his wife about problems and noticed that their discussions turned out better. His behavior changed his view of their relationship (he was more hopeful), his wife (she was more reasonable), and himself (he liked himself better when his actions were more measured, reasonable, and empathic). With these changes in perspective and outcomes, he became more optimistic about their relationship and worked harder to hear his wife's perspective. (Behavior → Beliefs → Behavior)

Interventions should be underpinned by an empathic understanding recognizing the person's potential and best motives; thus, effective interventions are framed in an affirming, constructive, and hopeful manner rather than a cold, hostile, and rejecting one (May, 1967). Remembering exceptions to the problem and the client's strengths and positive intentions can make it easier to link empathy and interventions. Clinician C used an unstable attribution about the future, which was more hopeful: Antonia doesn't "*yet* know" what she can do to handle Tomas better, implying that she will be more successful in the future.

> **Clinical Applications**   Maja is working with her client Morgan, who is questioning her sexual identity. Morgan has not come out to her family, in part because they frequently make homophobic comments and jokes. Despite these comments, she loves them deeply, enjoys their time together, but feels hopeless about being accepted by her family. What could Maja say to reframe Morgan's perspective on her family's inability to accept her? If she thinks Morgan's reactions are at least partly due to internalized homophobia, how could Maja reframe Morgan's reactions?

Interventions to Help Clients Change

We should remember that if a situation cannot be changed, there is no point in worrying about it. If it can be changed, then there is no need to worry about it either, we should simply go about changing it.

—Dalai Lama

As described earlier, changes in perceptions can lead to changes in behavior and vice versa, so the distinction between these two classes of interventions is arbitrary. Nonetheless, it can be useful to consider how some styles of intervention lead to different ways of thinking, whereas others more directly address behavior, and still others focus specifically on emotions. Where and how to best intervene depends in part on the nature of the problem, but also clients' preferences (American Psychological Association Presidential Task Force on Evidence-Based Practice, 2006).

Interventions for Changing Behaviors

As described in Chapter 8, many clients entering treatment have not yet identified a problem and committed to change. In fact, Prochaska and Norcross (2010) estimated that, depending on the population, only 10% to 20% of clients are in Action, another 30% to 40% are in Contemplation, and between 50% and 60% are in Precontemplation. Given this, they suggested clinicians should assess clients' stage of change early in treatment and be cautious about assuming that all clients are ready to address the identified problem (e.g., quitting drinking).

Clinicians can move beyond dichotomous ways of thinking about change (e.g., drinking or not drinking) to thinking about change as a process, with many smaller steps on the way. With clients in Precontemplation, clinicians can empathize, accept, and validate clients' experience, gradually helping them perceive the negative consequences of their behavior (Goldfried, 2007). When clients move slowly, it can be very helpful for clinicians to be patient and accepting, especially when this patience is balanced by gentle encouragement. In fact, clinicians' negative feelings (e.g., disengagement and negative countertransference) can interfere with treatment and may even lead to clients' deterioration (Fuertes, Gelso, Owen, & Cheng, 2013).

Clients in Contemplation can be encouraged to explore the costs and benefits of changing as well as barriers to change (Norcross et al., 2011; Prochaska & Norcross, 2010). Even when clients are not ready to take action on the identified problem, they may be ready to take smaller behavioral steps that prepare them for more challenging interventions (e.g., identifying at-risk situations, monitoring stress levels, developing a more positive support system, using positive coping strategies; G. K. Brown et al., 2006). Identifying barriers to treatment and making small, positive steps towards the goal, rather than being meaningless, may be essential to treatment, as they can increase clients' hopefulness and their probability of change on the identified problem (Norcross et al., 2011; Prochaska & Norcross, 2010).

Effective treatment triages the problem, addressing the most pressing issues first. For example, although developing stronger coping skills is important for people who are suicidal, it may be more important to first stabilize them with emergency services and then only later helping them develop coping skills and natural supports (G. K. Brown et al., 2006).

Treatment barriers occur at all levels: psychological, environmental, family and culture role expectations, and therapy itself. Premature terminations are more frequent when clients perceive a weak therapeutic alliance and poor multicultural competence (K. N. Anderson et al., 2019). Regardless of the nature of the barrier, Prochaska and Norcross (2010) suggested that clinicians intervene first with symptoms and situations, as more "internal" interventions may require more work and can feel blaming, especially if introduced prematurely. If helping a client sleep and exercise regularly will be sufficient to decrease depression, then start there.

As described previously, when clinicians are solution-focused and strength-based, they can help clients access the strengths and resources they already have (Franklin, Zhang, Froerer, & Johnson, 2017). Clinicians can identify the positive intention behind the problem behavior (e.g., that "nagging" reflects the client's "caring" for the other person's needs). They can recognize the client's strengths and resources in other realms to transfer them to the problem realm. They can listen for exceptions to the problem and times when their clients are already handling the problem successfully. They can notice evidence of change across sessions, even changes that might otherwise appear insignificant.

Antonia 5: Tomas's moods continue to be up and down. Today, I just walked away from him when he got angry.

Jon 5: Hmm, that's interesting. (Huh?) One month ago, when he got angry, you got angry and in his face. What are you doing differently? [feedback, open question]

Antonia 6:   I hadn't thought about it in that way, but you're right. It *is* different. (pause) I've been meditating, like we've talked about, and so when he got angry, I was calmer and didn't take it so personally. I knew that I had to leave the room, though, as I still don't feel strong enough to handle his anger.

In recognizing and commenting on this change, Antonia identified the skills and strengths that she has developed (A6). Jon could have identified these changes for her. However, a general goal of treatment is to empower clients so they can continue the change process following termination from treatment. Therefore, it is more helpful, when possible, to have clients take ownership for treatment, identify their own goals, and recognize their successes (Goode, Park, Parkin, Tompkins, & Swift, 2017). Note how Antonia's meditation practice affects the nature of her interactions with Tomas and how this causes her to perceive herself differently.

In most cases, an important aspect of treatment includes developing good coping and problem-solving skills. Across time, clients recognize the ways that negative coping is both ineffective and makes problems worse (Aldwin, 2007). They explore ways in which coping strategies such as self-medicating; self-injuring; and engaging in minimization, denial, or rationalization are maladaptive, and begin to substitute more adaptive coping mechanisms. They explore more adaptive coping skills, including solving controllable problems using planful action and attempting to understand and accept problems outside their control. Clients with weak social networks develop stronger supports and thus gain empathy, advice, and tangible support, working through difficult or confusing feelings (Aldwin, 2007).

For example, people who are depressed are less likely to engage in health-promoting practices (e.g., Gonzalez et al., 2007); therefore, paying attention to basic health care practices can be an important aspect of treatment. These practices may include eating well, getting enough rest, exercising regularly, maintaining a healthy weight, using alcohol moderately or not at all, learning how to relax, pursuing hobbies and leisure activities, and taking vacations. A regular spiritual practice may be an important part of creating and maintaining a healthy mind and body.

In addition, people who are depressed often have both acute and more chronic social skill deficits (Petty, Sachs-Ericsson, & Joiner, 2004). People who are depressed who ruminate on negative life events are more likely to relapse (Farb, Irving, Anderson, & Segal, 2015), as are people with critical, blaming, and judgmental family members (Hooley & Miklowitz, 2017). Addressing these and other skill deficits in both clients and their family members can be an important aspect of treatment and decrease the risk of relapse after termination from treatment.

Maja is working with Morgan, who is questioning her sexual identity and feeling hopeless about being accepted by her family. Since her last visit home to see her family, when her family belittled a relative who "looks gay," Morgan disclosed that she has been engaging in frequent self-injury and is bingeing on alcohol three or more times per week. If Maja believes that these behaviors reflect Morgan's feelings of depression, what behavioral interventions might be helpful? How might she discuss her hypotheses with Morgan?

Interventions for Changing Beliefs

Depression is the inability to construct a future.

—Rollo May

As described in Chapter 5, a person's beliefs, values, and goals influence a wide variety of behaviors throughout the day; thus, intervening with meaning can have significant impacts throughout a person's life. When the underlying thoughts and perceptions are realistic and useful, emotional responses and behaviors are more adaptive, whereas when perceptions and thoughts are maladaptive, emotional responses and behaviors are more dysfunctional.

Challenging beliefs and developing new meanings. People face difficult issues in life and often treat the meanings they draw in response to these events as truisms rather than possibilities (Gray, Maguen, & Litz, 2007). Although their meanings seem intended to protect them, they often do so at an unacceptable cost: Their new meanings can often be too extreme and overgeneralized. Healthy strategies for creating adaptive meanings take a middle ground, noting the self-protective nature of the meaning but making it more moderate and adaptive (e.g., recognizing when one is unsafe but also identifying how one can stay safer).

For example, Drew was recently assaulted and raped at a party. He has been feeling increasingly paranoid and unsafe, sees the world as unpredictable and out of control, and expects to be hurt. In therapy, he states, "I never feel safe. I can't go anywhere or do anything without looking over my shoulder and wondering what is going to happen next." A variety of interventions can challenge his problematic beliefs and assumptions:

- Clinician A: "You feel like you're never safe, that someone is going to hurt you. (Yeah) Never??? (pause) That word seems awful extreme to me. You, too? (pause) Are there times when you feel safer?" [reflection of feeling, self-disclosure, closed questions]

- Clinician B: "It sounds like you feel small and helpless since the attack because you're afraid that someone will hurt you again. (Yeah) It takes a lot of *courage* to keep trying even when you're afraid, to come here every week." [reflection of feeling, reframe]

- Clinician C: "You're feeling unsafe [uh huh], maybe even a little bit crazy. (Yeah) You're always looking over your shoulder. Many people feel that way after an attack. That's not crazy; it helps you feel safe again." [reflection of feeling, normalization, reframe]
- Clinician D: "You're feeling unsafe. (Yes) Take a minute, close your eyes, and breathe more slowly, like we've been practicing. (long pause) OK, how are you feeling now? [Calmer. More in control] Ah! You *felt* unsafe and out of control (Uh huh), but still have ways of regaining safety and control." [reflection of feeling, directive, open question, feedback]

Drew began with an extreme statement that was unlikely to match real experience (i.e., that he is *never* safe). Each clinician responded to his statement with a reflection of feeling, then challenged his assumption in a different way. Clinician A addressed his extreme thinking (i.e., "never") and suggested more moderate and realistic language and thoughts. Suggesting Drew will always be safe is unrealistic, especially as he has been assaulted, but it is realistic to expect there will be times when he will feel safer. If Drew was unable to identify safer times, Clinician A could bring the discussion back into the here and now (e.g., "How do you feel right now?").

Clinician B addressed Drew's underlying assumption of personal weakness by presenting a reframe of the "problematic" behavior (i.e., "It takes a lot of *courage* . . ."). Drew assumed that his fears and anxiety were all-encompassing; his clinician suggested that they were part of his experience, but that he was courageous in asking for help. Clinician B might further suggest it would be foolhardy *not* to be afraid. Reframes can be powerful but should not be used to dismiss a client's feelings in a "yeah, but . . ." fashion. They should start with a validation of the client's feelings, with the reframe introduced only after the client feels understood, as Clinician B did.

Clinician C normalized Drew's reactions as a common part of the experience of attack survivors, then again used a reframe by suggesting this common response is also a healthy one (i.e., "it's a way of feeling safe again"). Like Clinician B, Clinician C could suggest that it would be foolhardy not to be afraid after being raped and assaulted. Like Clinician A, Clinician C could ask whether Drew is always looking over his shoulder or whether there are times when he feels safer. Normalization and information giving can be powerful strategies for people feeling crazy: "This is a normal reaction. Let's find a healthier way of responding to this, though."

Clinician D did something different by using a directive (i.e., "Take a minute, close your eyes, and breathe more slowly . . ."). Rather than only thinking about when he feels safe or unsafe, Drew explored his experience in the here and now and developed skills to regain a sense of safety and control. Clinician D could continue this exploration by having Drew practice his breathing in other settings and observing his feelings afterwards. Exploring Drew's experience in the here and now offered a new and corrective type of experience.

Treatment is an opportunity to reduce the size of discrepancies between life events and meaning system, develop a coherent and positive life narrative, and make sense of life in a hopeful and useful way (Park, Currier, Harris, & Slattery, 2017; Slattery & Park, 2012). Notice how each clinician helped Drew do this. Searching for new and more adaptive meanings is especially important when the problem cannot be repaired, such as after illness, loss, or trauma (Park et al., 2017). Asking clients to reframe their experience and identify positive consequences or meanings should only be done, however, after clients feel deeply heard and understood (Ivey & Ivey, 2014). People can feel that their feelings have been dismissed after premature reframes.

Helping clients find meaning and a more balanced perspective following a painful or adverse situation can be profound work, but clinicians need to be careful not to negate the client's experience and suffering. Opportunities to begin thinking about positive outcomes (e.g., stronger coping, better relationships, and deeper spirituality) as well as their fears about the future help clients to move beyond cycles of negativity. Discussions of this discrepancy (e.g., both possible losses as well as growth and advantages) should be undertaken considering the client's readiness to do so.

Developing more adaptive views of themselves and their future. An ultimate goal of treatment is to leave clients with a sense of self that is more benign and hopeful (Park et al., 2017). Rather than accepting the credit for changes made during treatment, clinicians encourage clients to own changes made in treatment, perceive their work as collaborative in nature, and develop a stronger sense of self-efficacy (Goode et al., 2017).

Clinicians can help people re-vision themselves and their lives in many ways. In fact, they should look for opportunities at all points in their clinical work and while working on other treatment goals. These four clinicians approached this same goal in different ways.

- Clinician A: "It seems you're handling this much differently than you did even 2 years ago—less reactive and challenging your thinking more rapidly. What do you think?" [feedback, open question]
- Clinician B: "You've focused on the ways that you are "broken," but I also hear you describe healthier and more adaptive ways of expressing your anger." [paraphrase, feedback]
- Clinician C: "I'm wondering what was most important for you today. What do you want to take from today's session?" [self-disclosure, open question]

When identifying strengths and giving positive feedback, clinicians use concrete and specific language. Rather than whitewashing problems, dismissing them, or playing Pollyanna, they notice the healthy intention and adaptive nature of the client's behavior, identifying and enlarging successes and exceptions to the presenting problem (Franklin et al., 2017).

Throughout treatment, clinicians can listen for their clients' descriptions of people who have been supportive of them (e.g., parents, grandparents, a favorite teacher, neighbor, or pets). These supports can be accessed physically if they are still alive and available, but they can also be "accessed" through positive memories or images (e.g., "When your pain is at a 6 or 7 on a scale from 1 to 10, imagine your grandmother's warm hand on your shoulder and listen to whatever words of wisdom she might offer"). Clinicians can supplement these natural supports with stories about contemporary or historical figures who are especially important to the client, including sports, religious, or cultural figures (Slattery, 2004).

Reducing rumination and avoidance. Following a loss or trauma, people often experience more negative emotions and fewer positive ones, and they may experience **intrusive thoughts**, or unwanted, involuntary thoughts, ideas, and images. Intrusive thoughts may become **ruminations**—obsessive thoughts or worries—and ruminations may either be a temporary state or a more permanent style of approaching the world (Wade, Vogel, Liao, & Goldman, 2008).

Ruminations and intrusive thoughts may attempt to reduce perceived discrepancies, for example, between a person's actual behavior and values (Briñol, Petty, & Wheeler, 2006; Gray et al., 2007). They can be adaptive when they help a person resolve a discrepancy but are maladaptive when ruminations do nothing to solve the problem (Nolen-Hoeksema, Wisco, & Lyubomirsky, 2008). In fact, ruminating often interferes with problem-solving. People who ruminate have lower levels of psychological well-being, report less life satisfaction, and are more likely to report feelings of anger, anxiety, and depression (Briñol et al., 2006; Wade et al., 2008).

Negative cycles of rumination, intrusive thoughts and avoidance can be stopped in one of several ways. Distraction can be useful in the short term, as it leads to more positive affect, which can help people to stay calm and problem solve more effectively (Nolen-Hoeksema et al., 2008). When distraction leads to long-term avoidance, however, outcomes are more negative. One strategy that may help people who obsessively ruminate is **meditation**, any of a number of internal practices that build calm, awareness, and nonjudgmental self-acceptance, often by turning one's attention to a single focus, such as the breath. One of the most commonly used meditations is **mindfulness meditation**, the calm, nonjudgmental awareness of one's internal states and surroundings. In mindfulness meditation, clients are encouraged to observe their thoughts, feelings, and sensations without judging them or becoming stuck in them. Becoming more mindful can be empowering when clients stop avoiding painful emotions and learn they can control their thoughts. Finally, as described earlier, rumination often interferes with problem-solving. Helping clients resolve a problem—when it can be resolved—can sometimes reduce rumination.

What Do You Think?

1. Consider Beth Schneider's drinking. In what ways do her beliefs about herself, her relationships with others, and alcohol maintain her drinking and prevent her from changing? If her doctor identified her drinking as a problem, and she was willing to work on it, how would you address the beliefs that serve as barriers? What if she was not seeing her drinking as a problem?

✳ ✳ ✳

2. Return to the story Dr. Corsini told about the impact of his feedback following an intelligence test (Chapter 6). How do you understand that story given the ideas discussed in this chapter?

Interventions for Changing Emotions

Perceptions influence actions, and actions in turn influence self-perceptions and perceptions of the world. This description, although useful, overlooks the role of emotions. Emotions strongly influence how people behave, set into play ways of thinking about events, and are in turn influenced by behavior and thinking. Each of these three domains influences how people make meaning of their experience (L. Greenberg, 2008; Ivey & Ivey, 2014).

Many people avoid negative emotions and feel overwhelmed by them. Negative emotions can be disruptive to functioning and have been described as resulting from maladaptive and catastrophizing ways of interacting with the world. From this point of view, cognitions causing negative emotions should be controlled or tempered (Beck, 1976).

Avoidance of emotions, even negative ones, can itself be problematic, just as avoiding negative thoughts can be (L. Greenberg, 2008). Emotions are a normal and healthy part of experience, signaling an event's importance. It is important to attend to the degree to which emotions are maladaptively expressed, regulated, or controlled. Even when clients are stressed, anxious, or depressed, clinicians consider whether these emotions are maladaptive signs of distress rather than normal reactions to working through difficult issues. They should also attend to when emotions are used for instrumental purposes, such as getting attention or diverting blame, and when they are used to avoid a deeper feeling (L. Greenberg, 2008). For example, anger may mask feelings of shame and loneliness after the loss of a relationship.

Leslie Greenberg (2008) concluded that clients have five emotion-focused tasks in therapy: (a) becoming more aware and accepting of emotions, (b) expressing emotions more adaptively, (c) regulating emotions better, (d) reflecting on emotions and the events associated with them, and (e) transforming negative emotions through their association with positive emotions. Mindfulness, leading to an accepting and nonjudgmental attitude, and meditation, which strengthens skills in tolerating and regulating emotions, can be especially useful for people with depression or other poorly regulated emotions (MacKenzie, Abbott, & Kocovski, 2018). Consider how you might approach working with the emotions that Sandra Uwiringiyimana describes.

Cases in Empathy

It Was All Too Much | Sandra Uwiringiyimana

Sandra Uwiringiyimana (b. 1994) was born in the Congo, where she was named after Agathe Uwiringiyimana, an influential woman and prime minister in Rwanda. Uwiringiyimana also means "one who believes in God." These parts of her name defined her and how she saw life.

In response to increasing violence against ethnic Rwandans, Sandra's family fled their village and were resettled in a refugee camp in Gatumba, Burundi. Sandra is a survivor of the August 2004 Gatumba massacre, where 166 people in their camp, mostly Tutsis, were murdered, including her 6-year-old sister. In the years that followed, her family moved from one place to another in both the Congo and Rwanda, frequently living in a single room. She eventually emigrated to the United States with her parents and two siblings in 2007.

Her family's immigration to the United States was not seamless. Cultural and linguistic differences made her transition to school difficult. They found a supportive church, but caseworkers who were to help with their transition did not seem to understand the family's needs. Sandra was placed in sixth grade rather than eighth, as she would have entered in Rwanda, a setback for someone

who worked hard in school. Sandra was teased and bullied by peers at her new school and was confused by the meaning of race in the United States: "In America [but not Africa], my skin color did define me, at least in other people's eyes. I was black. I was black first, and I was Sandra" (Uwiringiyimana, 2017, p. 170). In Congo, her mother had run her own business, and her father had always held good jobs. In the United States, her parents worked factory jobs to make ends meet: "It was a wake-up call for all of us: As refugees in America, we were at the bottom of the heap" (p. 145). Then her father was hit by a van while on his way to pay the electric bill. He was in a coma for 3 months.

At home, my siblings and I had to help Mom figure out the bills because she was busy working and didn't have time to learn English. She needed our help to translate. I was getting better at English. Sometimes it felt like I was the parent, teaching her things.

It was all too much. I grew angry at the world, furious at God. I lost my faith. I decided there was no God and that everything my parents had told me about him was a lie. I thought no one loved us and no one cared, least of all God. My family was falling apart. People from church would ask, "How are you doing?" I hated that question. How were we doing? We were doing terribly. I listened to people praying to God and thought: You're all fools. God won't help you.

   I decided I would never go to church again. I told myself that if my dad died, I would not cry. I would stop feeling anything at all. I was very angry. I hated my life. (Uwiringiyimana, 2017, p. 150–151)

Sandra felt isolated at school, but also at home because her family did not talk openly about her sister Deborah's death, the massacre, or the difficulties related to immigrating. As she said,

   We were all trying to work through our own challenges. Everything was new to all of us. I'll never forget [my older sister] Adele's experience with culture shock at a high school track meet. She was set to run in a competition, and then a gun went off to mark the start of the race. No one had told her to expect a gunshot. She thought someone was shooting at people. She ran off the field. (Uwiringiyimana, 2017, p. 152)

What Do You Think?

1. What meanings has Sandra drawn from her experiences in the massacre or since immigrating? How are these similar to or different from D'Ja Jones's or Reymundo Sanchez's?

2. How would you help Sandra address her feelings of loss and hopelessness? Why?

3. Survivors of an earlier genocide of Tutsis reported especially high level of post-traumatic stress disorder (25%), depression (21%), and suicidality (25%; Rieder & Elbert, 2013). How would these data affect your work with her? What kinds of interventions would you consider?

4. Therapists working with refugees need to be open to considering the high need that they may experience, as well as to address both concerns and work within their client's cultural values and beliefs. See Exhibit 9.2. How might you integrate these ideas into your work with Sandra? How might they be helpful in working with the Lee family (Chapter 4)?

5. If you were seeing Sandra in therapy, what would you say that would consider the contradictory messages and themes that she presented? How would you evaluate your response using Carkhuff's (1969) description of empathic accuracy (subtractive/accurate/additive)?

Identifying and Addressing Barriers to Change

Teachers open the door but you must walk through it yourself.

—*Chinese proverb*

Sandra Uwiringiyimana faced real obstacles, physical and psychological, in surviving the Gatumba massacre and the immigration process. Strong clinicians anticipate ambivalence about change, such as she experienced, and investigate barriers even for people who appear ready to change (Fraser & Solovey, 2007). Barriers can take many forms: Clients may not see treatment

Exhibit 9.2 Issues to Consider While Working With Refugees

Concerns

Often have high rates of depression (44%), anxiety (40%), and posttraumatic stress disorder (36%)

May have direct trauma exposure and experience forced loss of home, culture, family, and language

May perceive microaggressions from members of the host country

May receive culturally insensitive diagnoses and treatment from the medical and mental health communities

Illness beliefs and idioms from the home country may conflict with those of the host country

May feel ignored or that their autonomy over medical decisions was denied

Barriers

Illiteracy and other communication barriers

Homelessness, unemployment, and lack of transportation

Stigma about mental health diagnosis and treatment

Differing norms for accessing mental health services and lack of access to information about services available

Recommendations

1. Recognize the high level of need that the client may present, including the physical, cultural, and psychosocial stressors inherent in emigration process (e.g., trauma exposure and loss of home and family).

2. Consider barriers to accessing treatment, both physical and psychological.

3. Respond with cultural humility, in an open and respectful attitude that honors the client's cultural values, beliefs, and identity, and comfort level in discussing these.

4. Incorporate the client's cultural narrative into diagnosis, goal-setting, and treatment processes.

Note. Data from Adams and Kivlighan (2019) and Lindert, von Ehrenstein, Priebe, Mielck, and Brähler (2009).

goals and methods as relevant, may feel alienated from the agencies providing treatment, or may believe that clinicians perceive them pejoratively and as unable to change (K. N. Anderson et al., 2019; Caldwell, 2009; R. E. Lee, 2009). Clients may not have a reliable car, money for gas, or dependable child care. They may believe that asking for help and discussing problems is a sign of weakness. Clients and their partners, family, and friends may actively resist change because it may destabilize the system and relationships. They may even perceive the problem (e.g., child abuse, domestic violence, binge drinking) as normative and acceptable. They may feel hopeless, ambivalent about change, or unable to change. They may not have the skills to change or may not believe that they deserve good relationships, positive outcomes or a hopeful future.

Identifying and discussing barriers to change can make treatment smoother and setbacks easier to anticipate and respond to.

A client's resistance to change can be seen in missed sessions, lateness to sessions, avoidance of topics, passivity in treatment, and refusal to discuss issues in depth (Eubanks, Burckell, & Goldfried, 2018). Some clinicians respond to these challenging behaviors by becoming irritated, loud, or belligerent; however, confrontational and conflict-laden responses further increase resistance and interfere with treatment (Serran, Fernandez, Marshall, & Mann, 2003). Although it is helpful to pay attention to a client's symptoms, problems, and weaknesses, it is equally important to recognize exceptions to problems and nurture a client's strengths and resources (Franklin et al., 2017). Even a client's "resistance" can be adaptive and may suggest that the client does not have the necessary skills at this point, has significant reasons not to change, or is not confident enough in the clinician and change process (Beutler et al., 2001).

A client may be resistant to the intervention as framed, but Serran and colleagues (2003) suggested that clinicians should perceive the "resistant behavior" as a signal that treatment goals, interventions, or approaches are a poor fit to the client. When clients are resistant in treatment, clinicians can explore the client's experience of problems, acknowledge the client's perspective, or step back and work with clients on a goal that better matches the client's goals or is less challenging (Eubanks et al., 2018). Treatment is not done *to* clients, but *with* them (Bohart, 2001).

What Do You Think?

1. What barriers made it difficult for Lil Loco (a.k.a. Reymundo Sanchez, Chapter 2) to change? What might make it difficult for Sandra Uwiringiyimana to work toward individual goals in counseling? What made it difficult for Andrea Yates (Chapters 1 and 5) to stay on her medications? What would you do to address these barriers? What are the adaptive parts of their resistance to change?

Evaluating Treatment

You seldom listen to me, and when you do you don't hear, and when you do hear you hear wrong, and even when you hear right you change it so fast that it's never the same.
—Marjorie Kellogg

As described in Chapter 5, it can be useful to consider whether the clinician is accurately hearing the client's surface and deeper meanings (Carkhuff, 1969). Nonetheless, for any of a number of reasons, either psychological or environmental (or both), a client may miss the clinician's otherwise brilliantly framed empathic response or intervention.

Therefore, although it is helpful to think about the accuracy of the clinician's responses, it may be even more useful to consider the effectiveness of a session from the client's point of view. To what degree is the client accepting of or denying the reframe or intervention (Ivey & Ivey, 2014)? The rating system in Exhibit 9.3 can be useful in this regard. To what degree do the clinician's responses and interventions facilitate insight and behavioral change and advance treatment goals? To what degree do they strengthen the therapeutic alliance? These questions can be considered both at the end of a session and throughout it. As discussed in earlier parts of this book, paying attention to clients' nonverbal cues, the ways they develop themes in treatment (or fail to), and verbal indicators of disagreement can signal whether the therapeutic alliance is strong and whether the client is accepting of the clinician's interventions (Thomas, 2005).

What Do You Think?

1. Review interview transcripts from earlier in this book (Andrea Yates, Chapter 1 and 5; Sandra Bland, Chapter 3; Annie Rogers, Chapter 5; D'Ja Jones, Chapter 5). How would you rate the empathy of these therapeutic responses (Carkhuff, 1969)? How would you rate the productivity of these short transcripts using the scale in Exhibit 9.3? What did you conclude from this process?

Exhibit 9.3 Rating the Effectiveness of a Session or Intervention

Extremely helpful	Listening is accurate and insightful. Moves treatment in a productive direction. Promotes greater self-awareness, helpful ways of thinking about the "problem," or positive changes in behavior. Client hears and accepts message.
Moderately helpful	Listening is generally accurate. Moves treatment in a productive direction, but leads to limited self-awareness, helpful ways of thinking about the "problem," or positive changes in behavior.
Neutral	Neither contributes to nor detracts from treatment goals, therapeutic process and therapeutic alliance. Client may verbally accept interventions without changing.
Moderately harmful	Detracts somewhat from treatment goals, therapeutic process and therapeutic alliance. Clinician's responses suggest poor listening or lack of interest.
Extremely harmful	Damaging to movement on treatment goals, and interferes with the therapeutic process and therapeutic alliance. Clinician's responses sound blaming, judgmental, and critical. Client may deny or reject interventions.

Note. From *Technical and Conceptual Skills for Mental Health Professionals* (p. 382), by L. W. Seligman, 2004, New York, NY: Pearson Education. Copyright 2004 by Pearson Education. Adapted with permission. Includes additional data from Carkhuff (1969), Ivey and Ivey (2014), and Reichenberg and Seligman (2016).

Summary

Effective clinicians want their clients to continue to be successful after termination from treatment. Thus, they help to develop their clients' self-efficacy, assertiveness, hope, and problem-solving skills. Because many clients are initially unready to change, attending to their readiness is an important aspect of treatment. Motivating clients to change, particularly clients who are more highly resistant, requires a strong therapeutic alliance, characterized by unconditional acceptance and empathic, genuine, and nonjudgmental attitudes. Clients who feel understood are generally more receptive to clinical interventions. In general, these interventions should require a shift in perspective, although not one that is so large as to be unacceptable.

Changes in behavior often lead to changes in perspective and vice versa. Further, emotions influence actions and situational meanings and influence how people make meaning of their experience. This chapter described a number of interventions to create clinical change in behavioral, cognitive, and emotional realms.

Effective treatment recognizes and addresses barriers to change. Barriers occur for a variety of reasons but may manifest in passivity, poor motivation for change, or resistance. Treatment is done with clients rather than to them, thus it is important to consider the therapeutic alliance at stuck points and the ways that this "resistance" is adaptive.

Rather than paying attention to the quality of the intervention alone, effective clinicians evaluate the effectiveness of their work, especially how it strengthens the therapeutic alliance, causes clients to become more insightful, and leads to positive behavioral change.

For Review

Applying Concepts to Your Life

1. How do you feel when you believe you have not been heard? How do you react?

2. Have you noticed that changing your behavior in one way (e.g., quitting smoking, getting a new job) also changed the way that you perceived yourself or others? How has changing your thinking and perceptions (e.g., understanding someone) also changed your behavior?

3. If you have been "resistant" to change at some point, were there some positive aspects to your resistance? What were you trying to accomplish?

4. Pay attention to your own listening using the scale in Exhibit 9.3. How do you respond when you recognize that you are off track? To what degree is your response helpful?

Key Terms

discrepancy, 190   mindfulness meditation, 200
intrusive thoughts, 200   ruminations, 200
meditation, 200

Learn More

For more information about the concepts in this chapter, visit the *Empathic Counseling* companion website at http://pubs.apa.org/books/supp/slattery/.

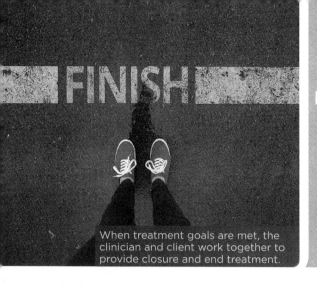

When treatment goals are met, the clinician and client work together to provide closure and end treatment.

10 Ending Treatment

Looking Ahead III➡

After reading this chapter you will be able to answer these questions:

1. What differentiates normal from premature terminations?

2. What do clinicians do to create a positive termination process?

3. What feelings do clients and clinicians report at termination? How might these affect the termination process?

4. What factors should be addressed in the course of planning discharge from treatment?

5. What strategies can clinicians use to decrease risk during termination from treatment?

I Felt Like I'd Been Beaten Up | Elyn Saks

Elyn Saks is an attorney who graduated from Yale University, specializes in mental health law, and is a dean at the University of Southern California. She had her first psychotic break when she was doing graduate work at Oxford University, although she had begun experiencing problems when she was 8 years old. She had three extended hospitalizations and has been in psychoanalysis and on antipsychotics for much of her adult life. She did analytic work with Dr. Kaplan for 13 years, although eventually she became unhappy with how the treatment was going.

I'd accomplished many successful life changes during that time. But he'd often been hard on me, and over time it had come to feel too hard, even punishing. He'd become more restrictive somehow—for example, he didn't want me moving around the office; he didn't want me to cover my face with my hands during our sessions, something I'd done with all my analysts to help me feel safe and contained. He kept saying that if things didn't change, he'd "terminate" me. "I'm going to terminate you." It was brutal to hear that, brutal for him to keep saying it. Was he doing it to elicit some kind of response from me? I didn't feel safe with him anymore; he was unpredictable, mercurial, even angry. Some days, I'd walk out of session feeling like I'd been beaten up.

"We're not getting anywhere," he'd say. "This isn't even therapy we're doing." (Saks, 2007, pp. 331–322)

Elyn asked for a consult with Dr. Freed, an analyst who had provided backup during Dr. Kaplan's vacations. Dr. Freed encouraged her to recognize the good work she had done with Dr. Kaplan and acknowledge that relationships, even good ones, have difficult periods. He strongly encouraged her to attempt to work things out. Per Dr. Freed's suggestion, Elyn reconsidered her decision to quit working with Dr. Kaplan, "[although] I wasn't sure I could; I wasn't sure I wanted to even try" (Saks, 2007, p. 322).

Elyn began to consider what had to change in order to get treatment back on track. Her list

did not seem onerous or impossible: "I needed him to stop saying we weren't getting anywhere. I needed him to stop threatening 'termination.' I needed a lessening of the physical restrictions" (Saks, 2007, p. 323). Dr. Kaplan refused to consider these requests.

That was their last session together, although Dr. Kaplan later called Elyn to work things out. Elyn began seeing Dr. Freed, but observed that

> Dr. Kaplan probably helped me more than anyone else in my life, and I love him today as much as I have ever loved anyone. For a long time, I carried inside me a palpable sense of loss. The decision to leave him was so awful, but I couldn't see any way around it; besides, it always felt like he's made that decision first. By refusing to negotiate with me, by threatening me and pushing me, he had in fact fired me. He'd rejected me, he'd betrayed me. (Saks, 2007, p. 324)

What Do You Think?

1. What did you think about Elyn's requests and Dr. Kaplan's reaction? What, if anything, would you do differently if you were in his shoes? Why?

2. What were Elyn's global beliefs and goals? How might they have influenced her decision to stop work with Dr. Kaplan?

3. Were you surprised that Elyn felt so many positive feelings about Dr. Kaplan given her decision to leave analysis with him? Why?

Normal Versus Premature Terminations

Death ends a life, not a relationship.

—Robert Benchley

Treatment can end in any number of ways. Both clinician and client may agree that goals have been met, or one of them may make a unilateral decision to end treatment because progress is not being made or the client is being actively harmed by treatment. Sometimes there are unavoidable clinician-related factors (e.g., illness, maternity leave, moves, job changes, or personal difficulties affecting one's competency). Sometimes treatment will no longer be covered under the client's **managed care**, the system of health care delivery that regulates the use of member benefits to contain expenses (Knapp, Younggren, VandeCreek, Harris, & Martin, 2013; Younggren & Gottlieb, 2008). Clinicians may end treatment due to a potentially harmful multiple relationship, a conflict of interest, or a loss of objectivity (Younggren & Gottlieb, 2008). Like Elyn Saks, clients can end treatment for any number of reasons, including feeling disrespected or believing that they are no longer making progress.

Normal Termination

Normal termination is "an intentional process that occurs over time when a client has achieved most of the goals of treatment, and/or when psychotherapy must end for other reasons" (Vasquez, Bingham, & Barnett, 2008, p. 653). Two things are especially important here: that the process is, in the best of circumstances, intentional rather than haphazard and, when possible, clinician and client together discuss ending treatment, when to do so, and how.

One obvious criterion for termination is when treatment goals are met. Despite the apparent clarity of this criterion, treatment goals can change across time, making it unclear when treatment goals have been met. Sometimes clients and clinicians set more modest treatment goals later in treatment, which may be more appropriate than initial, overly ambitious goals. In addition, the plan to end treatment when goals have been met assumes that movement on treatment goals only occurs during treatment. An equally valid goal of treatment could be to give clients the skills to make change, even though that change might not be seen or "complete" until after treatment is ended.

Most clinicians work on the goals that clients identify and end treatment when their clients are ready to end treatment or are no longer motivated to continue. Termination is often a collaborative process: Clients and clinicians discuss treatment, its successes and failures, the themes that developed over the course of treatment, and the ways that clients are now handling problems more successfully (Goode, Park, Parkin, Tompkins, & Swift, 2017; Shaharabani Saidon, Shafran, & Rafaeli, 2018). Depending on the length and type of treatment, sessions are often tapered as termination approaches. Sometimes clinicians maintain ongoing, albeit infrequent sessions, although the clinician's role is more like that of a lifeguard, intervening only "when absolutely necessary" (Goldfried, 2002, p. 371).

Premature Termination

Premature termination is when treatment ends before the client's treatment goals are met. This can happen for a variety of reasons and is fairly common. In fact, about 20% of clients drop out of therapy prematurely (Swift & Greenberg, 2012). While this rate of premature terminations is high, it is somewhat higher for people assigned to medication alone—about 1.2 times as high (Swift, Greenberg, Tompkins, & Parkin, 2017).

Sometimes, as described in Chapter 8, clients end treatment because clinician and client disagree on treatment goals (Hawley & Weisz, 2003). Sometimes clients have done all that they are able or willing to do at the time. Sometimes leaving treatment early reflects a problem in the therapeutic alliance (Olivera, Challú, Gómez Penedo, & Roussos, 2017): Like Elyn Saks, the client does not feel accepted or understood by the clinician. At other times the benefits of continuing in therapy are perceived as smaller than the anticipated financial or psychological costs.

One meta-analysis reported that trainees had more dropouts than did more experienced clinicians, and that more dropouts occurred in community settings rather than in studies completed in labs or controlled conditions. Theoretical orientation did not make a difference. Clients who dropped out of treatment tended to be younger, male, not in a committed romantic relationship, more poorly educated, or diagnosed with a personality disorder or an eating disorder (Swift & Greenberg, 2012). A study of clients found that although most dropouts reported leaving therapy because they felt better, a substantial minority also had more negative attitudes, including not finding therapy helpful, not feeling that it was going anywhere, not believing their therapist could help (Westmacott & Hunsley, 2010). On the other hand, clinicians believe the primary reason that clients leave treatment is that they are not ready to change (Westmacott & Hunsley, 2017). Clearly, it is important to help clients identify a problem they want to work on and help them recognize the benefits of changing.

Evidence on the role that race plays in premature terminations is conflicting. Early reviews suggested minority populations had high rates of premature terminations; however, a meta-analysis of more recent data concluded that race did not predict dropouts from treatment (Swift & Greenberg, 2012). Other studies have shown that poorer multicultural competence rather than therapeutic mismatch per se predicted premature terminations, as did low cultural humility (K. N. Anderson et al., 2019; Owen et al., 2016).

Clinicians' and Clients' Feelings During Termination

Many of us spend our whole lives running from feeling with the mistaken belief that you cannot bear the pain. But you have already borne the pain. What you have not done is feel all you are beyond the pain.

—St. Bartholomew

The end of treatment can be associated with many confusing feelings for clients and clinicians. Clinicians who monitor their feelings and handle them well can make the termination process easier for their clients and less risky for themselves.

Clinicians' Reactions

People entering the mental health fields differ in the strengths and weaknesses that they bring to the table. In many settings, clinicians need patience, a sense of commitment, a willingness to persevere through difficult periods, and an ability to recognize and work with intrapsychic dynamics. These skills may be especially important during termination, which can raise difficult issues for both clients and clinicians.

Unexpected terminations can challenge clinicians' comfort with their professional identity, raise concerns about loss and **abandonment** (i.e., abrupt endings to treatment that are neither clinically nor ethically appropriate), increase their needs for perfection and control, and raise doubts about the value of their work. Even normal terminations can bring up feelings of loss, guilt, shame, and abandonment, or pride, omnipotence, and excitement. Conversely, clinicians with high autonomy needs and expectations for independence may perceive a client's desire to extend treatment as evidence of continuing dependency needs and react with irritation or annoyance. Struggling with these feelings is not a problem, but acting without awareness is. At such points, they are more likely to project their own feelings and needs on their clients, lose the ability to use feelings in therapeutic ways, and act in ways that increase their clients' anxiety, dependency, and guilt. Clients of clinicians who adopt positive views of termination are more likely to have more positive outcomes (Bhatia & Gelso, 2017).

Clients' Reactions

Clients also differ in their reactions toward termination depending on their meaning systems, especially their attitudes about connections and loss (Shaharabani Saidon, Shafran, & Rafaeli, 2018). Some clients experience positive emotions during termination and use this period as an opportunity to explore and come to terms with other losses (Knox et al., 2011). Others are able to internalize feelings of competence and **transfer** (or **generalize**) their learned behavior to other parts of their lives. Conversely, some clients feel abandoned or rejected and may leave treatment prematurely and abruptly, rather than facing the pain that may arise during termination. One qualitative study of clients found that this outcome was most likely when clients entered therapy already experiencing grief and loss (Knox et al., 2011). In fact, clinicians may continue to "comfort" and "coach" their clients years after termination from treatment by means of messages that clients internalized during their treatment.

In some cases, client reactions may be a response to their clinicians' own attitudes about endings, in general, and termination from therapy, in particular (Bhatia & Gelso, 2017). Perhaps Dr. Kaplan's own personal needs, dynamics, and attitudes about treatment influenced his reactions to Elyn's decision to leave treatment. Clinicians may also inadvertently or unconsciously undermine their clients' positive reactions to termination by perceiving their reactions as resistance or avoidance of therapeutic issues. Empathic clinicians recognize both their clients' fears and hopes and use their assessment to create a positive termination process.

Clinical Applications	Charlene was actively suicidal for several months. She frequently called and emailed her therapist, Martin, throughout the day. Martin had expected that Charlene would require a much less intensive level of service when he conducted the initial intake. Martin worked full time at a university, and he no longer felt able to provide the level of care that he believed Charlene needed. Charlene was then involuntarily hospitalized, and Martin considered terminating Charlene's treatment. What recommendations would you give Martin about reducing his clinical risk during treatment?

✳ ✳ ✳

Consultation is meeting with supervisors or coworkers to solicit advice about difficulties in a clinical case. During a consultation with a colleague, Martin recognized that Charlene's suicidal feelings had increased as they approached termination. He also observed that he had become more anxious and pessimistic and less hopeful as Charlene had become increasingly suicidal. He recognized that some of his reactions may have been due to unprocessed feelings about his mother's suicide. What recommendations would you make at this point?

Goals for Ending Treatment Well

What you get by achieving your goals is not as important as what you become by achieving your goals.

—*Zig Ziglar*

In general, clinicians tend to focus on one or more of the following three tasks during termination: assessment of changes made, generalization of these changes to areas of the client's life outside of therapy, and resolution of issues in the therapeutic relationship (Shaharabani Saidon et al., 2018). These tasks can be mapped on two dimensions, the temporal focus and the focus of discussion. See Figure 10.1.

Consolidating and transferring skills from treatment to the real world (represented as "Consolidate" in Figure 10.1) is not emphasized in every theoretical approach (Ivey & Ivey, 2014; Norcross, Zimmerman, Greenberg, & Swift, 2017). Although it may be clear to us that they have made important changes, some clients have difficulty seeing these changes (Consolidate). One

FIGURE 10.1 Model of Termination Tasks and Goals

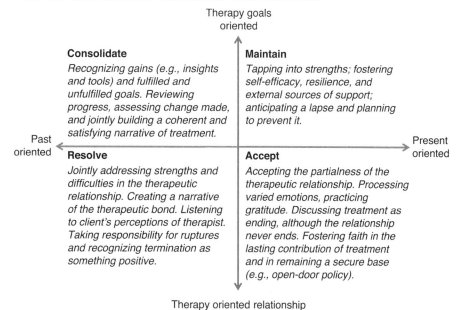

Therapy goals
oriented

Consolidate

*Recognizing gains (e.g., insights
and tools) and fulfilled and
unfulfilled goals. Reviewing
progress, assessing change made,
and jointly building a coherent and
satisfying narrative of treatment.*

Maintain

*Tapping into strengths; fostering
self-efficacy, resilience, and
external sources of support;
anticipating a lapse and planning
to prevent it.*

Past
oriented

Present
oriented

Resolve

*Jointly addressing strengths and
difficulties in the therapeutic
relationship. Creating a narrative
of the therapeutic bond. Listening
to client's perceptions of therapist.
Taking responsibility for ruptures
and recognizing termination as
something positive.*

Accept

*Accepting the partialness of the
therapeutic relationship. Processing
varied emotions, practicing
gratitude. Discussing treatment as
ending, although the relationship
never ends. Fostering faith in the
lasting contribution of treatment
and in remaining a secure base
(e.g., open-door policy).*

Therapy oriented relationship

Adapted from "Teach Them How to Say Goodbye: The CMRA Model for Treatment Endings," by H. Shaharabani Saidon, N. Shafran, and E. Rafaeli, 2018, *Journal of Psychotherapy Integration, 28*(3), p. 388. Copyright 2018 by the American Psychological Association.

of our clients, for example, complained that things were no different than when she entered treatment, but we saw a big difference: She had held a gun to her head during the first week of treatment and had had significant insomnia but now had only occasional suicidal ideation and insomnia. Clients need to recognize the progress they have made and see themselves as competent and capable (Norcross et al., 2017; Shaharabani Saidon et al., 2018). Rather than accepting all the credit for changes made during treatment, clinicians emphasizing this approach acknowledge that their work was collaborative in nature and encourage clients to own these changes (Goode et al., 2017).

When clinicians focus on helping clients maintain progress in the future (represented as "Maintain" in Figure 10.1), they help their clients transfer the changes made in therapy to other settings (e.g., identify ways of being assertive with their friends and family as well as with their clinician), experience a sense of self-efficacy and resilience, and identify strategies for relapse prevention. Clinicians with this focus help their clients self-disclose safely, challenge their negative cognitions both inside and outside of therapy, and discover ways to continue using these skills long after therapy has ended (Norcross et al., 2017; Shaharabani Saidon et al., 2018). Some approaches to change, including Alcoholics Anonymous and other substance abuse treatments, particularly emphasize this future-oriented approach to the termination process (e.g., identifying what they can do to stay sober).

When clinicians focus on the therapy relationship during termination (Shaharabani Saidon et al., 2018), they may consider the past ups and downs of treatment to acknowledge termination as a positive part of treatment (represented as "Resolve" in Figure 10.1). Alternatively, they may be more present-oriented and see therapy as a journey of change (represented as "Accept" in Figure 10.1). Such clinicians note that clients can continue to change on their own and return to treatment in the future without viewing this as a failure of the client or treatment.

Balancing Opposing Reactions to Termination

As discussed earlier, termination can be a positive process, but it can also be characterized by feelings of loss and even abandonment. Empathic approaches to termination recognize both of these poles: the changes and increasing competencies, but also the dependency, fears about relapsing, and anxiety about losing an important relationship. Some clients and clinicians may emphasize one pole over the other. For example, they may assume that a particular client is incompetent and will have difficulty continuing on her own—or collude to agree that a client is doing well, has no concerns about termination, and will have no difficulty staying on track. In most cases, both sets of concerns are present and should be addressed: that the client is strong and capable but, like other people, will have better and worse periods in the future.

Discussing these mixed and confusing feelings can help clients consolidate the changes they have made during treatment and develop positive stories about treatment, their work in it, and their relationship with their clinician (Epston & White, 1995). It can help them identify positive and growth-promoting ways of perceiving "negative" feelings.

What Do You Think?

1. How did Dr. Kaplan balance these opposing feelings and end-of-treatment tasks with Elyn Saks? What did he do well, and what did he do less well?

Relapse Prevention

Relapse rates from substance abuse are high (40%–60%), as is the case for people successfully treated for depression with antidepressants (about 80% within 2 years; DeRubeis, Siegle, & Hollon, 2008; National Institute on Drug

Abuse, 2012). As a result, an especially important task of termination is **relapse prevention**, a process of reducing the probability of a relapse (represented as "Maintain" in Figure 10.1). Relapse prevention includes transferring newly acquired skills to other situations, identifying strategies for maintaining skills across time, and identifying high-risk situations. One way to identify high-risk situations is to monitoring **well-being**, a holistic state of being healthy, happy, and satisfied with life (Gökbayrak, Paiva, Blissmer, & Prochaska, 2015; Norcross, Krebs, & Prochaska, 2011; Norcross, Zimmerman, Greenberg, & Swift, 2017).

As described in Chapter 8, the frequency and impact of lapses can be reduced by (a) eliminating triggers to the problem behavior (e.g., boredom, loneliness, stress, and environmental stimuli associated with the behavior) and (b) challenging negative cognitive and emotional reactions to lapses. In some cases, it can be useful to help a client's family reframe the meaning of lapses because they may also believe that a lapse signals a return to the full-blown syndrome that brought the client into treatment. In general, clients with serious mental illnesses are at higher risk of relapse when family members are perceived as critical, high in expressed emotion, or distressed (Hooley & Miklowitz, 2017; Masland & Hooley, 2015) and at lower risk if familial warmth is high (López et al., 2004). Furthermore, the importance of warmth and lack of criticism within the family may depend on culture. For example, one study of people with schizophrenia found that low familial warmth predicted relapse for Mexican Americans, whereas for European Americans, high criticism was a better predictor of relapse (López et al., 2004).

| **Clinical Applications** | Amber has a history of binge drinking throughout her adult life. Her husband and daughters are frustrated by her drinking, and although she has been abstinent for 15 months and responding well to cues that triggered her drinking, they are afraid that she is never going to be able to stay dry. What messages would you give her and her family at the end of treatment? How would you frame these messages? How would this family's culture affect your framing? |

Ethical Considerations During Termination

This life is yours. Take the power to choose what you want to do and do it well.
—Susan Polis Schutz

As with other clinical decisions, our ethical guidelines and aspirations can guide our decision-making regarding termination. The American Psychological Association's (APA's; 2017a) ethical standards are that we (a) make reasonable efforts to create orderly transitions when they are predictable, (b) end treatment when it no longer seems helpful, (c) can end treatment if endangered by our client, and (d) provide reasonable referrals and step-down services.

Although APA (2017a) describes the minimum standards for treatment, strong terminations do more than exceed that minimum (Knapp et al., 2017). Coming to a mutual agreement about termination respects autonomy and promotes beneficence because clients who experience positive endings are more likely to return if needed; it also promotes *general* beneficence because such agreements have a positive impact on the field and community: Clients who experience positive outcomes are more likely to recommend treatment to others. Further, those discussions are especially productive when clinicians ask clients about how they will recognize they are ready to end treatment and acknowledge their expectations (Olivera et al., 2017).

Identifying ways to avoid premature terminations is also consistent with the ethical principle of nonmaleficence. Although many clients have unreasonable expectations for the length of treatment, educating them about the change process and typical lengths for therapy significantly increases how long clients expect to be in treatment and how long they stay (Swift & Callahan, 2008, 2011). When clients receive their preferred treatments, only about half as many drop out of treatment. This orientation to and education about treatment could take place during the informed consent process.

As expectations about change account for about 15% of the variance in treatment outcomes, clinicians can help clients develop reasonable and positive expectations to decrease premature terminations (Swift & Greenberg, 2015). In addition, nearly 30% of the variance in treatment outcomes is related to the strength of the therapeutic alliance, which is predictive of lower rates of dropouts from treatment, meaning that paying attention to the therapeutic alliance across time is important—clinically and ethically (K. N. Anderson et al., 2019; Swift & Greenberg, 2015).

Although clinicians do not need to continue seeing their clients forever and Dr. Kaplan did not need to continue seeing Elyn Saks, clinicians should balance their duty to their clients, their right to terminate treatment under some circumstances, and their clients' right to avoid being abandoned (Younggren & Gottlieb, 2008). When clients and clinicians disagree about when it is time to end treatment, it can be helpful for clinicians to describe their viewpoint (e.g., what can still be accomplished, what barriers may be discouraging clients or causing anxiety, what can be done to meet specified goals) in respectful and empowering ways. For example,

> You've made considerable progress toward your goals—your relationships, your parenting—but this is a very difficult time for you, and you're considering stopping therapy. We can approach this in a couple of different ways. We could explore ways of handling your anxiety about these issues better, or we can decide that we have done enough for now.

> You know what you need better than anyone, though, and I trust that you know when to stop coming here. Some people discover that therapy starts the change process—like rolling a snowball downhill—and that they continue to make changes after therapy has ended. Others find they want to come back at some later point—sometimes for a quick tune-up, sometimes to work on things that they didn't feel ready to work on previously. Regardless, my door is always open.

Notice that this clinician clearly identified the changes already made and strategies for responding to her client's anxieties about treatment, while also supporting the client's autonomy and other end-of-treatment goals. She briefly addressed relapse prevention, opened the door for future treatment, supported the client's self-determination, and was empowering.

Managing Risk During Termination

When clinicians end treatment in ways that are not ethically or clinically appropriate, licensure and ethics boards, courts, and clients perceive this ending as abandonment (Younggren & Gottlieb, 2008). Failing to do any of a number of actions that are part of normal, competent practice—to discuss the termination process, to facilitate transfer to step-down services, or to inform clients of coverage and emergency services when out of town—could put clinicians at increased risk of lawsuit or disciplinary action (Knapp et al., 2013). Similarly, ending treatment against a client's wishes while the client is actively suicidal or homicidal is likely to be reasonably perceived as abandonment (Knapp et al., 2013).

The best-case scenario for termination is one in which clients feel understood and well-treated, goals have been met, and termination is discussed with and agreed to by both client and clinician (Olivera et al., 2017). However, these ideal circumstances are not always possible. Some clinicians work in settings or under reimbursement plans that set firm session limits. Similarly, some insurance plans cap the number of allowed sessions. Terminations triggered by these structural considerations are called **forced terminations**. Clinicians have the right to end treatment under such circumstances: Although they must refer clients to other services, if appropriate, and stabilize clients in crisis, clinicians are not obligated to offer long-term pro bono treatment (Younggren & Gottlieb, 2008).

Even relatively abrupt terminations can be appropriate and ethical. Clients who violate reasonable expectations for treatment, including those who come to sessions intoxicated or frequently miss appointments, indicate that they are not actively committed to treatment. Similarly, clients who have violated their clinicians' rights, threatened them in any way, or engaged in significant boundary violations have "actually terminated the relationship already" (Younggren & Gottlieb, 2008, p. 502).

What Do You Think?

1. Although the clinical risk in Elyn Saks's termination from treatment is more subtle than that in some scenarios described elsewhere in this text, what does Dr. Kaplan do that increases his risk of ethical complaint or legal action? What, if anything, could he have done to decrease this risk?

Wise clinicians can manage their risk in the infrequent case of abrupt or unilateral terminations (Knapp et al., 2013; Younggren & Gottlieb, 2008), some of which are listed in Exhibit 10.1. Rather than jumping to conclusions about the meaning of their clients' problematic behavior, they discuss their concerns with their clients. They talk with their clients about the problems they are facing, consult with colleagues, consider how to handle problems respectfully, and carefully document their concerns and thought processes.

The risk of legal action or ethical complaint is low when clinicians have engaged in good clinical practice. Clinicians decrease risk when they give reasonable notice of the interruption or end of services, make good faith efforts to facilitate their clients' transfer to other appropriate services, and are thoughtful and respectful of clients' needs (Knapp et al., 2013). Providing a careful informed consent process and describing the clients' rights and responsibilities at the beginning of treatment—as well as the consequences

Exhibit 10.1 Questions to Consider in the Course of Both Normal and Abrupt Terminations

1. Have we collaboratively discussed and agreed on the goals and process of therapy and the termination process? Have we continued this informed consent process across time?

2. Is our termination process consistent with that described during our discussions of termination?

3. Having identified an appropriate decision and termination process, am I following it in a consistent, yet respectful manner?

4. Is the termination process consistent with my theoretical model?

5. Is the termination process respectful of my client's presenting problems and ongoing needs? Did I offer reasonable options for aftercare?

6. If problems arose in treatment, did I discuss these in consultations or supervision? Did these consults conclude that the proposed termination process was appropriate and consistent with my ethical guidelines and the standard of care?

7. Have I carefully documented my termination process, especially for abrupt terminations?

Note. Data from Vasquez, Bingham, and Barnett (2008) and Younggren and Gottlieb (2008).

of failing to meet reasonable expectations—can make clinical decisions more understandable to clients and a decision to terminate treatment less problematic (Younggren & Gottlieb, 2008). Depending on the clientele with whom one works and one's theoretical orientation, informed consent processes might include discussions of financial responsibilities, missed appointments, and phone coverage during vacations. Clinicians may appropriately taper frequency of treatment, provide reasonable aftercare recommendations, and assess potential harm to self and others. Good clinical practice varies with theoretical orientation but should be justifiable within it. For example, clinicians offering long-term depth therapies who regularly terminate treatment abruptly without examining issues of loss raised by termination are not practicing within their approach's standard of care.

When termination from therapy will be abrupt or unilateral, clinicians should first discuss the process in supervision or consultations (Knapp et al., 2013, 2017; Younggren & Gottlieb, 2008). Furthermore, especially when termination is difficult, clinicians should carefully document factors influencing the decision to terminate, recommendations made during consultations, the client's mental status during the termination process, and the nature of aftercare recommendations.

Clinicians may ultimately draw conclusions about termination with which their clients disagree. They may believe, for example, that they do not have the competence to work with the client and presenting problem, while their clients may argue that this does not matter. Younggren and Gottlieb (2008) clearly concluded that it is unwise to waver about termination in response to clients' badgering or concerns. Doing so can undermine treatment and reinforce manipulative or self-defeating behavior. Even in such situations, the process should not be mean-spirited or disrespectful; instead, it should be empathic, considerate, and warm, yet firm.

Clinical Applications	Charlene told Martin that she wanted to stop treatment. Martin was feeling tired and overwhelmed that day and didn't initiate a conversation about this request. What do you think about his response? What would you want to say to him?

Strategies for Helping Clients Own Their Change

Perhaps because psychologists focus on and attempt to decrease clinical risks, clinicians often overemphasize how termination can be experienced as a loss, which "subtly reinforces the dependency of the person seeking assistance on the 'expert knowledge' of the therapist" (Epston & White, 1995, pp. 339–340). Instead, termination can be an important period in which to explore the ways in which clients have solved and overcome problems both in and out of therapy and begin seeing themselves as experts on their own lives and change process. Clinicians can use questioning as an integral part of this process, helping their clients be curious about the change process, own their change rather than attributing it elsewhere, and feel more empowered and in control (Epston & White, 1995). To accomplish these goals, clinicians can ask questions such as:

- "Imagine that I have a client with problems similar to the ones you used to have. What advice would you give this person given what you know now?"
- "If I'd met you at an earlier point in your life, what would I have seen that would have let me know that you would make the changes we've seen?"
- "As you think about the work we've done together, what are the most important things you've learned about yourself and your relationships?"
- "How will what you've learned here continue to influence the decisions you make in life and how you see yourself? Using these skills, where will you be in 5 years?"

Many clients enter treatment assuming that change is done *to* them rather than *by* them. Sometimes they believe that their clinicians have a magic wand (or crystal ball or time machine). Notice how Epston and White's (1995) questions create new meanings by firmly postulating that the client (with the aid of the clinician) made the change, had the necessary skills to change, and will be able to continue to expand this change process.

The Discharge Summary

I wanted a perfect ending. Now I've learned, the hard way, that some poems don't rhyme, and some stories don't have a clear beginning, middle and end.

—Gilda Radner

Whether or not discharge from treatment was mutually agreed upon, clinicians should write a **discharge summary**, a brief report summarizing the entering and ending client diagnoses, the course of treatment (e.g., number of sessions and cancellations, interventions used), and factors contributing to the success or failure of treatment. Discharge summaries should be clear and respectful and draw supportable conclusions while remaining tentative about aspects of the client's situation that are unclear. Discharge summaries are sometimes later requested by a third party (e.g., attorneys, physicians), and thus they should not include gratuitous information. For example, a mother's history of incest as a child would probably be inappropriate for the discharge summary for a child diagnosed with autism spectrum disorder, unless the mother's poor psychological status affected the implementation of treatment goals. The discharge summary can be relatively brief, but should describe progress, as well as issues that are still outstanding (Younggren & Gottlieb, 2008). For Elyn Saks, one might say the following:

> Ms. Saks is frequently paranoid and delusional, especially when experiencing a significant stressor or positive or negative life change. She occasionally has auditory and visual hallucinations. During her worst periods, she stops eating, sleeping, and bathing; her thoughts and speech becomes disorganized and paranoid; and she believes she has killed many people. Despite these problems, she has good friends, a healthy and supportive marriage, and a successful and challenging career.
>
> Ms. Saks continues to use psychotic thoughts as ways of avoiding the bad feelings that everyone experiences; nonetheless, she is increasingly able to see them as unconsciously motivated and meaningful. She is often resistant to taking antipsychotics, believing that she should be strong enough to handle stressors on her own. She increasingly recognizes that the more she accepts she has a mental illness, the less it defines and controls her.

Discharge summaries should also include posttermination recommendations, such as referrals for step-down services.

> Ms. Saks is doing better than when first seen, but we have met an impasse and are at odds on the nature of continuing treatment. She has, however, agreed to see Dr. Freed for ongoing analysis and to continue taking antipsychotic medications, as prescribed. We agreed to meet twice weekly for a month to process her transition to Dr. Freed.

The more problematic the termination process, such as that of Elyn Saks, the clearer the documentation of that process should be in the client's chart (Knapp et al., 2013; Younggren & Gottlieb, 2008). Documentation should include the rationale for ending treatment, names of clinicians and other resources consulted about termination, steps taken by the clinician to end treatment in a competent and ethical manner, and recommendations made for aftercare.

Clinical Applications	Although Martin acknowledged that his feelings of stress and anxiety were only partially related to Charlene, he recognized that he did not have the time, technical skills, or emotional competence at this point in time to continue working with her, especially because, while in the hospital, she had disclosed that she experienced frequent dissociation, extensive self-injurious behavior, and chronic suicidality. What issues should he consider as he prepares to transfer Charlene to a more appropriate level of outpatient care? What referrals and recommendations would you consider?

Summary

Treatment follows a pattern, with different issues addressed at the end of treatment than at either its beginning or middle. In particular, these include transferring skills to other settings, increasing client ownership of the change process, and preventing a relapse. These tasks may occur in the midst of confusing feelings of excitement and hopefulness, as well as loss and abandonment for both client and clinician. Termination should consider the pitfalls clients might face while fostering hopefulness about continuing changes begun in therapy.

All clinical interventions are associated with some risk. Clinicians can, however, decrease their risk of ethical complaint or legal action at these points: They can respond respectfully and empathically to the clients' needs and concerns, request consultations, and document their decisions and decision-making process well, including careful discharge summaries.

For Review

Applying Concepts to Your Life

1. If you've been in therapy before, think about the range of feelings you had when it ended. If you have not been in therapy, how did you feel during an important transition in your life (e.g., a move, graduation, end of a relationship)? How did you handle these feelings?

2. If you've been in therapy before, how did your clinician handle the end of treatment? Were the concerns raised in this chapter addressed well? If you have not been in therapy, think about another type of transition. If that transition was relatively difficult, what could have made it work better?

Key Terms

abandonment, 213

consultation, 214

discharge
   summary, 222

forced
   terminations, 219

generalize, 213

managed care, 210

normal
   termination, 211

premature
   termination, 211

relapse prevention, 217

transfer, 213

well-being, 217

Learn More

For more information about the concepts in this chapter, visit the *Empathic Counseling* companion website at http://pubs.apa.org/books/supp/slattery/.

Part V Professional Issues

This final part of the book addresses three important issues for all therapeutic work. First, clinicians must conduct their work in an ethical manner. We explore the role of ethics in anticipating and preventing problems while remaining respectful and empathic. We emphasize key concepts from the American Psychological Association's Ethics Code and present a process for ethical decision-making. Second, clinicians must document their work in clinical reports. Just as empathy is critical when assessing and treating clients, it is also critical when writing clinical reports that may eventually be read by the client or a third party. We explain how to document treatment in a respectful, sensitive, and accurate way. Finally, clinicians must attend to their own self-awareness and self-care in empathic counseling. We discuss how to assess one's own competence on a regular basis, recognize potential problems such as burnout, and use effective coping strategies to remain effective and empathic over the long run.

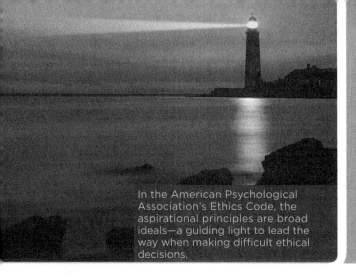

In the American Psychological Association's Ethics Code, the aspirational principles are broad ideals—a guiding light to lead the way when making difficult ethical decisions.

11 Ethics

Looking Ahead IIII➡

After reading this chapter you will be able to answer these questions:

1. What ethical standards and aspirational goals guide ethical clinical work?

2. What strategies can clinicians use to identify and prevent risk of ethical problems?

3. How do self-knowledge and self-awareness help clinicians remain ethical?

4. What is a positive approach to ethics and how does it different from simply preventing and responding to ethical problems?

Cases in Empathy

A Band-Aid for Complex Problems ▎ Dr. Helper

Most clinicians enter the field to help people. Even clinicians committing an ethical violation are likely to have had good intentions and meant to be helpful (Pope & Keith-Spiegel, 2008). This positive intention is seen in the story of Anonymous (2000)—called Dr. Helper here—a psychologist who was "helpful" after making a deathbed promise to take care of a client's wife, Edna, and their children. Dr. Helper began seeing Edna as a client, hired her as office staff when she needed work, saw himself as part of her family, bought her jewelry, and eventually started a sexual relationship with her, although he was married to someone else. Eventually Dr. Helper ended his affair with Edna. In the end, Edna eventually felt used, exploited, and abandoned. Dr. Helper's wife divorced him, and the Licensure Board censured him. He concluded, "I failed because I didn't know how to limit care" (Anonymous, 2000, p. 3).

What Do You Think?

1. What specific problems do you see with Dr. Helper's responses? Why?

2. If you had made this deathbed promise, what are some more ethical ways of responding to this promise? What strategy would you use to choose among these responses?

The Aspirational Principles

Ethics is nothing else than reverence for life.

—Albert Schweitzer

As we discussed in Chapter 1—and throughout this book—effective treatment includes both behaving in positive and ethical ways and avoiding harmful acts. In this chapter, we expand our earlier discussions of ethics, put them in a broader context, and consider ways to understand these more fully.

The American Psychological Association's (APA's; 2017a) *Ethical Principles of Psychologists and Code of Conduct* includes both aspirational principles and standards. The **aspirational principles** in this code of ethics are nonbinding, broad ideals informing a clinician's ethical decisions. They were developed to "guide and inspire psychologists toward the very highest ethical ideals of the profession" (p. 1062). These five principles are that clinicians do good (**beneficence**); avoid harm (**nonmaleficence**); support their clients' ability to think and act freely for themselves (**autonomy**); behave in a faithful, honest, and trustworthy manner (**fidelity**); are accurate, honest, and truthful in their work (**integrity**); and promote fairness in the community and in clinical settings (**social justice**). Knapp, VandeCreek, and Fingerhut (2017) also argued that we should consider our responsibility to the public at large.

Consider Dr. Helper's work with Edna (Anonymous, 2000). He seems to have been trying to be helpful (beneficence), but it is less clear that nonmaleficence, autonomy, and fidelity influenced his decision-making. He entered a series of situations that had a high probability of leaving Edna feeling exploited and appeared to ignore considering the long-term consequences of his actions. Ethical clinicians weigh both the best and worst possible outcomes of their proposed act (Pope & Keith-Spiegel, 2008).

Dr. Helper did not follow the guiding principle of fostering autonomy. He seemed to believe that *he* should solve Edna's problems and meet her needs as they arose. When she needed a therapist, he agreed to see her rather than encouraging her to find another therapist (one who hadn't treated her late husband). When she needed a job, he hired her. When she was feeling alone, he stepped in as friend, family, and lover. His actions may have been well received, but encouraged dependency; instead, ethical clinicians **empower** their clients (i.e., support clients to recognize, accept, use and develop their personal and political power to meet their goals). Clinicians can empower clients by helping and encouraging them to identify strategies for meeting their own needs.

Dr. Helper used a definition of fidelity similar to that of the American Nurses Association (n.d.), which defines fidelity as "loyalty, fairness, truthfulness, advocacy, and dedication to our patients. It involves . . . keeping a commitment and is based upon the virtue of caring" (p. 2). The APA's (2017a) definition is consistent with this one, but it is broader, focusing on more than our clients' immediate needs. It recognizes conflicts of interest that could lead to perceptions of exploitation, as Edna experienced, and acknowledges that a client's best interests may require a referral to other professionals and institutions.

Even when writing about these events after the fact (Anonymous, 2000), Dr. Helper seemed to have had little insight into the motivations that led him to engage in behaviors that most clinicians would identify as very risky. His failure to look at and question his motivations and decisions hurt Edna, his family, his career, and our profession.

The Ethical Standards

The aspirational principles describe goals to guide clinicians' behavior, but they can be difficult to apply to specific situations. In contrast, the **ethical standards** are a set of requirements involving more specific expectations for the field, violations of which can lead to disciplinary censure. Clinicians face four basic ethical issues throughout their careers: informed consent, competence (technical, multicultural, and emotional), confidentiality, and multiple relationships. The APA Ethics Code standards are briefly described here, along with examples of applications of these standards. However, clinicians should also regularly read their professions' code of ethics to understand and apply these standards more fully and carefully (e.g., American Association for Marriage and Family Therapy, 2015; American Counseling Association, 2014; APA, 2017a; National Association of Social Workers, 2017).

Informed Consent

Informed consent is a voluntary agreement to participate in a procedure on the basis of understanding its nature, its potential benefits and possible risks, and available alternatives. Clinicians provide clients with sufficient information to make knowledgeable decisions about their treatment (Barnett, Wise, Johnson-Greene, & Bucky, 2007). Clients should be informed about **confidentiality** and its limits (i.e., a clinician may reveal information about client identity, diagnosis, or treatment to a third party only when the client gives permission or when the clinician is legally required to do so). Clients should also be informed about fees, availability of emergency services, and the involvement of third parties (e.g., the court or an employer). They have the right to know about other available treatments as well as the benefits and potential side effects of these treatments.

The informed consent process generally starts in the first session but should continue across time as additional questions emerge (M. A. Fisher & the Center for Ethical Practice, 2008). For example, during an initial session, when reviewing her informed consent forms with a client, a clinician might describe how she makes decisions about referring clients for medication and then explain this process more fully later if that client's depression did not respond well to psychotherapy alone.

Why is informed consent important? The informed consent process fosters the therapeutic alliance, client autonomy, and rational decision-making while reducing the potential for exploitation and harm (Snyder & Barnett, 2006). Giving clients the opportunity to give informed consent to treatment demonstrates respect for them and creates a collaborative process that empowers clients to meet their goals (**empowered collaboration**; Knapp et al., 2017).

Clinical Applications

Marion came to treatment with a phobia of birds that had her increasingly housebound. After a review of the literature, her therapist, Kenn, decided to use the technique of flooding in treatment (i.e., exposing her to a very high level of the feared stimulus), although he decided not to tell her beforehand. He concluded, "If I told her, she wouldn't do it!" What ethical concerns do you have about his decision? Are these balanced by the possible benefits?

✳✳✳

Sharlynn was actively suicidal and threatened to take 150 mixed pills. She was unwilling to agree to go to the hospital. Dee, her therapist, told Sharlynn what she was going to do at each step as they considered options for keeping her safe. What do you think of her actions? Are there other things that she should do to remain ethical in this situation?

Competence

Competence includes knowledge and skills as well as the attitudes, values, and judgment necessary to implement them well (Barnett, Doll, Younggren, & Rubin, 2007). There are multiple kinds of competence. **Technical competence**, the knowledge and skills to perform a therapeutic task well, is gained through formal reading, coursework, or training in an area of specialty; skill is developed through ongoing supervision and consultations with qualified clinicians. Maintaining competency also requires that clinicians recognize their current **emotional competence**, the ability to perform without bias or psychological distress clouding judgment or impairing their ability to act effectively. Effective clinicians address issues that can cloud their judgment (e.g., bias, distress, substance use and abuse, mental and physical illness). Both technical and emotional competence can vary across time.

The degree of expertise needed to become competent depends in part on a clinician's initial levels of general clinical competence as well as the unique skills required in an area. A social worker who provides individual psychotherapy might have the technical competence to offer vocational counseling—depending on the complexity of the vocational issues—but might not be competent to do a custody evaluation. Although he might have the technical skills to do a custody evaluation in English and Spanish, if he failed to recognize the complications of language and culture when evaluating a Mexican immigrant, his actions might not demonstrate **multicultural competence**, which includes the skills and knowledge that are appropriate for, and specific to, treating a given culture. Even if he was skilled in performing custody evaluations with Mexican Americans and has a good translator, his emotional competence might drop during the course of his own contentious divorce.

Competence is a state that can be achieved but must be maintained and enhanced in the face of ever-changing personal contexts (Barnett, Doll, et al., 2007). Competence increases with increasing skill development but can drop when a clinician is under stress (Knapp et al., 2017). Thus, maintaining competency requires ongoing professional development, self-care, and regular assessments of one's emotional health and level of skill.

Why is competence an important issue? When clinicians work without the specific competency to perform specialized tasks (e.g., forensic work, neurological assessments, or family therapy), they offer a lesser quality of service and, as a result, compromise the client's mental health and the reputation of the profession. Clinicians who do not maintain their level of competence are also more likely to be sued or be the subject of ethical complaints. Behaving ethically and competently is an important risk management strategy for protecting one's reputation and preventing lawsuits (Knapp, Younggren, VandeCreek, Harris, & Martin, 2013).

Clinical Applications

Darcy is going through a divorce. She has been monitoring her stress levels, cut back on accepting referrals to work with couples, and reentered personal therapy but is still seeing clients and believes herself effective, as does her supervisor. What factors might affect her competence? How would she recognize her current level of competence?

✳ ✳ ✳

Nadya is a talented child therapist working with children with autism. She receives more referrals than she can handle. In trying to meet this need, she often skips completing case notes, rarely reads the newest research on autism, and hasn't been to a continuing education workshop in 4 years; nonetheless, the referrals pour in. How do you see Nadya's competence?

Confidentiality

Confidentiality is a broad right that allows clients to discuss sensitive issues safely without worry that this information will be disclosed to someone else. In general, nothing about clients' presence or activity in treatment can be shared without their specific permission to do so; however, a number of situations limit confidentiality, including state and legal mandates to report child or elder abuse and imminent dangerousness to self or others. In addition, clinicians must discuss treatment issues with their supervisors and share some information with insurance companies to receive payment. These limits to confidentiality should generally be discussed early in treatment and further discussed at later points if other disclosures are necessary (C. B. Fisher & Oransky, 2008; M. A. Fisher & the Center for Ethical Practice, 2008).

Although clinicians may have permission to disclose some information, this permission should be limited to information relevant to the source. For example, interventions that will address a child's attention and focus in school would be appropriate to share with the school, while a parent's diagnosis of an illness would not be, unless it was specifically related to difficulties a child was having in school. For example, disclosing a parent's trauma history in this situation is probably gratuitous and possibly damaging.

Sometimes rules about confidentiality seem absurd to outsiders. Family members may know that a client is receiving therapy but hit a brick wall when calling to see how treatment is going. Unless the client has provided specific permission to release this information, clinicians must respond noncommittally (e.g., "I can neither confirm nor deny that she is a client here"). This prohibition protects those people who want to keep their mental health care private, although it does not prevent them from disclosing aspects of their own treatment to others or giving their clinician permission to disclose their information. They own the information and can choose where and how to share it.

Why is confidentiality important? Confidentiality creates a safe environment that helps clients disclose and explore material that they may not have shared before (M. A. Fisher & the Center for Ethical Practice, 2008). Describing these limits on confidentiality during the informed consent process can foster the therapeutic alliance and the client's autonomy and rational decision-making. Should a disclosure be required at a later point, having already shared the limits of confidentiality reduces a client's perception of being exploited (Snyder & Barnett, 2006).

Clinical Applications	In the course of hospital rounds, Sophie talked to Dr. Wu about her client Liza's status and her response to a new antidepressant. Dr. Wu asked whether Liza's symptoms stemmed from her history of sexual abuse (to guide his prescribing process). Liza had given Sophie permission only to disclose her symptoms and her response to the antidepressant, not to discuss her history of incest. What should Sophie do?
	✳✳✳
	Daria and her son were eating lunch at a local coffee shop when a former client came up and began talking about the breakup of his marriage. Is this ethical? What should Daria do? Why?

Multiple Relationships

Multiple relationships occur when clinicians engage in more than one relationship at a time with a client, each with conflicting goals, needs, and expectations (e.g., becoming his or her friend, employer, teacher, business associate, sex partner or lover, in addition to being his or her therapist). Any second relationship or obligation that exploits clients to further the clinician's personal interests at the expense of the client's—or that appears to do so—is problematic. This second relationship can cloud the clinician's ability to make objective and sound decisions and can create expectations that interfere with treatment (Gottlieb, Robinson, & Younggren, 2007; Knapp & Slattery, 2004; Slattery, 2005).

Multiple relationships differ in their impact on treatment and their degree of clinical risk. **Boundary violations** are behaviors deviating from professional norms, with high potential for negative consequences for the client (e.g., sexual relationships, bartering). Boundary violations can have explosive consequences, are associated with increased risk of ethical complaints, and should always be avoided (Gutheil & Gabbard, 1993; Knapp et al., 2013). In contrast, **boundary crossings** are behaviors deviating from the strictest professional norms, including small self-disclosures. Boundary crossings are less risky and can even be desirable under some circumstances, such as when occasionally extending a session's length for a client who is in crisis or self-disclosing material to help clients meet their therapeutic goals (Barnett, Lazarus, Vasquez, Moorehead-Slaughter, & Johnson, 2007).

Boundary crossings can be difficult to avoid in some settings but, like boundary violations, can create unclear expectations, muddy communication processes, and sometimes leave clients feeling exploited. Some treatment decisions may create a "slippery slope"; once stepped on, there is an increased probability of additional and perhaps increasingly harmful unethical acts.

Clinicians should carefully consider decisions to deviate from professional norms before the fact or as soon after the fact as possible (Barnett, Lazarus, et al., 2007; Pope & Keith-Spiegel, 2008). Consultations with colleagues, supervisors, or the clients themselves can be helpful. Pope and Keith-Spiegel (2008) suggested making decisions about boundary crossings by imagining both the "best possible" and "worst possible" outcomes, considering the published literature, and paying attention to uneasy feelings, doubts, or concerns that surface during the decision-making process.

Why is avoiding multiple relationships—especially boundary violations—important? Although a number of writers have suggested that boundary crossings may have some benefits (e.g., Dybicz, 2012), one (now dated survey) found that about 50% of professionals who had previously had a sexual relationship with a professor, clinical supervisor, or therapist reported negative consequences from that relationship (Lamb & Catanzaro, 1998). For some, the consequences decreased with time, but about twice as many people reported that consequences became more negative with time. Whether the second relationship begins before, during, or after the therapeutic relationship, multiple relationships can be destructive to both parties, as well as to their families, friends, and the profession. The reputations of both that particular clinician and the field as a whole are compromised by boundary violations.

Clinical Applications

Not wanting to be rude, Daria invited her former client, who was clearly shaken while talking about the breakup of his marriage, to join her and her son as they finished lunch. What do you think of Daria's actions? If you see a problem, how could she have handled this more ethically?

✳ ✳ ✳

Belle lives in a small community where it is traditional for people to give holiday gifts to friends, teachers, and other people for whom they are thankful. She received a child's drawing and a number of plates of cookies. She also received a lovely engraved watch like the one that she had been wanting but couldn't afford. Would accepting the drawings and cookies be ethical? Would accepting the watch be ethical? Why or why not? What should she do?

Sensitivity to Differences

Competent, effective clinicians are sensitive to race, culture, class, gender, sexual orientation, religion, and other contextual factors. Such sensitivity improves the assessment, diagnostic, and treatment processes and strengthens the therapeutic alliance. Clinicians sensitive to issues of cultural differences offer services that are user-friendly and user-appropriate; respect differences in values, belief systems and habits; are sensitive to cultural differences; decorate their offices in a way that reflects their openness to people of other cultures; and consider cultural issues as they develop goals and treatment plans (Slattery, 2004).

Sensitivity to differences has multiple dimensions. For example, an agency in a Latinx neighborhood may hire Spanish-speaking staff and encourage other staff to develop their language skills and understanding of Latinx culture. The waiting room may have magazines, notices, and paperwork in both English and Spanish. The staff's awareness of Latinx culture may help them recognize that apparent boundary problems may instead reflect *personalismo*, a preference for and expectation of personal rather than role-limited relationships (Añez, Silva, Paris, & Bedregal, 2008; see also Exhibit 2.2 in Chapter 2 of this volume). The staff name and discuss oppression, prejudice, and discrimination as it affects their clients' lives and treatment (Sue & Sue, 2016).

This attitude of respect is a general one rather than specific to a particular racial or ethnic group. The many questions to consider regarding sensitivity to differences include the following: Is the office really accessible? In addition to having a ramp or elevator, does the office offer a path between furniture that is wide enough for wheelchairs? If young children are seen, are chairs and decorations child-friendly and child-proofed? Will male clients feel comfortable in a pink, frilly office? Will Jewish clients feel welcome in an office decorated for Christmas holidays?

Clinical Applications	At his fourth therapy session, Beau disclosed that he is gay, although he indicated clearly that this was neither a problem nor related to his history of recurrent depression. Nonetheless, Marcee, who believes homosexuality is a sin, began to push Beau on this issue. He was offended and made a complaint to her supervisor. What would convince you that Marcee's actions were ethical? Unethical? What could she do at this point to behave more ethically?

✳ ✳ ✳

Hank, who only speaks English, hesitantly accepted a client who only speaks Mandarin, although he did so because there is no Mandarin-speaking counselor in their community, the nearest one being 2 hours away, and this client does not drive. He found a translator who was acceptable to his client. Was it ethical to accept this client? Why or why not? What else should he consider?

Why is being sensitive to differences important? This sensitivity is a practical demonstration of psychology's values of respect, beneficence, nonmaleficence, and justice (Hoop, DiPasquale, Hernandez, & Roberts, 2008). Without this sensitivity, treatment may be derailed because clients have difficulty believing their clinicians understand them and expect they are unwilling to make the effort to do so (Pope & Keith-Spiegel, 2008). Because of the power differential between clients and clinicians, clinicians who are culturally insensitive may impose culturally oppressive views that interfere with developing empathy, undermine the therapeutic relationship, and lead clinicians to set inappropriate and disempowering goals.

Balancing Client Rights With Ethical, Legal, and Other Requirements

Because our every action has a universal dimension, a potential impact on others' happiness, ethics are necessary as a means to ensure that we do not harm others.

—Dalai Lama

The Consumer Bill of Rights, ratified by nine national associations of mental health providers, clearly described clients' rights in treatment (Cantor, 1998). These rights include to be treated with dignity and respect, to receive competent treatment, and to be actively involved in setting the direction of treatment. Clients have the right to be informed about costs, anticipated risks, and alternative treatments, and to make decisions based on this information. They have the right to have their culture respected. They have the right to keep their treatment confidential and to have disclosures occur only with their permission.

On paper, some of these rights seem clear and unarguable; however, they become more complicated in the real world. This section describes real-world examples outlining the potential conflicts that clinicians need to resolve and further describes the range of ethical and legal considerations that clinicians must consider.

Legal Requirements

Ethical standards and legal requirements often address the same situations; however, conflicts frequently arise. As a result, decision-making in clinical settings often involves many shades of gray. While ethical principles are derived from moral decisions about "right" and "wrong," legal considerations are based on a complex mix of historical precedents, social norms, and moral decisions that have evolved over many years through legislation and court cases.

Mandated reporting. Confidentiality is clearly an ethical standard that must be diligently maintained except under certain mandated situations, such as **mandated reporting** of child or elder abuse, or when the client voluntarily gives up confidentiality. These limitations should be clearly outlined during the informed consent process.

Even in situations where the need to violate confidentiality is legally mandated, such as reporting abuse or ensuring the safety of a suicidal client, making such determinations is often unclear. For example, clients often talk about wanting to hurt themselves or someone else. When is such talk "letting off steam," and when is it an urgent indication that the client intends harm? Some clinicians may discourage such discussions, fearing that if they know too much, they will have to have their client hospitalized. Effective and empathic clinicians allow clients to express and explore their thoughts and feelings fully while remaining vigilant for signs that they may need to take some action. Further, rather than considering only whether suicidality and other kinds of dangerous behaviors should be disclosed, answering this question should always include considerations of when and how to make such a disclosure. When possible, disclosures should be discussed with clients first, reflecting the clinician's respect for their freedom, dignity, and autonomy during a difficult period (Pope, 2015).

Laws and legal precedents covering mandated reporting of child and elder abuse differ across states, as do requirements to report dangerous driving and confidentiality afforded children and teenagers. Outlining these variations in state law is beyond the scope of this book; more detail is provided in state publications and on state websites. Clinicians should learn the rules in their state and maintain ongoing competence on changing interpretations of these issues.

Clinical Applications

While in prison, Ralph, who has a significant history of abusing alcohol, told his counselor that he had been "clean" (abstinent) for months; however, another client told the therapist that not only was Ralph still drinking, but he was making and selling alcohol. Now that his therapist knows this information, can she use it in therapy, and if so, how? Should she confront the client? Should she divulge the source of her information? Their informed consent said that the therapist would not share clinical information with the prison administration unless prison security was compromised. The warden might agree security was compromised, but their consent did not address these questions about what would happen in therapy. What factors might influence her decisions?

✳ ✳ ✳

Jacqui (age 15) was brought to treatment because she was being "disrespectful" at home and her grades were falling at school. Her mother wanted to know from Juanita whether Jacqui was doing anything "dangerous," although Jacqui wanted her privacy and forbade Juanita from disclosing any information. Further muddying the issues, children, their parents, and clinicians may differ in their identification of problems (Shirk, Karver, & Brown, 2011). Family dynamics may underlie children's symptoms, and thus helping children and teens learn to communicate with parents in safe and effective ways is often important. How can one be ethical, empathic, and effective under these circumstances?

* * *

Tiona was referred for treatment by Child Protective Services after she left bruises on her two daughters. Tiona accused the agency of being racist (she's African American), noting that this style of parenting was the way that she, as well as her family and friends, were raised. "It worked for me!" What ethical issues are raised by this case? How would you work with her on these issues?

* * *

When might intentionally searching for a client on the Internet be appropriate? Should the client consent first? Why?

Duty to warn. The landmark case *Tarasoff v. Regents of the University of California* imposed a duty to warn identifiable victims of a threat. In this case, Prosenjit Poddar, a client at a university counseling center, told his psychologist that he intended to kill his ex-girlfriend, Tatiana Tarasoff. Dr. Moore took this threat seriously and unsuccessfully attempted to hospitalize Poddar, who then dropped out of treatment (Bersoff, 2014). Dr. Moore consulted with his supervisor and contacted the university police; Poddar told them that he would stay away from Tarasoff. Dr. Moore's supervisor ordered him not to break confidentiality to warn Tarasoff; however, Poddar subsequently killed Tarasoff.

Tarasoff's parents sued the Regents of the University of California, the campus police, and the Health Service employees for failing to warn their daughter of the danger. The California Supreme Court concluded that when "a patient poses a serious danger of violence to others, [the therapist] bears a duty to exercise reasonable care to protect the foreseeable victim of that danger" (quoted in Ewing, 2005, p. 112). Protecting an intended victim can be accomplished in a number of ways, including warning him or her; however, seeking a voluntary hospitalization of the would-be perpetrator, addressing the issue in therapy, or changing the frequency or focus of treatment may often be enough (Bersoff, 2014; Knapp et al., 2013). This duty to warn does not extend to situations where the potential victim is unidentifiable (e.g., a general threat or a potential new sexual partner of someone diagnosed with HIV).

Although violence of this magnitude rarely occurs, the *Tarasoff* case raised a number of issues. First, it placed limits on a client's right to confidentiality:

A client's confidentiality is trumped by a serious threat of violence. Bersoff (2014) noted that it is unclear at what point confidentiality should be broken: a death threat? An assault? An emotional assault? Second, feelings of betrayal by breaks in confidentiality are reduced when clinicians describe limits to confidentiality during the informed consent process and again if threats are made. Third, clinicians are protected from legal consequences by accurate assessments and careful documentation of both assessments and conclusions (Knapp et al., 2013). Finally, the *Tarasoff* ruling suggests that the ethical aspirations of doing good and avoiding harm do not refer only to good and harm for the client but also for the larger community.

Similar problems occur in other settings. When should clinicians break confidentiality to tell parents that adolescent clients are engaging in dangerous behaviors? When they are having unprotected sex? Using recreational drugs? What impact will breaks in confidentiality have on the therapeutic relationship and the adolescent's developing autonomy and responsibility? Clinicians can use the informed consent process to discuss what information can be disclosed and how disclosures will occur (Behnke, 2007). Such discussions can be used to foster the adolescent's autonomy and relationship with parents.

Client autonomy can facilitate treatment and recovery (S. H. Schwartz et al., 2012), but as the *Tarasoff* decision has indicated, autonomy should be balanced by other considerations, including others' safety. As seen in the discussion in the next box, clients who are involuntarily hospitalized still retain the right to refuse treatment (Schopp, 2001). Unfortunately, allowing people in the court or prison system the right to refuse psychiatric treatment has extended their de facto imprisonment in some cases well beyond what they would have served for the crime with which they were charged (Heilbrun & Kramer, 2005).

Cases in Empathy

How Could They Fail to Protect Our Family From Her? ▮ Andrea Yates

On June 20, 2001, when she was 36, Andrea Yates took each of her five children (aged 7, 5, 3, and 2 years and the youngest 6 months) into their bathroom. She drowned them in the bathtub, then laid four of the five on their beds, covering them with sheets. Later, her husband, Rusty Yates, said, "We didn't see her as a danger . . . How could she have been so ill and

the medical community not diagnose her, not treat her, and obviously not protect our family from her?" (quoted in Roche, 2002a, para. 51). His question remains an important one.

Andrea had a significant psychiatric history: She had a psychotic episode, two hospitalizations, and two suicide attempts after the birth of her youngest son. She had experienced depressive episodes earlier in her life following the breakup of a relationship, after her father's heart attack, and probably after she miscarried in 1998. She reported that she believed she had been bulimic in college.

Although many women are "blue" after childbirth, few are depressed, and even fewer psychotic. Andrea's symptoms were significant and outside normal postpartum responses. When she was hospitalized after her son's birth, she said,

> I had a fear I would hurt somebody. . . . I thought it better to end my own life and prevent it. . . . There was a voice, then an image of the knife . . . I had a vision in my mind, get a knife, get a knife. . . . I had a vision of this person being stabbed . . . the aftereffects (as quoted in Court TV, 1999, p. 1)

Her first vision followed the birth of her oldest son, but she "blew it off." She had similar visions about 10 times, although there were discrepancies in the stories she gave across time.

Andrea's symptoms extended beyond the delusional guilt, obsessive thoughts, and homicidal and suicidal ideation focused on in the media. In 1999, her doctors reported she was "essentially mute," "withdrawn and suspicious," with "severe psychomotor retardation" (Starbranch, 1999, p. 2). She had self-inflicted scratches on her arms and legs and "frequently" picked at her scalp or pulled her hair as "a nervous reaction" (Court TV, 1999, p. 2). She told Dr. Resnick, a psychiatrist for her defense, that she believed there had been a surveillance camera monitoring her bad mothering for months. Their television occasionally talked to her:

> Well . . . they'd ate some candy one morning and we had the TV on . . . cartoon . . . and— and just flashed a scene where the comic— the cartoon characters were talking to us . . . and they were saying, "Hey, kids, stop eating so much candy." It was just a flash and then back to the program. (A. Yates, in O'Malley, 2004, p. 155)

She also told Dr. Resnick that she heard Satan's voice, "a deep, growling voice, [that] said my name" (p. 155). Dr. Starbranch referred to her as one of "the five sickest—and most difficult to get out of psychosis—patients that I've ever treated" (Starbranch, in O'Malley, 2004, p. 177).

Andrea's relationship with the psychiatric establishment was mixed at best. After her hospitalizations in 1999, Dr. Starbranch told her another pregnancy might cause an even worse episode of postpartum depression. Nonetheless, Andrea refused Zyprexa when she learned it was an antipsychotic and was intermittent in taking any of her medications. This reluctance may have been related to a deep mistrust of psychiatric medicines and a desire to breastfeed. She described Haldol, the drug her husband thought worked miracles, as a "truth serum" that caused her to lose control (Roche, 2002b). She was discharged from intensive outpatient treatment and stopped taking her medications and seeing her psychiatrist and social worker.

When she was hospitalized in 2001, Andrea had to be forcibly put into and dragged from the car. In this hospitalization, her medications were frequently adjusted up and down, leading her husband to speculate that reducing the Effexor caused her psychotic break (Yates, 2004). As is often necessary, Dr. Saeed began treating her before receiving her medical records. When he finally read them, he concluded, "No new info" (Roche, 2002b, p. 49). Although it took 10 days for her to start feeding herself again and she was essentially mute in the hospital, he concluded that there was no evidence of psychosis and removed the antipsychotics because he thought she was experiencing some facial akinesia, an occasional side effect of Haldol.

Andrea drowned her children 37 days after being released from the hospital, 13 days after last taking Haldol. She had seen her psychiatrist only 2 days before the murders.

What Do You Think?

1. What ethical questions, if any, are raised by this case material? What, if anything, would you, as a clinician treating Andrea Yates, do differently? Why?

2. What rights did Andrea have relative to treatment? What about her family and the public? How would you balance these competing rights and make these decisions?

3. How would the aspirational principles outlined at the beginning of this chapter guide your thinking?

Worksite Requirements

A clinician's workplace comes with a unique set of conditions. Each setting has its own intake system, strategies for managing treatment, and guidelines for making and documenting clinical decisions. These policies place specific constraints and expectations on clinicians, some of which may, at times, create difficult situations, tax their empathy, compromise their effectiveness, or test their ethical decision-making.

Clinical Applications

Mae (age 10) was throwing tantrums and being oppositional at home, although not at school. Her therapist, Soozie, believed that these problems were related to marital issues and family triangles and alliances. Soozie's agency does not provide family therapy (although Soozie has considerable training and expertise in it), and her supervisor suggested individual treatment instead. Should Soozie compromise the type of treatment she offers or refer Mae's family to another facility? Does it matter whether referral to another agency negatively affects Soozie's ability to maintain productivity, which is another agency requirement? What if the family's ability to pay for services requires them to remain at this agency?

✳✳✳

College counseling centers often do a number of things to respond to limited resources, including limiting the number of sessions allowed, referring students to off-campus providers, and using waiting lists. Frances began treating a student, Leon, using a brief treatment model, but discovered that his problems were much more significant than were apparent in initial assessments and were likely to require longer term interventions. What options should she consider?

✳✳✳

Bubb hates doing paperwork and frequently gets behind in it to maintain the high levels of productivity his agency requires. Often he even neglects to write timely **progress notes**, which are brief and informal notes made by a clinician immediately after a session summarizing the content and process of the session as well as diagnostic impressions When Bubb's supervisor discovered he was behind in his documentation, she pulled him off his caseload for a week and asked him to complete his back paperwork, requiring him to write progress notes for sessions from as far back as several months ago, which he does not remember. What should Bubb do? Why?

Financial Considerations

Financial considerations are worth highlighting. Discussing money in therapy makes many clinicians uncomfortable, yet for most, clinical work is their livelihood, making such discussions essential. Few clinicians enter the field primarily because of their love of spreadsheets, billing, and accounting. In fact, although these are dated numbers, only 21.4% of clinical, counseling, and social work programs responding to a survey offered basic marketing as part of their training (Daniels, Alva, & Olivares, 2002), and even fewer mentioned basic finance training (18.4%). More recent discussions of competencies for doctoral-level practitioners focus on specialty-specific skills, multicultural training, and ethics and do not refer specifically to financial decision-making (cf. Beacham et al., 2017; Rozensky et al., 2015). These numbers reflect the interests and biases of clinicians in the field.

Balancing ethical standards while remaining empathic and effective can introduce financial complexities. Both clinicians in private practice and those working for agencies and nonprofits need to pay attention to how they will maintain productivity and **billable hours** (the number of hours of clinical service that will be paid by clients and insurance companies) while also being ethical, empathic, and effective. For many clinicians, that may mean focusing on those services where managed care or private pay clients will pay for their work. They may choose to see additional clients rather than developing client handouts, reading professional journals, or obtaining consults from other providers working with a client. They may need to think about when they will see **pro bono** (i.e., work for a reduced fee) clients and under what circumstances. In fact, clinicians with heavy managed care involvement work longer hours, provide more direct contact hours, and report less satisfaction with their work than clinicians with less involvement (Cantor & Fuentes, 2008; Rupert & Baird, 2004). This is a prescription for burnout.

Small or poorly funded agencies may have such tight budgets that they are unable to purchase the most current versions of psychological assessments. Limited resources may prohibit adequate supervision of sufficient length or quality. Budgetary restrictions may require high levels of productivity that are manageable for some clinicians, yet impossible for others who are otherwise strong—at least if they are going to retain their ability to be empathic and competent.

Further, how does one maintain productivity and competency given the changing research and theory in the field (Phelps, Bray, & Kearney, 2017)? Each profession or state has its own standards for continuing education for licensed professionals. Still, it could be argued that one would be minimally prepared by performing only the required continuing education rather than reading additional literature, discussing professional issues with colleagues on an ongoing basis, or consulting about issues as they arose.

Clinical Applications	Fees and client copayments should be specified early in the provision of service, and discussion of them should be a normal part of the informed consent process (Pomerantz & Handelsman, 2004). The Basset family readily agreed to the fees charged by their family therapists but became reluctant to pay them when Mr. Basset lost his job and health insurance and the family faced bankruptcy. Although they were highly motivated and more stable than when they first entered treatment, their fighting still escalated into violence about twice a month. What should their family therapy team do? When, if ever, should clients' financial situations influence the type or length of services they receive?

Limitations of Time and Energy

Problems arise in that one has to find a balance between what people need from you and what you need for yourself.

—Jessye Norman

A clinician's work is never completely finished: More time and attention might be extended to clients, more preparation could be done before sessions, more reading and training could improve competencies. Maintaining the ability to perform clinical work competently depends on ongoing professional development. Nonetheless, development requires time (which might not be reimbursed) and a willingness to identify professional development as an ongoing priority. Further, clinicians have their own needs to attend to, their own lives to live. Clinicians' struggles to balance their own needs with their involvement with clients, ensuring that they are functioning competently, can become an ethical issue. Regular and ongoing self-awareness and self-care are essential aspects of maintaining competency (Knapp et al., 2017). All clinicians should consider how they are going to maintain their competency and expertise while meeting their individual and family needs.

**Clinical
Applications** There are a number of ways to think about the problems that Lia Lee's doctors had in working with the Lee family (Chapter 4). One possibility is that her doctors were overextended and rushed. Because they did not recognize their limits, they did not listen to the family as well as they might have otherwise. What could you do to maintain a competent practice even when you are busy?

✳✳✳

Several writers have argued that, under some circumstances, deviations from standard professional boundaries can be helpful but that such deviations should be thoughtfully considered and discussed with colleagues, supervisors, or clients before the fact or as soon after the fact as possible (Barnett, Lazarus, et al., 2007; Kolmes & Taube, 2014). What factors would you use to evaluate whether attending a client's wedding would be ethical, empathic, and effective? Would thinking about your own stress levels and time constraints be factors you would consider? Why or why not?

Supervisory Issues

Supervisors need to balance many different concerns, some of which may be of greater or lesser importance depending on whether the agency's mission is primarily training or if it offers clinical services and only secondarily offers training and supervision. As a result, supervisors may emphasize training and professional development or productivity to differing degrees.

A multiprofessional, international research project found that greater support and autonomy in the workplace was strongly associated with clinicians' levels of satisfaction with their career development (Orlinsky & Rønnestad, 2005). Higher career satisfaction was also associated with more client growth, greater perceptions that their clinical work promoted client healing, and, perhaps surprisingly, greater breadth and depth of case experience. Conversely, clinicians who experienced more work-related frustrations (e.g., cancellations, slow client growth, client suicides) were least satisfied with their careers.

**Clinical
Applications** Theo, a newly hired supervisor, is considering what tasks to assign to his new interns. On the one hand, he knows that the training process will be most successful if he assigns interns a range of client problems and modalities of treatment, but on the other hand, he wants his interns to have a positive experience (also correlated with career development). Furthermore, he wants his agency to provide high-quality care. How could Theo respond to these tensions among the

needs of his interns, those of his agency's clients, and the agency's reputation? What other factors should he think about?

✳ ✳ ✳

Fernanda is supervising Bubb, who is several months behind in his paperwork. She recognizes that Bubb is a talented therapist, but she is also worried that they have no documentation for hundreds of billable hours. She is concerned that they may get audited and would be unable to document their provision of services. She is also worried about what might happen in the admittedly infrequent case of a client suicide and how this might leave Bubb, her, and the agency open to a lawsuit. Further, she is hesitant to continue supervising someone who cuts such corners in his work. What might she consider in attempting to resolve these problems?

Making Decisions in Response to Ethical Dilemmas

As Pope and Keith-Spiegel (2008) concluded, even good people can make ethical mistakes and blunders. Ethical and competent clinicians, however, engage in a decision-making process that actively decreases the probability of mistakes. They ask themselves, "What if I'm wrong about this? Is there something I'm overlooking? Could there be another way of understanding this situation? Could there be a more creative, more effective way of responding?" (p. 641).

To remain ethical, clinicians use a decision-making process that identifies the problem and ways of responding to it, evaluates possible options, and considers the outcome after taking action (Knapp et al., 2017). See Figure 11.1. Such a process helps clinicians anticipate problems beforehand and increase the probability of a good outcome. Even if Dr. Helper had agreed to take care of his client's family, directly offering material and emotional care was only one of many available options. He might have offered to do grief work with Edna, helped the family identify services to address their ongoing needs, or located another therapist to help them build needed vocational and communication skills following his client's death. He might have requested a consult to help him identify the likely costs and benefits of each option.

Although anyone can make mistakes, having a well-developed personal moral code, a strong grounding in one's professional ethics, and a good decision-making process for preventing and responding to ethical problems can help a clinician skillfully handle ethical dilemmas (Handelsman, Gottlieb, & Knapp, 2005). The balance of this chapter describes strategies for developing these skills.

FIGURE 11.1 Five-Step Ethical Decision-Making Model

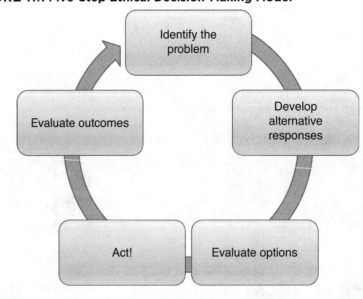

Risk Management

Clinical risk is the risk of disciplinary complaint or legal action during clinical practice. Every clinical intervention incurs some risk of disciplinary complaint or legal action, although that risk is usually fairly low. Some acts, however, are inherently risky, including sexual misconduct, nonsexual dual relationships, problems with fees and insurance, child custody, confidentiality and competency (Knapp et al., 2013). Recognizing risk factors and reducing clinical risk before a problem develops is an important strategy for **risk management** (i.e., reducing the clinical risk incurred during evaluations and treatment).

Knapp and his colleagues (2013) described clinical risk as a function of three types of variables: client, context, and clinician. See Exhibit 11.1. As this formulation suggests, Dr. Saeed's treatment of Andrea Yates was risky because his actions were below professional standards when he failed to request her previous hospital records and inadequately assessed her risk of harm to herself and others (client, context). Dr. Park Dietz made errors in his forensic evaluation for Andrea Yates's first trial; these errors ultimately led to overturning the initial decision in this case. This forensic assessment was inherently risky because it was a very visible and controversial murder trial (context factor). Dr. Dietz also experienced greater risk due to problems in his technical competency, including his misuse of evidence according to Texas mental health law and his suggestion that a *Law & Order* episode had inspired the murders, when such an episode had not aired (Hays, 2002). Perhaps acute stress levels

---

Exhibit 11.1 Factors Impacting Risk of Ethical Complaints or Legal Action

1. **Client factors.** The client's diagnosis, especially personality or dissociative disorders; risk to self or others; history of child abuse; history of legal involvement; and wealth
2. **Context.** Especially settings and interventions with greater legal exposure (e.g., large group practice or hospital), fewer clinical and legal resources (e.g., solo or small group practices), type of service (e.g., custody evaluation), and when there is a multiple relationship (e.g., friend, relative, or sexual partner)
3. **Clinician factors.** Depends on the clinician's knowledge, skills, emotional resources, and experience at a particular point in time, and the match between these and a particular client

Note. Data from Knapp, Younggren, VandeCreek, Harris, and Martin (2013).

---

and his feelings about a mother killing her children compromised Dr. Dietz's emotional competence while completing this assessment and increased his risk during the evaluation (clinician factor).

Clinicians can engage in a number of strategies to decrease their risk of ethical complaint or legal action. They can perform a careful assessment of risk factors and make sure that they have the requisite competency and personal and emotional skills to perform a particular intervention or work with a given client. They can examine their context, identify factors increasing their risk and those that decrease that risk, and manage these risk factors in this setting. They can request peer consultations or supervision when they identify potential problems. They can document their decisions and actions carefully, including their rationale for decisions (Knapp et al., 2013). They can listen to and respond to their clients respectfully and empathically. As Younggren and Gottlieb (2008) concluded, "satisfied consumers have no reason to file complaints or lawsuits" (p. 501).

Preventing and Responding to Ethical Problems

Science cannot resolve moral conflicts, but it can help to more accurately frame the debates about those conflicts.

—Heinz Pagels

No chapter or book can offer answers for all ethical dilemmas. The American Counseling Association (Glosoff & Kocet, 2005), for example, noted that there will often be "reasonable differences of opinion regarding which values, ethical principles, and ethical standards should be applied when faced with ethical dilemmas" (p. 6). Because clinicians are unlikely to read about and consider all ethical dilemmas beforehand, they should have a strategy for responding to dilemmas that will stand up to public scrutiny (Knapp et al., 2013). Having such a strategy is one of the most important risk management strategies for protecting one's reputation and preventing lawsuits.

Competent and effective clinicians prevent potential problems proactively, are willing to recognize difficult feelings about clients (e.g., anger, fear, disgust, sexual attraction), and use these difficult feelings as signals of potential problems. They understand that these feelings can have negative consequences, but also that they can be a therapeutic resource when addressed rapidly and well (Knapp et al., 2017). Clinicians also pay attention to behaviors and emotions that suggest that they may have moved into nontherapeutic roles, including those of parent, friend, host, guest, or caretaker (Slattery, 2005). A family therapist who regularly disciplines the children during sessions rather than letting the parents do so, for example, may have moved into a parental role, which can undermine treatment.

Clinicians might attend the same synagogue as their clients, their children and their clients may be on the same sports team, or they may see their clients at the local coffee shop. Many good clinicians work in settings other than the traditional outpatient office (e.g., client's homes, schools, prisons, nursing homes, or group homes), challenging traditionally defined boundaries of clinical care (Knapp & Slattery, 2004). Work in these settings may be motivated by the client's health or transportation barriers, opportunities to practice and generalize skills learned in treatment, or the desire to meet the needs of underserved populations. A clinician's challenge in these settings is determining when a boundary crossing is reasonable and meets therapeutic goals and when it is problematic (Gutheil & Gabbard, 1993).

Paying attention to behaviors or settings that are at cross-purposes with clinical work can prevent unethical behavior. Some treatment behaviors are consistently identified as inappropriate by clinicians, including engaging in sexual activity, accepting large gifts, bartering, and borrowing money (Pope, Tabachnick, & Keith-Spiegel, 1988). Some settings are associated with expectations that are likely to interfere with treatment. These behaviors and settings may confuse the nature of the relationship—is it professional or more personal?

Boundary crossings can have different meanings and consequences depending on client, clinician, and context factors. Although a clinician's greeting in a public setting might be meant as kind and respectful, some clients may perceive it as intrusive and a break in confidentiality. One client could see an offer to help him remove his coat as kind, while another could see that offer as seductive. Staying ethical requires recognizing clinical risk associated with a given action; remaining aware of the impact of the individual, setting, and situation; and choosing how to act given that assessment (Knapp et al., 2013; Pope & Keith-Spiegel, 2008).

Once a clinician recognizes a problematic situation, consider the best and worst possible outcomes (Pope & Keith-Spiegel, 2008). For example, Dr. Helper's actions had a range of possible outcomes, both positive and negative (Slattery, 2004). He had intended to help Edna and her son during a difficult time, but his actions prevented her from developing the skills and relationships that she needed, caused her to feel exploited, led to his divorce, and damaged his profession. Had he considered other ways of meeting his therapeutic goals, he might have chosen another approach. Was he really the only person who could offer Edna a job, serve as her support system and family, provide treatment, and become her lover? His decisions were shortsighted solutions that attempted to meet her needs directly rather than empowering her to identify strategies for meeting her needs both then and in the future.

Boundary crossings may have neutral or even positive consequences. When it appears that outcomes may be harmful, however, clinicians should discuss the situation with a supervisor, then openly and nondefensively with their clients (Knapp & Slattery, 2004; Pope & Keith-Spiegel, 2008). Listening to and taking clients' viewpoints seriously has the potential to strengthen the therapeutic relationship even under difficult circumstances.

Toward a Positive Approach to Ethics

A man who has committed a mistake and doesn't correct it is committing another mistake.

—Confucius

Codes of ethics have historically been approached from a defensive posture—that is, what should not be done. Legal and ethical standards in the ethics codes describe minimal expectations and identify behaviors leading to disciplinary action when violated and "should not be confused with clinical, ethical, or moral responsibilities" (Pope, 2015, p. 353). Focusing only on the ethics code can cause clients harm if clinicians view the ethical standards as a list of rules to follow and then respond out of fear (Knapp, Gottlieb, & Handelsman, 2018). Many people experience anxiety when thinking about ethics, but this anxiety can interfere with cognitive functioning and lead to poorer decision-making (Kouchaki & Desai, 2015).

Rather than only meeting minimal qualifications, a more positive approach to competency, for example, includes striving for the highest standards of competence on an ongoing basis (Knapp et al., 2017, 2018). When possible, clinicians can look for ways to enhance the nature of their relationships with clients, supervisees, and colleagues rather than only avoiding boundary violations and exploitive relationships. They can involve clients in decisions throughout treatment rather than just at its beginning and develop trustworthy relationships rather than only avoid making prohibited disclosures. Instead of only avoiding being prejudiced or discriminating, they would demonstrate cultural humility, learn about other cultural viewpoints, develop case conceptualizations using this knowledge, and promote fairness throughout their work (Knapp et al.,

2017; Sue & Sue, 2016). As they consider their clinical records, they may ask whether there are better ways of writing them (Pope, 2015).

Every action—scheduling new clients, working with colleagues, and deciding how time outside of work is spent—can be considered through a moral lens (Knapp et al., 2018). In the course of an intake, for example, a clinician could encourage collaboration on a treatment plan (autonomy) and understand the role of culture in their client's presentation (competency and social justice). Consider how the other cases discussed in this chapter might be handled differently using a positive approach to ethics rather than only following a defensive posture.

When treated individually and in isolation, the aspirational principles and ethical standards can lead to an overly simplistic and caretaking approach to practice. For example, avoiding collecting information on child abuse (to avoid further traumatizing a client) can itself be harmful because avoiding these discussions can suggest that being abused is shameful (Becker-Blease & Freyd, 2006). Treating clients as though they are fragile or incompetent can harm because this kind of treatment can create a self-fulfilling prophecy. In contrast, openly discussing abuse, violence, loss, and oppression can be both distressing and helpful.

When balanced by the aspirational principles, the ethical standards provide a rich, thoughtful, and respectful way of doing clinical work. Clinicians can foster autonomy in decisions about end-of-life care, for example, while also recognizing that clients from another culture may perceive the process of decision-making differently than they do. For many middle and upper-class European Americans, responding to a cancer diagnosis is often primarily an individual decision; however, clinicians working with other races, classes, and cultures might consider how treatment and other decisions will affect the family as a whole. Nondisclosure of a cancer diagnosis might be seen as paternalistic in the United States, but in other countries (e.g., Italy, Vietnam, Russia), such nondisclosure might be seen as an act that maintains hope and an ongoing sense of aliveness and connection (Candib, 2002).

Summary

As this discussion has suggested, behaving ethically requires an awareness of the ethical standards and the research findings regarding ethical behavior. Beneficence, nonmaleficence, autonomy, fidelity, integrity, and social justice are aspirational goals of ethical work to strive for. The ethical standards, on the other hand, describe actions to enact and avoid. The five standards discussed at length in this chapter include informed consent, competency, multiple relationships, confidentiality, and sensitivity to differences.

Ethical practice should be more than merely applying ethical standards in a rote manner (Handelsman et al., 2005). Clinicians might consider alternative actions and anticipated consequences, including probable clinical risk. When considering actions with a greater inherent risk, clinicians might attend to emotional responses to clients and motivations for engaging in questionable behaviors. They should recognize and respond to relevant legal statutes, state laws mandating reports of child or elder abuse, court rulings about how to respond to dangerous clients, their personal moral code, agency requirements, and client diagnosis and treatment plan.

Unethical behaviors have wide-ranging, short- and long-term consequences. The profession loses credibility when clinicians betray the public trust. Clients and their families and friends may not seek needed treatment, or, if they do request treatment, may be skeptical about services offered. Clinicians may lose their licenses and livelihood, even though their intentions were good. Empathic, open, nondefensive communications and an ongoing process of reflection can decrease the probability of missteps (Pope & Keith-Spiegel, 2008).

Finally, clinicians should not only consider requirements for ethical behavior but also ways of striving for the highest standards of ethical behavior on an ongoing basis, what we refer to here as **positive ethics**. Pursuing positive ethics may mean considering every act from a moral lens and anticipating both positive and negative consequences to the degree possible.

For Review

Applying Concepts to Your Life

Begin extending your thinking of ethics beyond this book:

1. Write your "ethics autobiography" (Bashe, Anderson, Handelsman, & Klevansky, 2007). Consider your motivations and goals for entering the helping professions. What personal values and ethics guide your behavior? What experiences have influenced your ethical decision-making?

2. Write an anger, conflict, and violence autobiography (D. Kossmann, personal communication, October 3, 2008), paying attention to your experiences and their meanings in your family and relationships. Use this autobiography to identify forms of anger, conflict, and violence to which you are especially sensitive, your typical responses to these feelings, and factors limiting your ability to respond well. What possible consequences might your knowledge of these have (both positive and negative)?

3. As you watch movies or read novels depicting counseling or therapy, think about the clinician's behavior. If you believe the clinician behaved unethically, what would have been more optimal and ethical? If you think about ethical behavior as stepping off onto a "slippery slope," what could that clinician have done better?

Key Terms

aspirational
  principles, 228
autonomy, 228
beneficence, 228
billable hours, 242
boundary
  crossings, 233
boundary
  violations, 233

clinical risk, 246
competence, 231
confidentiality, 232
emotional
  competence, 231
empower, 229
empowered
  collaboration, 230
ethical standards, 229

fidelity, 228
informed consent, 229
integrity, 228
mandated
  reporting, 237
multicultural
  competence, 231
multiple
  relationships, 233

nonmaleficence, 228
positive ethics, 251
pro bono, 242
progress notes, 242
risk management, 246
social justice, 228
technical
  competence, 231

Learn More

For more information about the concepts in this chapter, visit the *Empathic Counseling* companion website at http://pubs.apa.org/books/supp/slattery/.

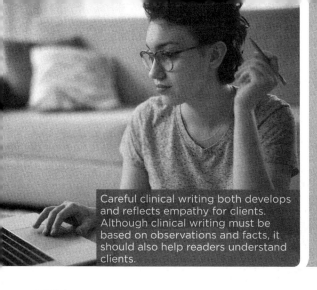

Careful clinical writing both develops and reflects empathy for clients. Although clinical writing must be based on observations and facts, it should also help readers understand clients.

12 Writing Empathic Clinical Reports

Looking Ahead

After reading this chapter you will be able to answer these questions:

1. Why is clinical writing important?
2. Describe how different types of clinical writing serve different purposes.
3. What characterizes effective clinical writing?
4. How is empathy important to clinical writing?

Cases in Empathy

You Start Seeing Yourself as Deserving | D'Ja Jones

Chapter 5 introduced you to D'Ja Jones,[1] the 32-year-old African American college student and mother of three who is in therapy working on her feelings of trauma and loss. In what follows, she discusses her abusive ex-boyfriend and compares him with her current, nonabusive boyfriend:

Jones: I think probably the most . . . craziest thing was thinking to myself as this man [her ex-boyfriend] was *stomping* me, that he had on shoes that I had bought him, and he's stomping me with shoes that I bought him. And that, I don't know why, that as I'm laying here on the ground and

he's just stomping the crap out of me, I don't know why that filtered through my mind, but it did. And it stuck with me. And to this day, I've had boyfriends, you know, I've had boyfriends that I'm just like, "If you're shopping and getting some shoes, can you get me a pair of shoes?" No. Like, to this day, I will never buy another man's shoes . . .

Slattery: But that's *this* story, how about . . . [moving hand to the left, from one story to another]

Jones: How did I get here?

Slattery: Yeah. Are you able to tell a different . . .?

Jones: I am.

[1] D'Ja is a pseudonym. We have also changed some identifying details to protect her confidentiality in this book, which is intended for a broader audience than the video.

(D'JA JONES continued)

Slattery: Your story *here* was "everybody I know betrays me . . ."

Jones: Yep, that was my story.

Slattery: "Or leaves me."

Jones: Or leaves me or abuses me, um . . .

Slattery: [motioning between stories again] But there's a longer . . .

Jones: Yeah, I think that what got me here was—children are amazing because they love you unconditionally, and that helped.

Slattery: And then you start seeing yourself as deserving of . . .

Jones: You do, to a point, but um it was never *kids* who had betrayed me.

Slattery: Right.

Jones: It was always grown-ups.

Slattery: HmHmm.

Jones: Especially men.

Slattery: HmHmm.

Jones: And so for my [current, nonabusive] boyfriend to come in and—geez, I threw so much at this man and whatever I threw, he took it and kept on with me. So, for me to have somebody . . .

Slattery: *Thank* you.

Jones: Right, so for me to have somebody, a *grown-up*, a man love me unconditionally, that was everything. It took a while to penetrate . . .

Slattery: (Draws a deep breath)

Jones: . . . But when once it *did*, it gave me the strength, and it gave me the steps, the first steps that I needed to take to gain back my own self-respect, my own self-worth, my own self-esteem, my own moral compass with who I wanted to be as a woman, and that's how we get here. Because he gave me space to just be messed up . . .

Slattery: To be *you* . . .

Jones: . . . To be messed up, to be a complete, utter mess, and take my time with finding my way back to *who* I was supposed to be and get back on the right track. My kids constantly there. I can yell at them, I can punish them, I can tell no to something, and later they'll still tell me they love me and give me a hug and kiss. And that was *amazing* to me and something worth preserving, and something worth keeping. So, I felt that I needed to do what I needed to do to keep that, because reality is eventually this man was going to get tired, eventually these kids are going to *clue in* that they're not getting back what they're giving out. That was my huge motivation.

Slattery: You knew there was something important here.

Jones: Yes.

Slattery: And if you didn't make a change . . .

Jones: Drastic change.

Slattery: . . . That you were going to lose the things that were most important to you.

Jones: Right.

Slattery: And you did.

Jones: And I did. (APA, 2020, minutes 24:42–28:43)

What Do You Think

1. What things does Dr. Slattery do well—or not so well—in this section of their session?

2. What do you *know* about D'Ja Jones based on this transcript? What can you *guess* about her based on this transcript? How do you recognize the difference?

3. Given what you know or guess about her, write briefly about D'Ja.

4. Consider how your meaning system influences what you include and omit from what you write about her. How does your meaning system influence your word choices and description?

What Do We Know?

People rarely directly provide the answers to our referral questions. A woman may say that she feels depressed, but given the vague way that most people use the word *depressed*, her meaning remains unclear. Does she mean that she is sad today, blue most days, or considering suicide? Are a man's symptoms of multiple sclerosis making it impossible to continue working? He may describe his experience carefully but may underestimate or overestimate symptoms for several reasons (e.g., not wanting to admit problems, not remembering problems).

Clinicians have to make observations and then draw thoughtful inferences from what we see and hear. The **observation** process is the careful, close examination of an object, process, or other phenomenon for the purpose of collecting data about it or drawing conclusions. The type of data collected from observation is **sensory data** (i.e., information that can be seen, heard, felt, tasted, or smelled). In contrast, an **inference** is a conclusion based on observations and reasoning. Different people may observe the same phenomenon but make different inferences about what the observation means. In a clinical context, different clinicians may hear the same verbal statements from a client and see the same nonverbal body language but draw different inferences from what they see and hear.

Which of the following are observations about D'Ja Jones, and which are inferences?

- She is talkative, open, and feels comfortable in this session.
- She has had a significant history of loss, trauma, and betrayals.
- She has a history of difficulty trusting others, especially adult men, but believes that she is more open to others now.
- She blames herself for the abuse, which affects her self-respect, self-worth, self-esteem, and moral compass.
- She has tended to think dichotomously about other people.

Most of the things on this list we might feel pretty confident about, but thoughtful clinicians consider other conclusions too. Although D'Ja was certainly talkative in session, was she open, honest, and comfortable? Although some people talk more when they are comfortable, others talk less. What did she talk about and what did she choose not to talk about?

Most of the other items on this list are inferences. We know what D'Ja reported here, but we don't, for example, know whether she lost her moral compass or felt like she did. We also don't know if her description of her life is stable or more mood-dependent. When we are aware of our inferences, and when we evaluate their veracity, they become **hypotheses**, empirically testable propositions about some fact, behavior, or relationship, usually based on theory, which state an expected outcome resulting from specific conditions or assumptions.

What other information can help clinicians evaluate these hypotheses? Most clinicians pay attention to discrepancies between what people talk about and how they talk about it. For example, D'Ja generally talked about feelings of trauma, anger, and depression but did so in the past tense or, when she discussed these in the present tense, was able to identify ways of handling these symptoms adaptively. Her **affect**, or overtly displayed emotion (as opposed to mood, which is more internal and subjective), was relaxed, and she appeared confident rather struggling to discuss her history. Clinicians may also collect information in a psychosocial history or gather a genogram or timeline. They can administer formal assessments of mood, other psychiatric symptoms, or specialized assessments addressing the issues a client brought to the table. Finally, additional sessions or contacts with other informants (e.g., parents, teachers, employers, partners) can help clinicians put client reports in a larger context and make sense of the things they describe.

Clinical Applications	Ross stopped to think about Davyd, the child he worked with earlier in the day. Davyd (age 9) is HIV-positive and has lived with his aunt since his mother's murder. Davyd has begun picking his nose until it bleeds and flicking blood at adults at his school, which he does more frequently around his math teacher, but rarely at home. Ross is aware of what he sees (observations) and what he thinks these observations mean (inferences) and has been generating propositions that he can test over the course of treatment (hypotheses). What observations, inferences, and hypotheses do you see?

Why Clinical Writing Is Important

I write entirely to find out what I'm thinking, what I'm looking at, what I see and what it means.

—Joan Didion

Writing is an important aspect of most clinical jobs, often taking 25% or more of a clinician's work time, and is an overt reflection of one's otherwise-invisible clinical skills. Clinicians write intake evaluations, session notes, psychological evaluations, and discharge summaries. They also may write letters to the court, probation department, or school, for example.

Careful clinical writing both develops and reflects empathy for clients. Why is empathy important for clinical writing? An empathic approach to developing a clinical assessment has consequences for the clinician's work, the client, and readers. Potential readers of clinical reports include the clients themselves, as well as family members and other professionals working with the client (e.g., schools, courts). Empathy strengthens the therapeutic relationship, leading to stronger and more helpful disclosures from clients. Although clinical writing must be based in observations and facts, it should also help readers understand clients, who may feel crazy to themselves and others (e.g., Raymond Corsini's story, Chapter 6). When clinical reports express a truly empathic understanding, then readers are more likely to understand clients, engage with them, and respond empathically themselves.

This chapter describes clinical writing, especially how it differs from other technical or less formal kinds of writing. In general, this writing is more formal, objective, and detailed, and conclusions and recommendations are carefully supported with data (observations). Because clinical writing systematically organizes information from a number of realms, it can help clinicians avoid confirmation biases and facilitate empathy—both their own and that of others who read the clinical reports.

Clinical writing aims to answer a question and obtain recommendations for the future; however, readers want to know the basis for these recommendations so that they can evaluate their validity for themselves. As a result, most clinical writing starts out by presenting observations and inferences gathered in response to the particular referral question, then forms a clinical assessment of the problem and offers treatment recommendations. This logical organization increases the report's effectiveness and usefulness. Referral questions reflect the referral source's concerns. For example, D'Ja Jones and her psychiatrist might each have different questions underlying their referral. Her psychiatrist might wonder whether D'Ja would benefit from being on medication, while D'Ja wonders whether her history of trauma will interfere with her ability to pursue her career goal, which is to enroll in a clinical psychology graduate program and then become a clinician.

Clinicians should specifically address their referral source's questions. Their writing carefully documents their thinking to help the writer and readers work together as a team, even though time and distance may prevent face-to-face contact. Because writers and readers may not meet, clinicians should be especially careful that their writing is clear and unambiguous.

D'Ja may tell her family what she thinks of her clinician, but no one other than the two of them will directly see their clinical work. Instead, other parties' evaluations of clinicians' work are often based on their writing and their skill to communicate clearly, knowledgeably, and empathically about their work. Readers conclude that the clinician possesses strong clinical skills when reports are well written, well organized, logical, and complete; when the clinical assessment is contextualized, respectful, and empathic; and when conclusions follow observations and are consistent with current theory and research. A clinician's professional reputation is valuable and should be protected and fostered.

Record keeping is required by professional organizations, insurance companies, and state and federal laws. Records document that treatment occurred and was provided with good judgment, meeting the profession's standards of care (Knapp, VandeCreek, & Fingerhut, 2017). Careful, thoughtful documentation can protect clinicians from malpractice claims, ethics violations, and license reviews (Knapp, Younggren, VandeCreek, Harris, & Martin, 2013). Records can also help clinicians identify progress, remember and track symptoms and issues, and develop assessments.

Effective clinical writing takes several forms; each is related to its specific function in clinical work. Some of these forms are discussed in what follows (i.e., brief report and SOAP note), and others are discussed in elsewhere in this volume. Both the form and the content of the writing address the specific purpose of the writing product and respond to the referral question.

Clinical Applications	Leah quickly develops a strong therapeutic alliance with her clients and generally gets positive outcomes and feedback from them. She hates doing paperwork, however, and is frequently weeks behind it. Leah's last client Monday reported that he had some suicidal ideation but that he had no plan to complete suicide. He hanged himself Tuesday morning. Leah had not completed her notes for their Monday session when her supervisor talked to her on Wednesday. What do you think about this situation in terms of effective clinical practice and ethical work?

Brief Reports

He doesn't watch, he notices.

—Thomas D'Evelyn

Although your brief "report" for D'Ja may have been good, it probably was less well developed than the reports written by most counselors, therapists, social workers, and caseworkers. Most reports are between three and 10 single-spaced pages in length, depending on their purpose, perhaps an amount of detail that initially seems impossible for new clinicians. As described in Exhibit 12.1, they often include unusual behavior during the session, cognitive processes, mood and affect, consistency between verbal and nonverbal behaviors across time, style of relationships and relating, client's goals, willingness to change, and more. These build a three-dimensional picture that communicates the clinician's understanding of the client, the presenting problem, and resources or obstacles to treatment. A very brief report based on D'Ja's first session can be found in Exhibit 12.2. Note the descriptions of mental status in this report and compare these to the description of Malcolm Little in Exhibit 6.4.

Exhibit 12.1 Questions to Address in a Report

The questions that follow will not be relevant to every referral question, but they may be helpful to consider. Certainly, your report would be far too long if each were addressed!

Referral question:

❑ Why was client referred for appointment?

❑ Referral questions should be addressed in the report's summary and recommendations should be supported by observations throughout.

Background and demographics:

❑ Describe client in terms of all information influencing the referral question or treatment: age, gender, race, language spoken (if not the native language of the community), immigrant status and acculturation, and custody status (for children of divorced/separated parents).

❑ What background conditions may be relevant to the referral? Include history of violence, family history of substance abuse or mental health problems, and previous treatment history.

Physical appearance:

❑ Does client appear healthy? Are there signs of physical illness or physical limitations?

❑ Is client well-nourished, undernourished, obese? Tall, short or average for age?

❑ Is client well-groomed or, in the case of a dependent child or adult, well cared for?

❑ What is client's general manner of dress? Casual? Formal? Appropriate, careless, or inappropriate for the setting?

❑ Describe the posture and gait? Unremarkable? Tense? Rigid? At ease? Stooped? Slumped?

Symptoms:

❑ What symptoms (e.g., anxiety, depression, inattention, anger, obsessions and compulsions, hallucinations or delusions) are reported? With what frequency and severity?

❑ How long has client had symptoms? Have symptoms remitted in the past? To what does client attribute change?

❑ What formal and informal treatments have been used? Which were effective? In what ways?

❑ When are problems absent? What times of day? What situations? With what people?

❑ What kinds of stressors have been reported? How severe?

❑ What are client's coping level and normal strategies like? Normal? Resilient? Exhausted? Overwhelmed? Deficient skills?

❑ What supports exist? Family? Friends? Congregation? Coworkers? Social services? Are supports adequate, inadequate, broad and well developed, or enabling?

Exhibit 12.1 Questions to Address in a Report *(Continued)*

Cognition:

❏ Is client conscious and alert? Oriented by four (i.e., recognizing who and where they are, the date, and the purpose of meeting)?

❏ Is client able to attend? Distractible? Is client able to concentrate and persist at tasks?

❏ Were problems and strengths in short-term or long-term memory observed? How? Was information never coded, lost, or distorted? Are defects a consequence of dementia, a defense mechanism, problems in encoding or retrieval, or level of intellectual functioning?

❏ What was client's fund of information like? Was it consistent with client's level of education? Has fund of information dropped (either by self-report or history)?

❏ Does client perceive reality in a typical manner? If not, are perceptions positive and adaptive or otherwise (e.g., optimism or pessimism)? Are these defensive distortions or psychosis?

Speech:

❏ What is the flow of speech like? Unremarkable? Loud? Quiet? Mute? Blocked? Pressured? Paucity of ideas and content? Flight of ideas? Tangential?

❏ Is the session's language the client's first or primary language?

❏ How are grammar and word choice? Unremarkable or diverging from standard English? Were words used or pronounced inappropriately? Fluent, thoughtful, and a well-developed vocabulary?

❏ How coherent were client's communications? Does B follow A? Are discontinuities evidence of creativity and enthusiasm or a psychotic disorder? How do you know?

❏ What sorts of preoccupations (if any) characterize the person's thought processes? Death and dying? Current stressors? Mental health? Religion? Relationships? Escaping the situation? Sex? Drugs? Physical illness?

❏ Is client a relatively concrete or abstract thinker? Can client follow metaphors? Understand new ideas? Follow the implications of ideas?

Interpersonal presentation and behavior:

❏ What sort of rapport was established? Did it change across the course of the session? In what manner?

❏ Was client open and honest? How do you know? If there were changes during the session, when did they occur?

❏ What was eye contact like? Unremarkable? Fleeting? Avoided? Absent? Staring? When did it change?

❏ How did client present? As withdrawn? Threatened? Vulnerable? Awkward? Shy? Friendly? Stubborn? Competent?

❏ What is client's self-esteem like? Are strengths recognized and valued? Where is it strongest? Weakest? Physically? Intellectually? Relationally? Socially? Vocationally?

Exhibit 12.1 Questions to Address in a Report *(Continued)*

❏ How does client relate to others? In a warm, trusting manner? Aggressively? Dramatically? Help-seeking? Dependent? Aloof? Self-protective?

❏ Is client socially mature? Does client recognize and follow social norms?

❏ Does client have good common sense? Make good decisions? Engage in behaviors that are maladaptive and self-destructive?

❏ What are interpersonal boundaries like? Is client so reserved that little information is shared or is there an expectation that everything can be asked about or touched?

Mood and affect:

❏ Are self-identified moods consistent with interpersonal presentation? Are moods responsive to external stimuli? Appropriate to the situation or topic in form and intensity?

❏ How labile is affect? Flat and unresponsive? Restricted? Normal and responsive? Broad and demonstrative? Labile and unpredictable?

❏ What are client's dominant and subdominant moods? Depression? Anxiety? Fear? Anger? Joy? Calm? Surprise? Pride? Guilt? Shame? Relaxation? When do moods change? Do mood states seem (by self-report or report of others) typical of other situations?

❏ Is anger or aggression directed inward or outward? With what consequences?

❏ How are mood states expressed? Pacing? Fidgeting? Body tension? Verbal outbursts? Changing the subject?

Behavior:

❏ Is client on time, late, early?

❏ Does client do anything unusual in the course of session (or omit something that is typical)? When? How does this relate to your referral question?

❏ What is the person's activity level like? Unremarkable? Slow? Repetitive? Restless? Agitated? Tremor?

Change process:

❏ What are client's goals? Are they clear and realistic? Does the client perceive them as achievable?

❏ How motivated is the person to change? Does the person believe change is possible?

❏ Does client perceive advantages to changing? What obstacles are identified? Does client perceive obstacles realistically?

❏ Does client possess insight into symptoms and problems? Are problems perceived as internally or externally caused? Does client identify problems as controllable?

❏ What is client's self-efficacy about these particular problems and problems in general? When has client changed successfully in the past—both for this problem or issue and others? What made change possible?

Note. Data from Zuckerman (2019).

Exhibit 12.2 Hypothetical Report on First Session With D'Ja Jones

Intake Report

D'Ja Jones is an attractive and well-groomed 32-year-old African American college sophomore and mother of three. She reported a significant history of loss, trauma, and betrayals that has interfered with her relationships, especially with men. She has previously addressed these concerns during 3 years of psychotherapy but would like an objective second opinion, as she was concerned that her history might cause her problems if she attends a clinical or counseling program.

Ms. Jones was oriented by four and focused rather than distractible during our session. Short- and long-term memory were unremarkable. She is believed to be of above-average intelligence and reports being a conscientious student with very high grades who is considering applying to graduate school in the near future. In her descriptions of events reported, she was able to consider positive and negative aspects of a situation, while admitting that she had been unable to do so in the past.

Ms. Jones has good communication skills. She spoke rapidly and openly about a range of feelings and events, both good and bad, using frequent verbal underlining for emphasis. Her speech generally followed standard conventions of spoken English, although it was also peppered with occasional vernacular (e.g., "most clumsiest"). Her posture was relaxed and open, and she made good eye contact.

We had a good therapeutic relationship, which improved across the course of the session. Initially, Ms. Jones appeared to be composed and agreeable in her communications, telling stories in response to questions, although later she seemed more spontaneous and allowed more give-and-take in interactions. She was open to positive frames of her behavior.

Ms. Jones reported a history of feelings of depression, periods of depression, and relationships that undermined rather than supported her, although denied current symptoms. Her affect was normal range and appropriate to the situation, and she did not appear anxious or depressed, even as she discussed her history of loss and trauma; instead, she seemed confident and pleased with the progress she has made. She talked with pleasure about her academic success, improved parenting, and active involvement in her children's Parent Teacher Organization. She perceives considerable support from her partner and children, who she believes are motivating her to be her very best, both as a student and as a person.

Ms. Jones has a significant history of trauma and loss (e.g., domestic violence, financial abuse, and deaths of her mother and grandmother), and clearly identified a history of symptoms that would have interfered with her goals in the past. She is considering entering a master's program in clinical or counseling psychology after she graduates but wants to be sure that she is academically and personally prepared for graduate school. She accurately attributes blame for problems to extended family or boyfriends who either failed to support her or who actively stole from or abused her. On the other hand, she also accepts responsibility for her role in problems and believes that she had been naïve and had used poor coping skills during this period. She reports high grades, good coping skills, better life choices, and fewer symptoms. She reports wanting to make a difference.

At present, Ms. Jones perceives herself as active and capable of meeting academic and personal goals. She recognizes where she has been, but also how far she has come. She perceives significant social support from her nuclear family, recognizes and uses more adaptive coping strategies, and sees herself as having regained her self-respect, self-worth, and moral compass. Given these changes, it is reasonable to believe that she has the skills, insight, and motivation to become a successful member of the counseling community.

Note. Data from transcript and video of the session (APA, 2020).

As described in Chapter 6, observations should be careful, contextualized, and gathered from diverse sources and settings. Inferences should be based on multiple observations, evaluated relative to several explanations, and drawn only after considering and challenging possible biases and weighing evidence supporting and challenging those explanations.

What Should Be in a Report?

In general, clinicians strive to provide a brief but well-reasoned and complex picture of the client. This picture provides information relevant to the referral question, but rather than only exploring one side, should examine all explanations relevant to the request. For example, will D'Ja's history of trauma interfere with or drive her success in the field? The report should gather data addressing this question and draw a conclusion, even if that conclusion is that more information is needed.

A strong report is insightful and useful. People enter treatment because of confusion about what is happening. D'Ja reported a significant trauma history. The last two paragraphs of the report in Exhibit 12.2 directly address D'Ja's concerns about whether she would be able to succeed in graduate school.

A strong report is clear and specific, avoiding **Barnum statements**, which are statements that appear to be specifically about one person's characteristics but in fact apply to almost everyone. For example, note how the following statement appears to be individualized but is so general as to describe almost anyone. Astrologers, mind readers, and palm readers often use such statements.

> Although you need others to like and admire you, you tend to be critical of yourself, often fearing that you are failing to meet your goals. Although you have some weaknesses, you are generally able to compensate for them. You have considerable untapped potential that has not yet been turned to your advantage. Sometimes you have serious doubts about whether you have made the right decisions or done the right thing.

Barnum statements are often favorable ("considerable untapped potential"), vague ("some weaknesses"), and two-headed, including both favorable and unfavorable information ("need others to like and admire you, you tend to be critical of yourself").

Strong reports are respectful and **strength based**, which means that in addition to recognizing problems and concerns, they specifically document strengths and successes. They acknowledge positive intentions behind a person's actions (e.g., "Tomas reports frequently yelling at his family. His actions, although counterproductive, seem to be his way of caring for and engaging them, from whom he often feels disengaged."). No one makes mistakes all of the time, so a strong report notes these exceptions (e.g., "Although Tomas frequently argues with his wife, arguments are worse when they are tired or stressed. Most fights occur when one party feels dismissed.").

At first glance these statements look like Barnum statements, but the description of Tomas's behavior is more detailed and takes an explicit stand about his behavior and the cause of his problems. Strong reports are also different in being respectful even while identifying problematic behavior. Respectful statements are not gratuitous and unnecessary, but help strengthen the therapeutic alliance and identify treatment strategies building on these strengths (e.g., that his family should find more positive ways of engaging, build in time-outs when they are stressed or tired, strengthen coping skills, and improve listening skills).

What Do You Think?

1. Using the ideas in this section, what would you include in a clinical report for Andrea Yates (Chapters 1, 5, and 11)?

SOAP Notes

When you wish to instruct, be brief; that men's minds take in quickly what you say, learn its lesson, and retain it faithfully. Every word that is unnecessary only pours over the side of a brimming mind.

—*Cicero*

Clinicians write many kinds of reports, depending on the setting and their purpose. The form of intake reports, progress notes, treatment plans, reports to the court, and discharge summaries are different to match their specialized purpose. The report in Exhibit 12.2, for example, might be an intake report for D'Ja Jones's treatment file, or it could be used to formally address her concerns about entering graduate school.

Clinicians also keep notes about their sessions. These can take various forms. Although the following discussion focuses on one particular form, SOAP notes, these ideas also apply to other kinds of notes. **SOAP notes** are brief notes documenting the content of a single session in a very structured format: Subjective, Objective, Assessment, Plan. They also often include a session objective.

Session objective: Although not all agencies include a session objective, it is useful to include the primary objective, both to help other readers track the course of therapy and to keep the clinician on track with the treatment plan.

S: (Subjective) This includes the most striking and central aspects of a client's experience. It is often helpful to quote and use the client's own words.

O: (Objective) This section includes observations rather than inferences. These can include nonverbal behavior, changes in process, recent injuries or changes in symptoms, or summaries of brief assessment tools administered in session.

A: (Assessment) The clinical assessment should be supported by and follow from the S and O sections. Especially when issues of suicidality, homicidality, and abuse are present, clinical decisions and actions should be well documented. Why these decisions?

P: (Plan) What are the plan and objectives for the next session? What homework, if any, was given? When will the next meeting be? This plan should follow from the assessment section and match the next session's objective. Finally, sign and date the note.

An example of a SOAP note for a suicidal client is in Exhibit 12.3.

What Do You Think?

1. Return to the transcript of D'Ja Jones's therapy session and write a SOAP note. How does this note differ from what you might have written for another purpose, clinical or otherwise?

Exhibit 12.3 A Sample SOAP Note

Objective for session: Assess suicidality and stabilize client.

S: "I feel like no one cares and that no one really understands me. I'm not suicidal, though." "I'd never kill myself; I know how that hurts everyone else."

O: Client maintained a closed posture throughout session, with eyes averted. Affect was restricted; she spoke only in response to specific prompts about the proposed safety plan. Nonetheless, she placed ideas for the plan in her own words and tailored the plan to her situation.

A: Client has become increasingly depressed in the weeks since her mother's suicide. Although she also has a number of risk factors for suicide, most specifically, her mother's recent suicide, she denies serious suicidal ideation or plan. In addition, she has not attempted suicide since she stopped drinking 4 years ago, is aware that her suicide would "kill" her best friend and does not want to hurt her, is not using any substances, is not impulsive, and developed a good safety plan (see chart). Our strong therapeutic alliance and her supportive relationship with her best friend are additional protective factors.

P: Will not hospitalize at this point, although will continue to monitor suicidal ideation and adherence to safety plan and identify additional ways of stabilizing her. Homework: Monitor mood on scale of 1 to 10 throughout day, increasing contacts and requests for support from friend or brief phone contact with me when suicidality is above 6. Next: Tuesday, 12/26, 3 p.m. 12/19/19 Carmen D. Gabriel-Rodriguez, PhD, Licensed Psychologist

Recommendations for Guiding Clinical Writing

Practice, practice, practice writing. Writing is a craft that requires both talent and acquired skills. You learn by doing, by making mistakes and then seeing where you went wrong.

—Jeffrey A. Carver

Making observations and writing reports about others should be done carefully because the recorded observations and conclusions often have significant consequences for clients. Consider the following recommendations for writing about clients and clinical interviews.

Be succinct. Include only the most important aspects of the session including major session themes, changes in functioning, and concerns.

Be objective. Others watching the session should be able to agree with this description; conclusions should not be colored by the clinician's biases. Inferences should be supported and reflect an awareness of and rejection of competing conclusions.

Be strength-based. Writing in a strength-based manner is a good habit and increases the clinician's ability to be hopeful during sessions. Further, clinicians should consider that clients and other parties (e.g., family, attorneys, psychiatrists) may read what was written about them. Clinicians should not lie, obscure problems, or be vague; instead, be clear, honest, and respectful, while including strengths as well as weaknesses.

CYA[2]. Clinicians should document a client's suicidality, homicidality, and anything done to keep the client and significant others safe. Careful documentation of decisions and the decision-making process can reduce risk of ethical complaint or legal proceedings (Knapp et al., 2013; Younggren & Gottlieb, 2008). Dr. Gabriel-Rodriguez's reasonable and competent interventions documented under A in Exhibit 12.3 would protect her from legal suit and ethical complaint if this client had completed suicide after their appointment.

CYCA[3]. Not every piece of information needs to be included in a note. This is especially true for potentially embarrassing and irrelevant information, which should be included only if relevant to their work.

Be tentative about those things that are unknown. Clients will say many things, some of which are truthful, others that they may believe to be true. They will tell white lies and outright deceptions. When they say something that has not been confirmed elsewhere, especially if there may be some question about what they say, clinicians should make appropriately tentative

[2]Cover your a**.
[3]Cover your client's a**.

statements, prefacing their statement with verbs such as *reported*, *stated*, or *said*. For example, "Ms. Durrant reported that her husband became very suspicious and angry when she prepared a fancy dinner for the two of them." Her clinician does not know whether he became suspicious and angry or whether she just believed he did.

In addition to misrepresenting others' behaviors and intentions, clients may also intentionally or unintentionally inaccurately report their own thoughts, emotions, and behaviors. If Ms. Durrant *says* that she is very committed to treatment, unless there are other observations supporting this conclusion, the strongest statement one can make is, "Ms. Durrant stated she is very committed to addressing her use of alcohol at the present time." If her clinician believed she was very committed, he should give the evidence for his conclusion,

> Ms. Durrant appears very committed to addressing her use of alcohol at the present time. She reports wanting to do "whatever it takes" to stay clean, has attended every scheduled session, and has completed all homework carefully. Her husband and children are very supportive of her sobriety without either nagging or undermining her.

When no additional observations directly support the client's report, smart clinicians keep in mind that most people in substance abuse treatment programs are ambivalent about change. She has many reasons to deceive herself and her clinician.

Remember there are multiple hypotheses for any single observation. Wise clinicians consider all reasonable hypotheses for observations before drawing conclusions. They evaluate evidence both supporting their conclusions and countering them, while being fair.

> Although Ms. Durrant appears very committed to change and has been working hard in treatment, she has been in a very supportive setting and has not been exposed to triggers that have put her at risk in the past. Furthermore, she has many reasons to claim to be committed to change even if she is not, chief of which is her fear that her husband will leave her if he believes that she is using again.

Don't be afraid to draw reasonable conclusions. Despite these warnings, clinicians are paid to draw conclusions. They should draw reasonable and supported conclusions that are responsive to the referral question, while providing the evidence for their conclusions.

> Although Ms. Durrant continues to have occasional slips, she has worked hard in treatment, attending sessions regularly and going well beyond requirements for homework assignments. Because she has done well in treatment and has no history of neglecting her children, even when she has been drinking, her children should be returned to her as soon as possible. However, as her drinking has the potential to negatively impact her children, she should continue to be involved with treatment, and her treatment compliance should be considered in future custody decisions.

Be respectful. Empathic clinicians treat clients with respect, as people rather than objects. This does not mean that clinicians whitewash what they say; however, they should not demonize clients for having symptoms or making mistakes. They recognize and write about both their clients' weaknesses and their strengths. They observe exceptions to the problem, as exceptions are a more complete description of the situation and may offer opportunities for treatment. They use **person-first language**, which focuses on the person rather than the problem (American Psychological Association, 2019). When using person-first language, place the person first and the problem second because the person is more important than the disability or diagnosis (e.g., "women diagnosed with anorexia" rather than "anorexic women"). Avoid equating people and their conditions and descriptors that are slurs or have unnecessarily negative overtones (e.g., "child with cerebral palsy" rather than "cripple"). Instead, emphasize abilities (e.g., "uses a wheelchair" rather than "confined to a wheelchair") and recognize other aspects of the person.

> In the last 90 days, Ms. Durrant reports having "slipped" three times, consuming between one drink and a bottle of vodka on each occasion. Nonetheless, she reports calling her sponsor each time and has increased her attendance at AA meetings after each slip. She has noted which situations put her at risk and has been avoiding or changing these situations so they are less problematic. She has identified a series of coping mechanisms that she is using with increasing consistency to prevent relapses. She also reports now catching slips earlier in the cycle. Last week she called the Center when contemplating drinking, but before she had actually had a drink.

Exclude irrelevant information. Reports should clearly answer the referral question. Irrelevant information should not be included even when interesting. For example, it may be interesting and noteworthy that Ms. Durrant has a history of being sexually abused, but in discussing her ability to work well within a 12-Step Program, anything beyond a quick mention of her history is probably gratuitous and could be damaging. On the other hand, if clinicians believe that treatment will be compromised by Ms. Durrant's flashbacks and difficulties with trust, they would be remiss in not discussing her history.

Consider the audience. What Ms. Durrant's therapist needs to know is significantly different from what her children's teachers need. Just because Ms. Durrant is in treatment does not mean that she loses her right to privacy. In fact, disclosing protected health information without permission is both illegal and unethical and could leave clinicians open to a lawsuit.

Choose tense thoughtfully. Use past tense to describe things that have already happened (things that occurred in the session or before it). For example, "She appeared anxious during the session and frequently fiddled with her pearls. Despite this, she was open in disclosing problems." Use present tense to describe things that are currently happening (i.e., their current age, where they are employed). That is, "Ms. Durrant is a 46-year-old Native American mother of two, currently employed as a nurse practitioner at a local hospital."

Proofread carefully. Counseling and therapy usually occur behind closed doors. As a result, conclusions about the quality of clinical work are often based on clinical records and reports. When writing and the thinking in that writing are sloppy, readers generally assume the work is also sloppy and un-professional. Learning to write quickly and well is worth it!

Summary

Effective writing about clients takes several different forms; each is related to its specific purpose (e.g., a progress note, a report, treatment plan, discharge summary). Some of these forms have been discussed here, while others were discussed in Chapters 6 and 10. Both the form and the content of the writing address the specific purpose of the writing product and answer the referral question.

Clinical writing should be succinct, objective, and strength-based. SOAP notes, for example, are an especially succinct and objective style of writing used to document interviews and therapy sessions. Notes and reports should balance the needs of both the client and clinician. Clinical writing should include enough information to document competent interventions and assessments, without including unnecessarily embarrassing material that puts clients at risk. Consider multiple explanations and be appropriately tentative; yet draw reasonable conclusions, while acknowledging the limitations of those conclusions.

Readers draw conclusions about clinical abilities based on a clinician's writing style and inferences. Therefore, effective clinicians write carefully, accurately, and respectfully, addressing both referral questions and the needs and understanding of their audience. Clinicians' reputations depend on the quality of their clinical writing and are worth protecting.

For Review

Applying Concepts to Your Life

1. Observe how friends and family describe others over the next week. How do these descriptions differ from how clinicians would describe them? What descriptions from either professional or nonprofessional sources make you uncomfortable? Why?

2. As you begin working on your writing, pay attention to the aspects you do well, as well as those you would like to improve. How can you strengthen your writing? Develop a plan for improving your observational and writing skills.

Key Terms

affect, 256

Barnum
  statements, 263

hypotheses, 255

inference, 255

observation, 255

person-first
  language, 268

sensory data, 255

session objective, 264

SOAP notes, 264

strength based, 263

Learn More

For more information about the concepts in this chapter, visit the *Empathic Counseling* companion website at http://pubs.apa.org/books/supp/slattery/.

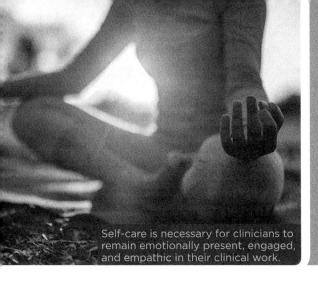

Self-care is necessary for clinicians to remain emotionally present, engaged, and empathic in their clinical work.

13 Self-Care

Looking Ahead ⅢⅢ➡

After reading this chapter you will be able to answer these questions:

1. What are the roles of self-awareness and self-care in empathic and effective work? Why are they important?

2. What dangers do empathic clinicians face in their work?

3. How do empathic clinicians effectively respond to their personal and professional ethics?

4. What types of coping strategies are best for dealing with stress?

5. How can we proactively prevent stress?

"How Do You Do It?" ❙ Sheila Carluccio

Sheila Carluccio posted the following on an electronic mailing list:

> I'm tossing this out for discussion as I have recently returned part-time to private practice after a long medical leave. Currently, I find myself trying to carefully balance client care, with personal care, with caring for my mother who is in the hospital after undergoing open heart surgery.
>
> One year ago my mother had a stroke which left her partially blind. At the time, I queried the listserv for psychologists in our area who might provide specialty treatment for medical issues in the geriatric population. I received not only recommendations for

referrals, but also a flood of warm, supportive responses from this list; many shared the difficulties they too faced caring for ill and elderly relatives. It was a difficult time, and my focus was about obtaining the best possible referrals for her.

But that's not why I am writing now. This time it's about *me*. This post is about balancing caretaking with self-care. About struggling to advocate for a hospitalized relative when you believe you see medical mishaps that may not endanger life but impact the quality of care they are receiving, struggling with feeling your emotions without acting out in such emotionally charged medical situations, struggling to be present to clients when an ill family member is on

(SHEILA CARLUCCIO continued)

your mind, struggling with guilt watching family members pour out their caretaking 24/7 because you're struggling with feeling *selfish* if you include self-care in that equation. Struggling with the ever evolving personal awareness that life is fragile and short and should not be wasted.

I hope I do not come across as *whining*. I know others here have been through much worse. I'd like to hear how they worked their way through self-care while remaining caring to personal and professional others. (S. Carluccio, personal communication, March, 2009)

What Do You Think?

1. What barriers to self-care does Ms. Carluccio identify? What impact does she see this situation having on her work as a psychologist?

2. What do you think of a clinician who, like Ms. Carluccio, asks these questions? Why? What about one who is stressed and distressed but who does not ask such questions?

3. If you've asked similar questions about yourself, how did you feel about doing so? When were you most likely to ask these questions?

Dangers in Providing Empathic Therapy

As soon as there is life, there is danger.

—Ralph Waldo Emerson

Providing effective treatment requires maintaining clear interpersonal boundaries between self and clients; remaining healthy, emotionally present, and engaged in clinical work; and helping clients deal with traumatic issues without vicariously experiencing trauma. To ensure these needs are met, good self-care is necessary. **Self-care** involves taking actions to protect or improve one's health and well-being.

What happens when clinicians neglect self-care? Clinicians who are out of balance in their personal lives may react impulsively toward clients whom they perceive as demanding, manipulative, or irritating. They may also engage in enabling behaviors that do not meet the client's long-term goals because they are unable to step back and recognize the big picture for treatment. Three particular risks that these clinicians face are blurred boundaries, compassion fatigue, and vicarious traumatization (Knapp, Younggren, VandeCreek, Harris, & Martin, 2013).

Blurred Boundaries

Ethical relationships are "associated with honesty and decency . . . and an absence of deceit, exploitation, misuse, injury, and violation of other people" (Zachrisson, 2014, p. 246). **Boundaries** provide a shared understanding that defines the roles for the clinician and client, the nature of their relationship, and the ground rules of therapy. These ground rules describe both the structure (e.g., time, place, money) and the content (what actually can and cannot transpire between clinician and client) of session time (Smith & Fitzpatrick, 1995).

Most clinicians would not intentionally engage in **boundary violations**, or behaviors deviating from professional norms with high potential for negative consequences for the client. For example, one boundary violation with extremely high potential to harm clients is when a clinician has sex with the client. Few newly licensed psychologists expect to have sex with a client over the course of their career, yet in one, now-dated study, about 9.4% of men and 2.5% of women reported having had a sexual relationship with at least one client over the course of their career (Pope, Keith-Spiegel, & Tabachnick, 1986). This study has not been replicated more recently, so we do not know the current incidence of client–therapist sexual relationships. Many also reported at least occasionally having had romantic or sexual feelings toward a client. Ethical and competent clinicians recognize sexual feelings, engage in regular self-care to reduce the risk of engaging in boundary violations, request consultations to prevent harm to clients, and keep current on ethical guidelines through readings, supervision, and trainings (Pope & Vasquez, 2016).

In contrast to boundary violations, **boundary crossings** are behaviors deviating from the strictest professional norms, including small self-disclosures. Boundary crossings are less inherently risky than boundary violations, but even boundary crossings can have dangerous consequences. They can undermine therapy by confusing the concrete with the symbolic, suggesting that clients' needs and desires can and should be met in therapy rather than in the client's "real" life, and thus increase the risk of boundary violations (Zachrisson, 2014). Boundary crossings may also increase the risk of engaging in boundary violations, or, conversely, clinicians engaging in boundary violations appear to engage in boundary crossings more frequently. One study found that clinicians reporting some types of boundary crossings (e.g., disclosing details of a personal stressor, crying in front of a client, giving the client unused sports or theatre tickets) were more likely to report engaging in sexual relationships with clients (Lamb & Catanzaro, 1998).

To reduce the risk of harming clients, clinicians should acknowledge when they are considering a boundary crossing, explore their motivations for the behavior, evaluate the suspected costs and benefits of engaging in it, and thoughtfully discuss such deviations from professional norms with colleagues, supervisors, or the clients themselves (Barnett, Lazarus, et al., 2007; Knapp et al., 2013). Clinicians may also recognize blurred boundaries when they have moved into nontherapeutic roles or are engaging in behaviors that are at cross-purposes with clinical work (Pope, Tabachnick, & Keith-Spiegel, 1988; Slattery, 2005).

Although ethical and competent clinicians can readily agree in theory that setting healthy boundaries is an essential part of good clinical work, identifying and implementing healthy boundaries in practice can be difficult because of the wide range of accepted theoretical models, interventions, and settings used in the field. Psychoanalytically oriented therapists may see self-disclosure and supportive work as ineffective, inappropriate, and outside acceptable boundaries, whereas clinicians working in community settings, offering teletherapy, visiting clients who are seriously ill or have transportation problems, or doing in vivo generalization of skills in the community may perceive different boundaries as effective and helpful (Slattery & Knauss, 2018; Slattery, Knauss, & Kossmann, 2018). Drawing effective boundaries, however, often requires particular attention to the ethical issues raised by the situation (e.g., informed consent, confidentiality, competency) and thoughtful consideration of the research and theoretical framework addressing such work.

Clinical Applications	Phyllis has been having difficulty with her teenaged sons (ages 14 and 15), who violate family rules and reject parental opinions. She has been thinking a lot about her client, Charlie (age 13), whose parents are critical and neglectful of his needs. He has been in crisis recently, and their sessions have begun extending beyond their normal limits. What should she consider as she evaluates whether these boundary crossings are helpful or problematic? What might she do if she believes the boundary crossings are problematic?

✳ ✳ ✳

Jonas has a client with significant agoraphobia who has difficulty making appointments. She has asked Jonas to offer therapy in her home. What should he consider before agreeing to do so?

Compassion Fatigue

Compassion fatigue, also sometimes called *burnout*, refers to a progressive loss of idealism, energy, and sense of purpose for the work of therapy and is characterized by emotional exhaustion, an increased depersonalization of clients, and a decreased sense of personal accomplishment. Clinicians experiencing compassion fatigue may feel hopeless, disengage from their clients, and experience symptoms of stress, depression, and anxiety (Wicks, 2008). Compassion fatigue is caused by work-related factors, such as excessive workload (although not necessarily more client hours), aggressive and threatening clients, clients with personality disorders, and overinvolvement with clients (Rupert, Miller, & Dorociak, 2015). Therapists experiencing compassion fatigue also complain about the difficulties of knowing whether they are being helpful, identifying available resources, implementing culturally relevant treatment modalities well, and developing the kinds of personal relationships they want (Alani & Stroink, 2015). On the other hand, a sense of control, workplace support, self-care, a sense of personal accomplishment, and job satisfaction are related to lower levels of compassion fatigue (Rupert et al., 2015).

Cases in Empathy

How Can We Avoid Being "Institutionalized"? ❙ Michael Partie

Michael Partie (2005) described providing clinical services to clients who are institutionalized. Clinicians who work in such settings are at high risk of compassion fatigue—which Partie referred to as clinicians becoming "institutionalized" themselves—unless they act to prevent this from happening.

> The people we support live in very small worlds, worlds often kept small by the manner in which we deliver services. Helping people expand the size of their worlds— socially, vocationally, physically, emotionally, recreationally, and existentially—must be a top priority. Institutionalization isn't about the kind of buildings or real estate one occupies, it's about the loss of power, movement, freedom, and vision.
>
> But how do we keep ourselves from becoming institutionalized?

> [In *A Leg to Stand On*, the neurologist] Oliver Sacks points out that the process [of institutionalization] is often unseen and unheard, and can overtake any of us unaware. Awareness and the will to resist institutionalizing influences in ourselves and in others is a good start. Reflecting on our own practices and questioning our assumptions can keep us from becoming lazy or lapsing into superstition. Celebrating successes—individual and group—can keep us positively focused. Practicing honesty and individual integrity, honoring the good work of others, courageously confronting our colleagues when needed, receiving praise with grace and correction with gratitude, and perhaps most important of all, approaching the lives of others with humility, are all ways we can keep our humanity as we help others to live full lives. (para. 9–11)

What Do You Think?

1. Have you ever felt yourself becoming more cynical or emotionally exhausted, losing your energy and sense of purpose—what Partie refers to as becoming "institutionalized"? If so, what about the situation put you at risk? What helped you recognize this process? What helped you break free?

2. Or, if you are feeling stuck now, what has helped during better periods?

Vicarious Traumatization

The expectation that we can be immersed in suffering and loss daily and not be touched by it is as unrealistic as expecting to be able to walk through water without getting wet.

—Rachel Naomi Remen

When clinicians work with clients who are victims or survivors of violence and other traumatic events, they are at risk for vicarious traumatization, sometimes called *secondary victimization*. **Vicarious traumatization** refers to a clinician's cumulative and progressive loss of meaning or sense that the world is a benevolent place as a result of exposure to clients' descriptions of trauma. Such exposure can lead to clinicians' distancing, insensitivity, and loss of trust in others, as their clients' experiences and meaning systems begin to adversely influence their own perspectives.

By definition, vicarious traumatization results from empathic engagement with clients' traumatic material. Empathic clinicians risk absorbing that pain into themselves by being open to clients' pain. For example, clinicians may incorporate their clients' painful stories into their own meaning system, leading to flashbacks, trauma dreams or intrusive thoughts, all symptoms of posttraumatic stress (Dunkley & Whelan, 2006). In a meta-analysis of 38 studies, risk factors for vicarious trauma included having a personal trauma history as well as a high number and percentage of traumatized clients on their caseload. However, social support and supervisory support appear helpful (Hensel, Ruiz, Finney, & Dewa, 2015).

Clinical Applications	Sam is a second-year graduate student who has recently been conducting therapy with a client with a history of childhood abuse. Since beginning this work, he has become more irritable and has been having problems sleeping. Should he should tell his supervisor? What else, if anything, should he do?

※ ※ ※

Sam read some research on vicarious traumatization and became curious about the roles of meaning and purpose in his life, particularly the impact of his recent weakening of his sense of meaning. What actions should he consider taking at this point, given this change?

Remaining Vigilant to Dangers in Providing Empathic Therapy

In dealing with those who are undergoing great suffering, if you feel "burnout" setting in, if you feel demoralized and exhausted, it is best, for the sake of everyone, to withdraw and restore yourself. The point is to have a long-term perspective.

—*Dalai Lama*

The American Psychological Association's (2017a) *Ethical Principles of Psychologists and Code of Conduct* prescribes that psychologists "strive to be aware of the possible effect of their own physical and mental health on their ability to help those with whom they work" (p. 3). As a result, clinicians regularly assess their emotional competence, in addition to their technical and multi-cultural competencies, especially as they influence clinical practice (Knapp et al., 2013; Wise & Barnett, 2016). Remaining ethical across time requires being vigilant to signs of changes in emotional competence within and across sessions, including blurred boundaries, increased cynicism and boredom, failures in empathic responding, and vicarious traumatization (Knapp, VandeCreek, & Fingerhut, 2017). Such self-awareness and self-care also promote clinicians' personal health and professional satisfaction (Pope & Vasquez, 2016). Because these dangers are ever-present for empathic clinicians, it is critical that clinicians learn about, recognize, and remain vigilant in their own work for signs of these problems. This vigilance requires a commitment to honest and ongoing self-evaluation and a willingness to make changes in their work when problems are detected.

Clinicians can recognize symptoms of burnout in their negative attitudes about clients and clinical work; increased fatigue, lack of energy, and mistakes; more anxiousness and fear at work; use of work to avoid negative feelings; and a loss in interest in things that had previously been engaging (Pope & Vasquez, 2016). Most, if not all, clinicians occasionally feel bored, exhausted, cynical, and nonempathic; however, ideally, clinicians will recognize these signs and intervene quickly. Finally, as described in Chapter 11, clinical risk can be thought of as a function of three variables (i.e., client, clinician, and context; Knapp et al., 2013). Clinicians can monitor these variables on an ongoing basis as a signal of times when they must be especially alert to problems.

Effective clinicians regularly assess skills, knowledge, emotional resources, and experience; moderate ongoing risk factors; manage stressors proactively; and reduce cognitive demands during crises. Many useful checklists and assessments are available to help clinicians recognize and prevent problems proactively—or at least as early as possible. See Exhibits 13.1 and 13.2. Clinicians may use meditation, reflective journaling, and informal and formal consultations with trusted colleagues to appraise their management of difficult clients and ongoing emotional competence (Thériault, Gazzola, Isenor, & Pascal, 2015). Different strategies may work for different clinicians or for the same clinician at different times; what is important is that clinicians recognize and engage in those activities that effectively maintain their emotional competence across time (Wise & Barnett, 2016).

Other Stressors in the Life of a Clinician

Although the empathy-related dangers just described have been identified as particularly problematic for clinicians endeavoring to remain empathic and balanced, it is important to note that clinicians face many other stressors. Some of these stressors are specific to the work of helping professionals, and others

Exhibit 13.1 Self-Care Assessment for Psychologists

Instructions: The items below contain statements about your personal and professional activities. Please use the following scale to indicate how often you engage in each activity.
How Often: 1 2 3 4 5 6 7
      Never   Always

1. I spend time with people whose company I enjoy. _____
2. I maintain a professional support system. _____
3. I take part in work-related social and community events. _____
4. I take breaks throughout the workday. _____
5. I participate in activities that promote my professional development. _____
6. I cultivate professional relationships with my colleagues. _____
7. I find ways to foster a sense of social connection and belonging in my life. _____
8. I am mindful of triggers that increase professional stress. _____
9. I seek out activities or people that are comforting to me. _____
10. I connect with organizations in my professional community that are important to me. _____
11. I make a proactive effort to manage the challenges of my professional work. _____
12. I avoid workplace isolation. _____
13. I spend time with family or friends. _____
14. I find ways to stay current in professional knowledge. _____
15. I share positive work experiences with colleagues. _____
16. I try to be aware of my feelings and needs. _____
17. I take some time for relaxation each day. _____
18. I avoid overcommitment to work responsibilities. _____
19. I monitor my feelings and reactions to clients. _____
20. I share work-related stressors with trusted colleagues. _____
21. I maximize time in professional activities I enjoy. _____

SCAP Scoring

Scoring of the five SCAP subscales:

Professional Support
Total Items: 2, 6, 12, 15, 20

Cognitive Awareness
Total Items: 8, 11, 16, 19

Professional Development
Total Items: 3, 5, 10, 14, 21

Daily Balance
Total Items: 4, 17, 18

Life Balance
Total Items: 1, 7, 9, 13

Note. Adapted from "Development of a Self-Care Assessment for Psychologists," by K. E. Dorociak, P. A. Rupert, F. B. Bryant, and E. Zahniser, 2017, *Journal of Counseling Psychology, 64,* p. 329. Copyright 2017 by the American Psychological Association.

Exhibit 13.2 Questions for Monitoring Professional and Personal Health

Match between person and clinician

- Who do you want to be as a person? As a clinician? To what degree are you meeting these goals?

- In what ways is your clinical work different than you had expected? How are these discrepancies rewarding or sources of stress?

- How do your emotional, relational, and work styles affect your clinical work? In what ways do the positive aspects of your style sometimes cause problems?

- Are your personal strengths, values, and goals a good match for your work demands? How do you handle those places where there is a poor match?

Stressors and supports at work

- How stressed are you at work? In what ways does this affect your work? Your relationship with coworkers?

- What challenges have you experienced in your professional life (e.g., mandated reporting of abuse, client suicide, client complaint)? How have you responded to these? What have you learned?

- To what degree does the number and type of clients you see, frequency of problems and crises, and degree of progress work for you? To what degree are you able to do the kinds of work that you value and at which you feel competent? What other rewards are you obtaining from your work?

- How are you feeling about your clients? To what degree are you able to be hopeful, respectful, and nonjudgmental? To what degree do you see your work with clients as enabling, irrelevant, effective or empowering?

- Are you experiencing stressors in your practice as threats or harm? Have you already experienced physical or psychological harm in your practice? How have you responded to this? Instead, are you feeling challenged by your clinical practice? When?

- How supported do you feel by colleagues in your agency, community, or state and national networks? Are you able to receive helpful peer support and consultations when needed? To what degree do you feel that your colleagues respect you and your work?

- If you have office staff, how supported do you feel by them? Are they able to help you where you especially need help? Is your office climate positive?

- How physically and emotionally safe do you feel at work? If you feel unsafe, what are you doing to feel safer? Are these accommodations helping you develop as a professional, or do they interfere with your personal and professional work?

- How financially safe are you feeling at work? Are you feeling that your financial future is safe and solid or that your client base is contracting and disappearing? Do you have a good retirement plan? A good health care plan?

- What concerns do you have about your future in the profession? What concerns do you have about the future of the profession? How are you handling these?

- If you have considered leaving your current position or the field, how have you handled your concerns?

Exhibit 13.2 Questions for Monitoring Professional and Personal Health (Continued)

Self-care

- To what degree are you monitoring your emotional competency and how challenges in your personal life affect your professional life?

- What messages did you learn from your family of origin about self-care? What messages about self-care do your friends and family give you now?

- What barriers to self-care do you recognize? When is self-care easier?

- What have you learned about your self-care needs (e.g., exercise, healthy diet, friendships, family time, religion and spirituality, psychological growth)? Are you on track with meeting these needs? If not, where would you want to spend more time?

- To what extent do your family and friends understand, value, and respect the work that you do?

- To what degree do you feel like you are able to maintain a healthy balance—for you—between your work and your personal life?

- To what degree do you feel like your life has a sense of meaning and purpose?

- To what degree do you feel like you are able to act within your values, both at work and in your personal life?

- To what degree do you feel like you are moving toward meaningful personal goals?

Note. Data from Norcross and VandenBos (2018), Pope and Vasquez (2016) and Wise and Barnett (2016).

are more ubiquitous in human life. Regardless of their nature, stressors can have a cumulative deleterious impact on clinicians' well-being and reduce their effectiveness in helping others. Dealing effectively with these stressors begins with recognizing them. Weiss (2004) identified four domains of stressors particularly relevant to counselors and therapists: client-induced stress, stress due to the work environment, self-induced internal stress, and stress related to events in the clinician's personal life.

Client-induced stress is a by-product of the nature of clinical work. For example, clinicians may encounter angry clients who throw tantrums or have outbursts; whose intense depression, suicidal ideation, or threats are frightening; who make accusations of incompetence or lack of caring; and who leave treatment prematurely (Weiss, 2004). Each of these types of clients raises difficult questions:

- What is the clinician's role, if any, in current problems? To what degree are the client's accusations accurate?

- Are assessments and interventions on track? Do they reflect the quality care that this client deserves?

- Is this client receiving the appropriate type and level of service? Does this client require a more intensive service than can be realistically offered in this setting?
- What changes, if any, would better stabilize this client?

Work environment stress derives from the settings in which clinicians work, including time pressure, excessive caseload size, organizational politics, unsupportive colleagues, poor supervision, excessive paperwork, and lack of control in the workplace (Hensel et al., 2015). In one study, clinicians working in agency settings reported lower levels of accomplishment and satisfaction and more stress than those in solo or group independent practice (Rupert & Kent, 2007), perhaps because those working in agencies have less control over their workloads, more exposure to managed care issues, greater time pressures, and more paperwork. Beginning clinicians may also experience additional stressors, including the pressures of obtaining licensure while also mastering clinical skills and obtaining the breadth and depth of experience needed to perform with adequate levels of competence.

Self-induced stress includes clinicians' expectations for themselves, which may be unrealistic, as well as fears of failure, self-doubt, perfectionism, need for approval, and emotional depletion (Weiss, 2004). Some levels of fear and concern can be normal and helpful (**adaptive**) because they can help clinicians recognize and prevent problems in treatment. However, excessive, unrealistic, and continuing fears and negative self-evaluations can themselves be problematic (**maladaptive**).

Event-related stress comes from many sources, including major life transitions, physical or medical problems, money pressures, and family issues (Weiss, 2004). Everyone is prone to these stressors, clinicians probably no more so than average. Such stressors, however, can increase the amount of stress experienced during professional stressors.

Clinical Applications	Phyllis has been having a difficult time with her sons and worrying excessively about her client Charlie. She believes that her supervisor is hypercritical of her, and she has become increasingly frustrated at work. Phyllis knows she has a difficult caseload and has been having a difficult time keeping up with her paperwork. What would you suggest she do?

✳ ✳ ✳

Harley is a supervisor of a small department in an urban community mental health center. Her staff has high caseloads and is paid poorly, neither of which she can control. What can she do to reduce their stress, increase their job satisfaction, and prevent compassion fatigue?

Personal and Professional Identities

I now know myself to be a person of weakness and strength, liability and giftedness, darkness and light. I now know that to be whole means to reject none of it but to embrace all of it.

—Parker Palmer

For many people, clinical work is "not only a job but also a calling, or vocation, a worthy profession that is chosen at least in part to provide a sense of meaningful activity and personal fulfillment" (Orlinsky et al., 2005, p. 11). A clinician's sense of meaning and purpose, values, and professional goals influences the nature of this calling and the trajectory of that vocation. To continue to flourish while doing this work, clinicians must develop clear personal and professional identities that foster ethical, empathic, and effective clinical work.

Clinicians should assess their strengths and weaknesses, skills, and emotional resources on an ongoing basis, with an awareness that these qualities will fluctuate depending on life stressors, ongoing professional development, and the particular intervention (Knapp et al., 2013). A careful personal skill inventory acknowledges that all characteristics are a double-edged sword: Strengths can also be weaknesses and vice versa (Bashe, Anderson, Handelsman, & Klevansky, 2007). A clinician may be proud of her empathy, for example, but also aware of how it sometimes interferes with her ability to be objective in her assessments. Another clinician may recognize that he sets strong personal boundaries and engages in regular self-care, yet finds it difficult to respond well to crisis calls outside of regular work hours. Recognizing these strengths and weaknesses can be one aspect of a proactive strategy for maintaining an effective practice.

Personal identity includes self-perceptions and defining values, goals, and characteristics. **Professional identity** may include some parts of personal identity but focuses more narrowly on the meaning and value given to membership in a field and adopting a theoretical or philosophical perspective, the tasks and goals that are central to that identity, and the ethical principles guiding that work. Professional identity influences not only what is done but also *how* it is done. Given their client population, work setting, theoretical orientation, agency policies, and so on, clinicians should develop a solid sense of the goals, values, beliefs, and theoretical assumptions that will guide their resolution of the clinical decisions that they must make throughout the day.

Clinicians' personal and professional values frame the nature of their practice and the quality of their work (Fowers & Davidov, 2006; Jennings, Sovereign, Botorff, Mussell, & Vye, 2005). Clinicians who identify as fair, honest, trusting, and open-minded will make different personal and professional decisions than those who hold other types of worldviews. In fact, master therapists tend to share a common set of personal and professional values: valuing and promoting relationships (i.e., relational connection, autonomy, beneficence, nonmaleficence) as well as expertise (i.e., competence, humility, professional growth, openness to complexity and ambiguity, and self-awareness; Jennings et al., 2005). Their focus on building relationships leads to and enhances their ability to practice ethically.

Ideally, personal and professional identities work together and support each other. If a clinician's personal identity is as a "caring person," but she defines caring in ways that are incompatible with her work with sex offenders (e.g., giving hugs and gifts and being available at all hours), she will likely become frustrated and at greater risk of burning out. A clinician who believes that poor people live in poverty due to their own poor work ethic but works in a community counseling center serving the working poor may have difficulty believing that his clients can change and be ineffective here; however, he might be very effective in another setting. Clinicians who act in an open-minded and accepting manner but who do not think and feel this way are unlikely to be seen as genuine, and their interventions are likely to be less effective. Finding a setting, a population, and a way of being a clinician that is consistent with and supported by one's personal identity (e.g., strengths, weaknesses, skills, values, goals) is likely to increase feelings of satisfaction and decrease the risk of burnout (Heinonen & Orlinsky, 2013).

Aligning Personal and Professional Ethics

The value of identity of course is that so often with it comes purpose.

—Robert R. Grant

Ethics and morals are important aspects of personal and professional identity. In the best-case scenario, clinicians' professional and personal ethics enrich one another (Fowers & Davidov, 2006; Knapp, Gottlieb, & Handelsman, 2018). Unfortunately, that is not always the case. Dr. Helper from Chapter 11 crossed multiple professional boundaries to "help" a dead client's wife. Would he have made different decisions if his professional ethics were more central to his decision-making process? Dr. Saeed from Chapter 11 decided to discharge Andrea Yates from the hospital primarily because of demands from managed care and limitations on time, not because of his personal and professional ethics.

Table 13.1 presents the ethical acculturation model. According to this model, when clinicians are working from both their personal values, which may be informed by their spiritual and cultural values, as well as their profession's ethics code and values, and they actively search for ways to integrate both sets of values ("integration" in Table 13.1), they have a richer and more sophisticated decision-making process to access during treatment and are

Table 13.1 The Ethical Acculturation Model

		Personal ethics	
		Low	High
Identification with professional ethics	Low	Marginalization	Separation
	High	Assimilation	Integration

Note. Adapted from "Training Ethical Psychologists: An Acculturation Model," by M. M. Handelsman, M. C. Gottlieb, and S. Knapp, 2005, *Professional Psychology: Research and Practice, 36*, p. 60. Copyright 2005 by the American Psychological Association.

more likely to adhere to the ethical standards (Knapp et al., 2018). Rather than choosing between these two apparently competing sets of ethics, they use both to inform their decisions and help them navigate difficult decisions.

Relative to clinicians in integration, clinicians working from only their personal values ("separation" in Table 13.1) or professional values ("assimilation" in Table 13.1) have more difficulty responding to ethical problems and are more likely to feel alienated from their values or their profession and to burn out (Handelsman, Gottlieb, & Knapp, 2005; Knapp et al., 2018). Clinicians with an "assimilation" stance may apply state law and professional ethical standards in a rote manner without understanding the standard's underlying principles or considering how they can guide competent treatment. To Handelsman and colleagues (2005), this is like "building a strong structure on a shaky foundation, and it may lead to empty, legalistic, and overly simplistic applications of our ethical principles" (p. 61). Clinicians making decisions based on personal ethics while ignoring professional ethics ("separation") may make "kind" gestures at the expense of clients' autonomy or confidentiality, be frustrated by the limitations of the ethics code, or believe that their personal values are stronger and more useful than those of their profession.

Finally, clinicians adopting a "marginalization" stance may be at even greater risk of ethical infractions because they are rudderless, without the guide of a personal moral code or professional ethics (Handelsman et al., 2005). Even generally ethical clinicians may be marginalized from personal and professional ethics during a personal crisis.

Effective clinicians see clinical issues (e.g., informed consent, confidentiality, dual relationships) from the point of view of empathic relationship building, for example, while also seeing them from their profession's ethical standards and principles. They consider the aspirational principles underlying the ethical standards (e.g., competence reflecting the overarching principle of beneficence), which may make it easier to follow the ethical standards (Knapp et al., 2018).

Coping Effectively With Empathic Hazards and Life Stressors

Our greatest glory is not in never falling, but in rising every time we fall.

—Confucius

While some clinicians may experience vicarious traumatization or compassion fatigue and begin engaging in unhealthy behaviors, problems are not inevitable. Other clinicians, just like other clients, may be resilient or even experience satisfaction, transformation, or growth from such work (Bartoskova, 2017; Molnar et al., 2017).

Effective coping begins with self-knowledge, accrued in an ongoing process of self-assessment and awareness (Knapp et al., 2013). These self-assessments should include recognizing the impact of work with challenging or traumatized clients, identifying personal risk factors and warning signs such as increased challenges or stressors in one's personal life, and health or mental health difficulties. During this process of self-assessment, consider asking questions such as the following:

1. When clients have symptoms like mine, what do I consider? What actions do I propose?

2. What is happening when I am feeling depressed or like a failure? Am I forgetting self-care? Have I been working with difficult clients without increasing my self-care? Has my client load decreased, causing me to worry about my income and job security?

3. When I am attracted to a client, how is this attraction related to problems with my partner or other parts of my personal life?

4. When I am feeling disillusioned, how are these feelings related to focusing on the less rewarding parts of work, such as paperwork and billing?

When self-assessment and self-awareness are not sufficient, seeking help from a trusted colleague or peer may normalize reactions, garner psychological support, change perspectives, increase resources, or decrease stressors. For some people, self-assessment may include sporadic or ongoing psychotherapy, which can provide additional objectivity and resources, deepen self-awareness, identify ways of handling difficult issues raised in the course of treating others, and ascertain when work is a way of avoiding issues in one's personal life.

Clinicians face a number of barriers to self-care beyond those of the general population (Alani & Stroink, 2015; Thériault, Gazzola, Isenor, & Pascal, 2015). They give the same reasons for inadequate self-care as anyone else might—lack of time, competing priorities, and lack of energy. In addition, clinicians often place the care of others ahead of the care of themselves, deny their own needs, and feel "selfish" or guilty when attending to their own care (Alani & Stroink, 2015). Although they may accept that personal psychotherapy is important to being an effective psychotherapist, they may have difficulty seeing how they can be helpful to others while they themselves are struggling. They may have difficulty shifting roles to become a client with its associated vulnerabilities and perceived loss of control. The mental health professions need to address the stigma that hampers clinicians from reporting and addressing the struggles they experience (Molnar et al., 2017).

Preventing Stress-Related Problems

Strive for excellence, not perfection. . . . You will make mistakes. . . . You cannot help everyone. . . . You will not know everything. . . . You cannot go it alone.
—*Knapp et al. (2013)*

The helping professions tend to focus on healing already-sustained damage. Although healing damage is necessary, clinicians must remember that the preferred approach is to prevent damage and promote health and well-being. This approach is preferable not only for clients but also for clinicians themselves. Clinicians can be proactive and create conditions in their work and in their lives that minimize exposure to stressors and equip them with effective resources to minimize the impact of stressors they encounter (Simms, 2017).

Probably the most important proactive strategy is having strong interpersonal bonds. Maintaining strong relationships with family and friends is critically important not only for living a healthy, happy life but also for building a system of social support that can provide instrumental, tangible, and emotional support, if and when the need arises, and help clinicians work through difficult or confusing feelings (Aldwin, 2007). Social support is the most reliable and powerful buffer when people encounter difficulties in life (Aldwin, 2007; Folkman & Moskowitz, 2004). Having strong relationships outside of the therapy room also reduces the need to turn to clients to meet needs for respect, admiration, and support.

Another proactive strategy is to structure life in ways that minimize stress. For example, clinicians can assess and address the aspects of their work life that are particular hassles and energy drains. They can schedule breaks, attend continuing education seminars to stay fresh, monitor the size and make-up of their caseloads, and set realistic expectations for themselves (Hensel et al., 2015; Molnar et al., 2017; Pope & Vasquez, 2016). Having good role models at work and outside of work can be quite helpful by providing opportunities for learning about a range of health-promoting behaviors including being assertive, nurturing emotional sensitivity, balancing work and personal lives, maintaining boundaries with difficult people, and integrating spiritual ideals in daily life (Zahniser, Rupert, & Dorociak, 2017).

Like their clients, clinicians can develop good coping and problem-solving skills. **Maladaptive coping** strategies are not only ineffective but can even make problems worse (Aldwin, 2007). Examples of maladaptive coping strategies include self-medicating with substances and engaging in minimization, denial, or rationalization. In contrast, **adaptive coping** skills are generally helpful and reduce stress. Examples of adaptive coping strategies include solving controllable problems through planful action and understanding and accepting those problems that are beyond a person's control (Thériault et al., 2015). Staying in good physical and mental shape helps people ward off stress and remain resilient and is as important for clinicians as for their clients (Simms, 2017; Wicks, 2008). A healthy lifestyle, at a minimum, includes eating well, getting enough rest, exercising regularly, maintaining a healthy weight, using alcohol moderately, taking time to pursue hobbies and leisure, and vacationing (Norcross & VandenBos, 2018; Simms, 2017).

A healthy mind and body can also be cultivated through regular spiritual practices. For some, this might involve traditional religious engagement. For others, spirituality might entail spending time in nature, actively promoting community change, practicing mindfulness, meditating, or doing yoga (Richards, Campenni, & Muse-Burke, 2010). For many clinicians, having a sense of meaning and purpose can be an important part of preventing burnout and other practice-related problems. Some clinicians decide that being effective goes beyond simply maintaining the status quo to actively working to make things better (e.g., Alani & Stroink, 2015; Sue & Sue, 2016). Finding meaning, purpose, and joy, despite being surrounded by pain at work, can be an especially important spiritual practice.

Above all, clinicians can proactively counter stress by improving their own perspective toward their work and their lives. Many recognize that striking a good work–personal life balance is a lifelong challenge and so approach life with a sense of humor (Rupert & Kent, 2007). They remain creative and resourceful, mindful of their ultimate reasons for engaging in therapeutic work in the first place, and celebrate strengths and successes (Alani & Stroink, 2015). They acknowledge that being a witness to the core struggles and triumphs of other human beings is a privilege and accept opportunities to expand themselves, continue to learn, grow personally and professionally, and serve as a role model and mentor (Weiss, 2004). They appreciate the variety in clients, presenting problems, and tasks they see, and find this variety rewarding.

Finally, rather than focusing exclusively on individual coping, we should also foster healthy workplaces to prevent compassion fatigue (Bober & Regehr, 2006; Killian, 2008). Such workplaces would limit exposure to people with trauma histories, provide social support (and encourage employees to obtain support from family and friends too), and offer opportunities to experience a sense of control in their workplace (Killian, 2008). Healthy workplaces encourage ongoing professional development as an important strategy for helping clinicians deal with work-related stressors (Norcross & VandenBos, 2018). Professional development comprises a variety of activities (e.g., workshops, formal education or training, supervision or consultation). A practice that includes other types of intellectually rewarding activities such as teaching, writing, service, and consulting can broaden a clinician's perspective and experience and enliven their mind and spirit.

As seen in the next case, clinicians do well in adopting a perspective of openness to their work and learning to view their mistakes as well as their successes as part of their own journey toward becoming an increasingly strong clinician (Cashman & Cushman, in press). They set reasonable goals for themselves, making reasonable and appropriate comparisons (relative to where they are rather than to the master clinicians they may have observed during training). They are open to learning from all sources (e.g., professors, mentors, books, movies, clients) and accept and learn from their mistakes.

Self-care should be tailored for the person and the person's stage of life (Norcross & VandenBos, 2018; Pope & Vasquez, 2016). What works well for one person may not work for another. The questions in Exhibit 13.2 can help clinicians assess their self-care process, recognize barriers to self-care, and develop more effective strategies for self-care.

Cases in Empathy

My Clients Have Taught Me a Lot I Anonymous

Mistakes can be an opportunity, if seen that way. One participant in Jennings and Skovholt's (1999) study of master therapists described how a mistake provided an opportunity for growth:

> My clients have taught me a lot. Early in my career, I saw a couple for a year, and what she complained about was his drinking. What he was basically saying was, "I wouldn't be drinking if you didn't bug me so much." And I knew absolutely nothing about

alcoholism at that point. They kind of faded out [of therapy], and I don't blame them when I look back on it because we didn't do much. A year later, she called me to make an appointment, came in, sat down, and said "I just want to tell you face-to-face how destructive you were to us." And that was one of the most powerful things that could have happened. I mean, I am forever grateful. It was incredibly hard to hear, but I had a sense that I had really done a lousy job and there was something about her being strong

(ANONYMOUS continued)

enough to come back. I was embarrassed. . . . It made a powerful impression. . . . I knew it was true and that I had a lot to learn. And I think that the other part was that I was incredibly impressed with the fact that she had the guts to do it. And I thought, you know, if she had the guts to do it, then I've got the guts to learn from it. . . . It colored my absolute commitment to learn about what I didn't know. (p. 7)

What Do You Think?

1. What can you infer about this clinician's meaning system? On what basis do you draw these conclusions?

2. People often have difficulty transforming their mistakes into something positive, as this master therapist did. If you can, think about a mistake from which you learned. How were you able to learn, rather than failing or becoming stuck?

3. Identify some goals for your own professional development. How are you going to go about meeting them?

Summary

Taking good care of oneself, both personally and professionally, is important in becoming and remaining an effective clinician. In this chapter, we described dangers of being an empathic clinician, including boundary blurring, vicarious traumatization, and burnout, and we considered how clinicians can remain vigilant for these dangers. We also described other sources of stress that clinicians often encounter and ways of coping with these stressors.

It is easy for clinicians to focus on either their personal or professional ethics as a guide to clinical practice. Effective clinical work depends on effectively integrating personal and professional ethics to support decision-making in response to ethical dilemmas and clinicians' personal and professional development.

Regularly engaging in good, proactive self-awareness and self-care practices as well as having effective safety mechanisms can reduce the probability of difficulties and enable clinicians to remain respectful and empathic even in the face of the inevitable stressors they will experience in their work and personal lives.

For Review

Applying Concepts to Your Life

1. With what kinds of people, problems, or situations do you have the most problems? When do you handle these best? What signs help you recognize when you're running into problems in your life?

2. What do you do to keep yourself healthy? Are there some ways you might improve in these areas? What can you do to begin putting these strategies into place right now?

3. What might interfere with your ability to regularly engage in self-care? What can you do to begin addressing these barriers and obstacles right now?

4. Perform a personal skill inventory, including your current skill levels across a wide variety of realms, competencies, attitudes, and personal strengths and weaknesses, especially as they might affect your clinical practice (Bashe et al., 2007; Knapp et al., 2013). What are your strengths and weaknesses? In which ways might your strengths function as weaknesses? In what ways might your weaknesses serve as strengths? What does this assessment suggest you should do to become an ethical and competent clinician?

5. Return to the "ethics autobiography" you wrote in Chapter 11. Consider how your history might support or challenge your new discipline's ethical standards and principles. What does your reflection suggest about your ethical acculturation? See Table 13.1.

6. Pay attention to your reactions to the ethical standards. When do you think they are unnecessary or too strict? When do you feel you know better about your clients' needs? What does this self-assessment suggest that you should do to develop as an ethical member of your profession?

Key Terms

adaptive, 281
adaptive coping, 287
boundaries, 272
boundary
  crossings, 273

boundary
  violations, 273
compassion
  fatigue, 274
maladaptive, 281

maladaptive
  coping, 287
personal identity, 282
professional
  identity, 282

self-care, 272
vicarious
  traumatization, 276

Learn More

For more information about the concepts in this chapter, visit the *Empathic Counseling* companion website at http://pubs.apa.org/books/supp/slattery/.

GLOSSARY

abandonment Treatment is ended by the therapist abruptly without being ethically or clinically appropriate.

accommodation Making reconceptualizations in a meaning system to incorporate new information. *See also* Assimilation.

accurate empathy A therapeutic lead that neither adds to nor subtracts from the client's meaning. *See also* Additive Empathy and Subtractive Empathy.

action A stage of change where clients are committed to changing and willing to accept the costs of change. Change is most rapid for clients in this stage.

adaptive Favorable; helpful.

adaptive coping Coping efforts that are generally helpful and reduce stress, including solving controllable problems through planful action and understanding and accepting those problems that are beyond a person's control.

additive empathy A therapeutic lead that recognizes and shares additional, underlying, often unspoken meanings, thoughts and feelings. *See also* Accurate Empathy and Subtractive Empathy.

affect Overtly displayed emotion, including overtly displayed mood, degree of emotional lability, and congruence between expression and subjective mood. *See also* Mood.

approach goals Goals focused on changes clients want to make. *See also* Avoidance Goals.

aspirational principles The ethical principles and goals that clinicians use to guide treatment, including beneficence, nonmaleficence, fidelity, integrity, autonomy, and social justice.

assimilation Integration of new information into existing meaning system. *See also* Accommodation.

assumption Underlying, often invisible and untested beliefs that guide behavior.

attribution A belief about the cause of behavior or of a person's quality or trait.

autonomy An aspirational principle guiding ethical decision-making, supporting clients' ability to make treatment decisions for themselves.

avoidance goals Less productive goals focused on what clients want to *not* do. *See also* Approach Goals.

Barnum statement A description of a person that appears to be clear and specific but in fact applies to almost anyone.

belief An assertion accepted as true. May be conscious or unconscious and about self, others, or the world. Part of meaning system.

beneficence Striving to do good for those with whom one works and

society as a whole. An aspirational principle guiding ethical decision-making.

billable hours Number of hours of clinical service billed to clients or insurance companies.

boundaries The "ground rules" supporting the client, clinician, and treatment, generally places limits on time, treatment setting, content discussed, and the nature of the relationship.

boundary crossings Behaviors deviating from the strictest professional norms (e.g., small self-disclosures). They may put clinicians at greater risk of engaging in boundary violations. *See also* Boundary Violations.

boundary violations Behaviors deviating from professional norms, with high potential for negative consequences for the client. *See also* Boundary Crossings.

case conceptualization A set of hypotheses about the forces driving a client's behavior and the causes and treatment of the presenting problem.

case conference Group discussions about a client's assessment and treatment that often include people from several disciplines, often all involved with the client.

clinical assessment The systematic evaluation and measurement of psychological, biological, and social factors in a person presenting with a possible psychological disorder.

clinical risk The risk of disciplinary complaint or legal action during clinical practice.

clinician A person trained to listen and provide guidance on personal, social, and psychological problems, especially from a psychological perspective. *See also* Psychotherapy.

closed question Questions quickly obtaining specific data and discouraging lengthy discussion, answered in a few words, and beginning with *do, does, is, could,* and *are.*

collectivism Group and family obligations are stressed more than self-reliance and independence or individual wishes, thoughts, and feelings. *See also* Individualism.

common factors Change agents that are shared by all effective therapeutic interventions. These include the therapeutic alliance, the clinician's personality, clinician–client match, catharsis, and an acceptable explanation of the problem.

comorbid Two disorders occurring at the same time.

compassion fatigue A progressive loss of idealism, energy, and sense of purpose and accomplishment at work, often with increased depersonalization of clients.

competence (a) Relative to ethics, a multidimensional and fluctuating attribute, often described as technical, emotional, and multicultural competence, and the attitudes, values, and judgment necessary to implement these well; or (b) in legal settings,

the accused's ability to make important decisions or to assist in his or her own defense in court.

confidentiality Ethical standard that client information will be disclosed only when clients give permission or when legally required to do so (e.g., duty to warn, mandated reporting).

confirmation bias Tendency to recall behaviors consistent with one's biases and overlook or forget behaviors inconsistent with these biases.

consultation Meeting with supervisors or coworkers to solicit advice about difficulties in a case.

contemplation A stage of change where clients are ambivalent about change, recognizing both the costs and benefits of change and having difficulty choosing to actively change.

content The material discussed in the course of treatment. *See also* Process.

context The broad range of influences on a person, including culture, family, history, political environment, trauma, and life events.

corrective emotional experience An experience in treatment that helps clients feel differently about themselves, their relationships, their past, or their future.

counseling *See* Psychotherapy.

counselor A person trained to listen and provide guidance on personal, social, and psychological problems, especially from a psychological perspective. *See also* Psychotherapy.

critical thinking Process of evaluating assertions and drawing

conclusions about them by identifying assertions, evaluating evidence supporting and countering assertions, identifying other explanations of this evidence, and choosing the most reasonable explanation.

cultural humility Willingness to listen to a client and client's cultural heritage with respect, openness, and curiosity.

culture The shared attitudes, values, beliefs, habits, traditions, norms, arts, history, institutions, and experiences of a group of people that, together, define their general behavior and way of life. Ethnicity, race, gender, class, age cohort, and sexual orientation, among other demographic groups, are frequently identified as cultural groups.

directiveness The degree to which the clinician has control over treatment goals and direction. *See also* Egalitarian.

discharge summary A brief report summarizing entering and ending client diagnoses, the course of treatment, and factors contributing to treatment outcomes.

discrepancy Either (a) the gap between where clients are and where they want to be or believe they should be or (b) the conflict between words and nonverbal behavior, actions, values or goals, which provides the content for a clinician's confrontation.

discrimination Unfair treatment of a group based on group membership. *See also* Privilege.

egalitarian Relationships where therapist and client share power over treatment decisions and goals. *See also* Directive.

emotional competence A type of competence, particularly the skill to perform a task without bias or distress clouding judgment or impair ability to act effectively. *See also* Technical Competence; Multicultural Competence.

empathy The accepting and hopeful understanding of another person from his or her unique point of view.

empowered collaboration Collaboration process empowering clients to meet their goals.

empower The process of supporting clients to recognize, accept, use, and develop their personal and political power to meet their goals.

encourager Microskill that encourages elaboration of ideas and emotions by repeating one or a few of the client's main words to focus attention on the ideas contained in those words.

enmeshed Permeable and unclear boundaries in a family. Two people may overidentify with and be unable to separate their emotional experiences from each other's.

ethical standards Ethical expectations that are part of a profession's code of ethics, violations of which can lead to disciplinary censure. *See also* Aspirational Principles.

expectancy confirmation Tendency to see behaviors that fit expectations and ignore evidence that would otherwise disconfirm it.

external locus of control Attribution of control over future outcomes to others (or society)

while recognizing little personal agency.

external locus of responsibility Attribution of responsibility for past circumstances to others or environmental factors; attributing blame to outside factors.

extrinsic Value of a behavior or goal comes from meeting some external need or value (e.g., belongingness, support, or prestige) rather than from the object itself. *See also* Intrinsic.

family genogram Assessment strategy visually organizing hypotheses about familial patterns and relationships that may contribute to problems or serve as resources for treatment.

fidelity Behaving in a faithful, honest, trustworthy, and responsible manner. An aspirational principle guiding ethical decision-making.

fixed mind-set Belief that qualities are traits and unchangeable. *See also* Growth Mind-Set.

forced terminations Terminations from treatment triggered by a program's or managed care plan's limit on sessions available.

functional analysis Assessment procedure in which antecedents to a behavioral problem (A), the behavior itself (B), and the consequences to the behavior (C) are systematically recorded to identify relationships between internal or environmental stimuli and behaviors.

fundamental attribution error Tendency to attribute others' behavior to internal and stable traits, while overlooking unstable, situational factors.

generalize To transfer learned skills to a similar but different situation or setting.

genuine Perceived as really listening and understanding rather than only pretending to do so. Generally, words, behavior, and values are consistent across time.

goal statements The client's long-term goals, often written in the client's own words.

goal Internal representation of desired processes, events, or outcomes. Part of meaning system.

groupthink The tendency to suppress or resist divergent thought processes or minority opinions when a group is working together to accomplish a task.

growth mind-set Beliefs that behavior is changeable and that one can learn from mistakes with effort and persistence. *See also* Fixed Mind-Set.

hypothesis An empirically testable proposition about some fact, behavior, or relationship, usually based on theory, which states an expected outcome resulting from specific conditions or assumptions.

implementation intention If–then plan describing specific actions the client will take toward goal and the circumstances under which they will be taken.

implicit bias Prejudice or stereotypes operating outside of conscious awareness, often as measured by the Implicit Bias Test.

individualism Needs of the individual are stressed over those of group or family. Individual wishes, thoughts, and feelings are emphasized over group responsibility and obligations. *See also* Collectivism.

inference Conclusion drawn from observations. Because meaning is added to the observations, two parties may disagree about what happened. *See also* Observation.

informed consent Both a formal and an ongoing informal process, whereby clinicians provide clients with information to make informed decisions about their treatment.

integrity Acting in accordance with psychology's principles, including accuracy, honesty, fairness, and truthfulness.

internal locus of control Attributions of control over future outcomes to oneself (e.g., to prevent future trauma).

internal locus of responsibility Attributions of responsibility for past circumstances to oneself.

intersectionality Overlapping social identities (e.g., race, gender, sexuality, class) contribute to the nature of oppression and discrimination experienced.

intervention The specific strategy that the client and clinician use to meet treatment goals.

intrinsic A behavior or goal has its own internal value rather than deriving from something else, like money or grades. *See also* Extrinsic.

intrusive thoughts Unwanted, involuntary thoughts, ideas, and images that may become obsessive and ruminative in nature.

joining The clinician's intentional or unintentional work to strengthen the therapeutic alliance.

just-world theory The belief that people get what they deserve and deserve what they get.

lapse A return of the problem behavior that the client sees as temporary and as an opportunity to learn, especially how to prevent the problem in the future. *See also* Relapse.

locus of control Location of a person's sense of control, either internal and controlled by the person, or external and controlled by outside factors including others, the environment, culture, or chance. Focus is on the control of present and future actions. *See also* Locus of Responsibility.

locus of responsibility Location of a person's sense of responsibility, either internal and controlled by the person him or herself, or external and controlled by outside factors, including others, the environment, culture, or fate. Focus is on responsibility for past events. *See also* Locus of Control.

long-term goal Primary treatment goal. *See also* Short-Term Goal.

maintenance A stage of change in which clients have met their goals and are working to maintain those changes. One focus of this stage is preventing a relapse.

majority culture The group in a society possessing greater power and whose language, religion, behavior, values, rituals, and social customs are seen as normative.

maladaptive Unfavorable; causes problems.

maladaptive coping Coping efforts that are ineffective and can even make problems worse, including substance use to self-medicate and engaging in minimization, denial, or rationalization.

managed care A health care system in which patient care is monitored by a company, sometimes limiting access to health care providers and services. It determines payments for services.

mandated reporting A legal requirement to make a report to a government agency under certain circumstances, especially in the case of child or elder abuse.

meaning system A framework for understanding the world, comprising beliefs, goals, values, and sense of purpose.

meditation Any of a number of approaches that build calm, awareness, and nonjudgmental self-acceptance, often by turning one's attention to a single point, such as the breath.

mental status evaluation A quick, semistructured assessment of functioning in several realms.

meta-analysis A research method that systematically combines results of research studies addressing a common set of hypotheses. Typically averages effect sizes across studies.

microaggressions Verbal, behavioral, or environmental racial slights that can be intentional or unintentional but communicate hostile and derogatory intent.

microskills The nonverbal and verbal building blocks that help clinicians join with clients, communicate empathy and understanding, and influence clients to change.

mindfulness meditation Calm, nonjudgmental awareness of one's body, thoughts, feelings, or actions rather than focus on past or future.

minimal encourager Simple sounds that help people feel heard or understood with few or no words.

miracle question Asks the client to imagine that a miracle occurred making the problem disappear and to identify how they would first recognize the miracle. Used to identify treatment goals and times and places when the client is already successful.

mirroring Subtly reflecting client's posture and movements to build rapport and empathy.

mood Refers to the client's "emotional atmosphere" and is internal, subjective, and relatively more sustained. Often inferred from the client's verbal tone and subjective report. *See also* Affect.

multicultural clinician Clinician who recognizes and accepts differences in cultural values, beliefs, and preferences; develops multicultural sensitivity, knowledge, and understanding; identifies attitudes, biases, and beliefs that influence his or her perceptions of and interactions with clients of other cultures; and uses culturally appropriate skills in clinical practice.

multicultural competence A type of competence, particularly the multicultural skills to perform a task so that it is appropriately tailored for working with a given population. *See also* Technical Competence; Emotional Competence.

multiple identities People belong to, identify with, and are influenced by multiple groups (e.g., ethnicity, race, gender, class, religion, sexual orientation, physical ability).

multiple relationship A relationship with a client beyond that of clinician that has incompatible or competing expectations, goals, or needs (e.g., being both therapist and friend).

nonmaleficence Avoiding doing harm. An aspirational principle guiding ethical decision-making.

normal termination When treatment is ended in ethical and clinically appropriate ways.

observation Sensory data (things seen, heard, felt, tasted, or smelled). Because no additional meaning is added, any two parties will agree it happened as described. *See also* Inference.

observer's paradox Simply making an observation affects the outcome; therefore, no one can ever know how a person would behave if the observer were not present.

open questions Questions eliciting major information and facilitating discussion; generally begin with *who*, *what*, *how*, *why*, or *could*.

oppression The process of arbitrarily and unjustly preventing a person from meeting his or her goals or potential. Can be overt or more indirect and subtle. *See also* Privilege.

paraphrase Microskill that promotes discussion by summarizing the essence of a client's message from a short period of time, both to demonstrate the clinician's understanding and to check out that understanding.

person-first language Places the person rather than a problem or condition first in a description to emphasize the person is more than the problem or condition.

personal identity Includes self-perceptions and defining values, goals, and characteristics.

placebo A treatment without an inherent biological effect in and of itself. A placebo's action is believed to come from the belief that the person is receiving an effective treatment.

positive ethics Rather than only meeting minimal ethical requirements, positive ethics includes striving for the highest standards of ethical behavior.

posttraumatic growth Growth following a trauma (e.g., changes such as increased awareness of values, greater spirituality, stronger interpersonal values, greater self-efficacy).

precontemplation A stage of change in which clients do not acknowledge that they have a problem and are therefore uncommitted to change.

prejudice Negative attitudes based on race, gender, ethnicity, or other group memberships.

premature termination Treatment ended before meeting treatment goals, generally against the clinician's advice.

preparation A stage of change in which clients are preparing to make active change by planning, getting information and support, problem-solving, and obtaining needed skills.

privilege Unearned advantages coming solely or primarily from group membership. Group members often assume privileges are deserved and appropriate. *See also* Oppression.

pro bono Literally, for the public good. Treatment offered without charge.

process The manner in which therapeutic material is presented or discussed (i.e., speed, place of introduction of material, style of interpersonal interaction, etc.). *See also* Content.

professional identity Includes meaning and value given to membership in a field; theoretical perspective; and values, goals, and ethical principles guiding one's work.

progress notes Brief and informal notes made by a clinician immediately after a session summarizing the content and process of the session as well as diagnostic impressions.

psychosocial history Assessment strategy of collecting current and historical information affecting client behavior and functioning in a wide range of realms (e.g., relative strengths and weaknesses, obstacles to change, resources and social supports, client meanings).

psychotherapy Process by which a clinician and client collaboratively resolve a personal, social, or psychological problem, often by exploring thoughts and emotions and by taking other perspectives.

racial identity Sense of group Identification, meanings associated with one's own and other races, and the salience of race to self-concept and individual identity.

racism Negative attitudes about a person based on race. A special case of prejudice.

referral question The question leading to a referral for evaluation or treatment.

reflection of feeling Microskill that communicates understanding by selectively focusing on feelings and emotions.

relapse A slip perceived as a full-blown return to the problem behavior. *See also* Lapse.

relapse prevention Reducing the probability of a relapse by helping clients consider slips as a lapse rather than as a relapse, develop coping skills and use them proactively, and identify triggers and either avoid them or handle them more effectively.

risk management Strategies used to reduce risk incurred during evaluations and treatment.

rumination Obsessive thought or worry.

scaling question Asks clients to indicate the degree to which a problem is occurring, often on a scale from 1 to 10. *See also* Miracle Question.

self-efficacy Belief in one's ability to do a particular action (e.g., to change).

self-fulfilling prophecy Others' expectations shape a person's self-perceptions and behavior.

sensory data Information that can be seen, heard, felt, tasted, or smelled. See Observation.

session objective Primary objective or goal for a treatment session.

short-term goal An immediate goal toward meeting long-term treatment goals. *See also* Long-Term Goal.

situational meaning Meaning assigned by a person to a particular event or experience. Includes appraisals as a loss, threat, or challenge, as well as causal attributions for why the event occurred, determination of the extent to which the event is discrepant with meaning system, and decisions about coping. *See also* Meaning System.

slip A return of the problem behavior, which can either be seen as temporary and an opportunity to learn (lapse) or permanent and without eventual positive consequences (relapse).

SMART-IC Acronym for goals that are specific, measurable, achievable, realistic and time-bounded, intrinsic, and committed.

SOAP notes Structured session notes describing the client's subjective experience (S), the clinician's observations (O), assessment (A), and plan (P) for the next session.

social justice Being fair and unbiased in treatment and promoting fairness in the community. An aspirational principle guiding ethical decision-making.

state An aspect of personality that is seen as more temporary and changeable.

strength based Evaluations and treatment that attend to strengths, successes, positive intentions, and exceptions to problems, in addition to weaknesses, mistakes, problems, and symptoms.

subtractive empathy A response that is off-track and misses or subtracts from understanding clients from their own point of view. *See also* Additive Empathy; Accurate Empathy.

summarization Microskill that quickly organizes a large amount of information to communicate and check understanding. Often used at a session's beginning or end and during changes in focus.

systemic Something operating on individual, interpersonal, institutional, and cultural levels, especially oppression.

technical competence A type of competence, particularly the knowledge and skills to perform a therapeutic task well. *See also* Emotional and Multicultural Competence.

therapeutic alliance The strength of the client and therapist partnership. About 30% of the variance in therapeutic outcomes is attributable to the client's perceptions of this alliance.

therapeutic relationship *See* Therapeutic Alliance.

therapist A person trained to listen and provide guidance on personal, social, and psychological problems, especially from a psychological perspective. *See also* Psychotherapy.

therapy model A theoretical framework describing causes of problems, how change occurs, and manner of assessment (e.g., behavioral or psychoanalytic).

timeline Assessment strategy recording all major events for clients and their immediate family, from birth to the present.

time orientation Perception of time as flexible or inelastic. Can be primarily focused on past, present, or future.

trait An aspect of the person, especially of personality, often believed to have a genetic basis.

trait negativity bias Tendency to focus on and give greater meaning to negative rather than positive traits. Negative actions are seen as more representative than positive ones.

transfer Either (a) to use a learned behavior in different settings (e.g., both the clinician's office and at home) or (b) to move from one setting or program to another.

treatment goals Either short- or long-term planned goals for treatment, generally chosen collaboratively between client and clinician.

treatment plan A plan identifying short- and long-term treatment goals, interventions planned for the treatment period, and, sometimes, anticipated date for goals completion.

triangle When there is an unstable relationship between two people, that relationship is stabilized by bringing in a third either for comfort or to redirect tension.

triggers Emotions, settings, and situations putting a client at risk of a relapse of problem.

unconditional positive regard Positive and nonjudgmental feelings toward client that are not contingent on the client's behavior, values, goals, or cognitions.

validation The need to have one's self-perception accepted or confirmed by others.

validity Extent to which an observation or assessment measures what it is supposed to measure.

values Transsituational goals serving as guiding principles. Influence a broad range of human behaviors and choices and prescribe modes of conduct. Part of meaning system.

vicarious traumatization Negative impact clinicians experience across time by listening to and engaging with descriptions of trauma.

well-being A holistic state of being healthy, happy, and satisfied with life.

YAVIS An acronym used to describe clients for whom traditional therapies are well suited: Young, Attractive, Verbal, Intelligent, Successful.

REFERENCES

Abdulrehman, R. Y. (2018, August). *Is the Christmas party killing cultural diversity/Reviewing institutional microaggressions at work.* Workshop presented at the annual convention of the American Psychological Association, San Francisco, CA.

Abelson, R. P., Frey, K. P., & Gregg, A. P. (2004). *Experiments with people: Revelations from social psychology.* Mahwah, NJ: Erlbaum.

Achenbach, T. M., & Rescorla, L. A. (2004). The Achenbach System of Empirically Based Assessment (ASEBA) for ages 1.5 to 18 years. In M. E. Maruish (Ed.), *The use of psychological testing for treatment planning and outcomes assessment: Volume 2. Instruments for children and adolescents* (3rd ed., pp. 179–213). Mahwah, NJ: Erlbaum.

Ackerman, S., & Hilsenroth, M. J. (2001). A review of therapist characteristics and techniques negatively impacting the therapeutic alliance. *Psychotherapy: Theory, Research, Practice, Training, 38,* 171–185. http://dx.doi.org/10.1037/0033-3204.38.2.171

Adams, J., & White, M. (2009). Time perspective in socioeconomic inequalities in smoking and body mass index. *Health Psychology, 28,* 83–90. http://dx.doi.org/10.1037/0278-6133.28.1.83

Adams, M. C., & Kivlighan, D. M., III. (2019). When home is gone: An application of the multicultural orientation framework to enhance clinical practice with refugees of forced migration. *Professional Psychology: Research and Practice, 50,* 176–183. http://dx.doi.org/10.1037/pro0000230

Ai, A. L., & Park, C. L. (2005). Possibilities of the positive following violence and trauma: Informing the coming decade of research. *Journal of Interpersonal Violence, 20,* 242–250. http://dx.doi.org/10.1177/0886260504267746

Alani, T., & Stroink, M. (2015). Self-care strategies and barriers among female service providers working with female survivors of intimate partner violence. *Canadian Journal of Counselling and Psychotherapy/Revue Canadienne De Counseling Et De Psychothérapie, 49,* 360–378.

Aldwin, C. M. (2007). *Stress, coping, and development: An integrative approach* (2nd ed.). New York, NY: Guilford Press.

Allan, B. A., Campos, I. D., & Wimberley, T. E. (2016). Interpersonal psychotherapy: A review and multicultural critique. *Counselling Psychology Quarterly, 29,* 253–273. http://dx.doi.org/10.1080/09515070.2015.1028896

Alspach, J. G. (2018). Implicit bias in patient care: An endemic blight on quality care. *Critical Care Nurse, 38,* 12–16.

American Association for Marriage and Family Therapy. (2015). *AAMFT Code of Ethics.* Retrieved from https://www.aamft.org/Documents/Legal%20Ethics/AAMFT-code-of-ethics.pdf

American Counseling Association. (2014). *2014 ACA Code of Ethics.* Alexandria, VA: Author. Retrieved from https://www.counseling.org/resources/aca-code-of-ethics.pdf

American Nurses Association. (n.d.). *Short definitions of ethical principles and theories: Familiar words, what do they mean?* Retrieved from http://www.nursingworld.org/MainMenuCategories/EthicsStandards/Resources/Ethics-Definitions.pdf

American Psychological Association. (2003). Guidelines on multicultural education, training, research, practice, and organizational change for psychologists. *American Psychologist, 58,* 377–402. http://dx.doi.org/10.1037/0003-066X.58.5.377

American Psychological Association. (2012). *Recognition of psychotherapy effectiveness.* Retrieved from http://www.apa.org/about/policy/resolution-psychotherapy.aspx

American Psychological Association. (2017a). *Ethical principles of psychologists and code of conduct.* Retrieved from http://www.apa.org/ethics/code/ethics-code-2017.pdf

American Psychological Association. (2017b). *Multicultural guidelines: An ecological approach to context, identity, and intersectionality.* Retrieved from http://www.apa.org/about/policy/multicultural-guidelines.pdf

American Psychological Association. (2019). *Guidelines for nonhandicapping language in APA journals.* Retrieved from https://apastyle.apa.org/manual/related/nonhandicapping-language

American Psychological Association (Producer). (2020). *Trauma and meaning* [DVD]. Available from https://www.apa.org/pubs/videos/4310015

American Psychological Association Presidential Task Force on Evidence-Based Practice. (2006). Evidence-based practice in psychology. *American Psychologist, 61,* 271–285. http://dx.doi.org/10.1037/0003-066X.61.4.271

Amrhein, P. C., Miller, W. R., Yahne, C. E., Palmer, M., & Fulcher, L. (2003). Client commitment language during motivational interviewing predicts drug use outcomes. *Journal of Consulting and Clinical Psychology, 71,* 862–878. http://dx.doi.org/10.1037/0022-006X.71.5.862

Anderson, C. J. (2003). The psychology of doing nothing: Forms of decision avoidance result from reason and emotion. *Psychological Bulletin, 129,* 139–167. http://dx.doi.org/10.1037/0033-2909.129.1.139

Anderson, K. N., Bautista, C. L., & Hope, D. A. (2019). Therapeutic alliance, cultural competence and minority status in premature termination of psychotherapy. *American Journal of Orthopsychiatry, 89,* 104–114. http://dx.doi.org/10.1037/ort0000342

Anderson, L. W., & Krathwohl, D. R. (Eds.). (2001). *A taxonomy for learning, teaching and assessing: A revision of Bloom's Taxonomy of educational objectives.* New York, NY: Longman.

Andrea Yates Confession. (2001, July 14). Clips 7 and 8. *Houston Chronicle.*

Añez, L. M., Silva, M. A., Paris, M. J., & Bedregal, L. E. (2008). Engaging Latinos through the integration of cultural values and motivational interviewing principles. *Professional Psychology: Research and Practice, 39,* 153–159. http://dx.doi.org/10.1037/0735-7028.39.2.153

Anonymous. (2000, March). Boundaries in therapy: The limits of care. *Pennsylvania Psychologist Update,* pp. 1, 3.

Anonymous. (2008, November 4). Psychotherapist body language. *AllExperts.* Retrieved from http://en.allexperts.com/q/Psychology-2566/2008/11/Psychotherapist-body-language.htm

Associated Press. (2002, February 21). Transcript of Andrea Yates confession. *Houston Chronicle,* p. 34.

Autin, F., Batruch, A., & Butera, F. (2019). The function of selection of assessment leads evaluators to artificially create the social class achievement gap. *Journal of Educational Psychology, 111,* 717–735. http://dx.doi.org/10.1037/edu0000307

Bai, S. (1999, May 2). Columbine High School: Anatomy of a massacre. *Newsweek.* Retrieved from https://www.newsweek.com/columbine-high-school-anatomy-massacre-166950

Banaji, M. R., & Greenwald, A. G. (2013). *Blindspot: Hidden biases of good people.* New York, NY: Delacorte.

Bandura, A. (1997). *Self-efficacy: The exercise of control.* New York, NY: W. H. Freeman.

Barnett, J. E., Doll, B., Younggren, J. N., & Rubin, N. J. (2007). Clinical competence for practicing psychologists: Clearly a work in progress. *Professional Psychology: Research and Practice, 38,* 510–517. http://dx.doi.org/10.1037/0735-7028.38.5.510

Barnett, J. E., Lazarus, A. A., Vasquez, M. J. T., Moorehead-Slaughter, O., & Johnson, W. B. (2007). Boundary issues and multiple relationships: Fantasy and reality. *Professional Psychology: Research and Practice, 38,* 401–410. http://dx.doi.org/10.1037/0735-7028.38.4.401

Barnett, J. E., Wise, E. H., Johnson-Greene, D., & Bucky, S. F. (2007). Informed consent: Too much of a good thing or not enough? *Professional Psychology: Research and Practice, 38,* 179–186. http://dx.doi.org/10.1037/0735-7028.38.2.179

Bartoskova, L. (2017). How do trauma therapists experience the effects of their trauma work, and are there common factors leading to post-traumatic growth? *Counselling Psychology Review, 32,* 30–45.

Bashe, A., Anderson, S. K., Handelsman, M. M., & Klevansky, R. (2007). An acculturation model for ethics training: The ethics autobiography and beyond. *Professional Psychology: Research and Practice, 38*, 60–67. http://dx.doi.org/10.1037/0735-7028.38.1.60

Beacham, A. O., Van Sickle, K. S., Khatri, P., Ali, M. K., Reimer, D., Farber, E. W., & Kaslow, N. J. (2017). Meeting evolving workforce needs: Preparing psychologists for leadership in the patient-centered medical home. *American Psychologist, 72*, 42–54. http://dx.doi.org/10.1037/a0040458

Beauchemin, E. (2004, August 1). Under foreign skies: Dr. Danny Brom. *Radio Netherlands.* Retrieved from https://www.radionetherlandsarchives.org/under-foreign-skies-dr-danny-brom-youre-a-trauma-freak-but-we-dont-have-trauma-here-in-israel/

Bebbington, K., MacLeod, C., Ellison, T. M., & Fay, N. (2017). The sky is falling: Evidence of a negativity bias in the social transmission of information. *Evolution and Human Behavior, 38*, 92–101. http://dx.doi.org/10.1016/j.evolhumbehav.2016.07.004

Beck, A. T. (1976). *Cognitive therapy and the emotional disorders.* New York, NY: International Universities Press.

Beck, A. T., Steer, R. A., & Carbin, M. G. (1988). Psychometric properties of the Beck Depression Inventory: Twenty-five years of evaluation. *Clinical Psychology Review, 8*, 77–100. http://dx.doi.org/10.1016/0272-7358(88)90050-5

Becker-Blease, K. A., & Freyd, J. J. (2006). Research participants telling the truth about their lives: The ethics of asking and not asking about abuse. *American Psychologist, 61*, 218–226. http://dx.doi.org/10.1037/0003-066X.61.3.218

Behnke, S. (2007, February). Adolescents and confidentiality: Letter from a reader. *Monitor on Psychology, 38*, 46–47.

Bélanger-Gravel, A., Godin, G., & Amireault, S. (2013). A meta-analytic review of the effect of implementation intentions on physical activity. *Health Psychology Review, 7*, 23–54. http://dx.doi.org/10.1080/17437199.2011.560095

Benish, S. G., Quintana, S., & Wampold, B. E. (2011). Culturally adapted psychotherapy and the legitimacy of myth: A direct-comparison meta-analysis. *Journal of Counseling Psychology, 58*, 279–289. http://dx.doi.org/10.1037/a0023626

Benjet, C., Azar, S. T., & Kuersten-Hogan, R. (2003). Evaluating the parental fitness of psychiatrically diagnosed individuals: Advocating a functional-contextual analysis of parenting. *Journal of Family Psychology, 17*, 238–251. http://dx.doi.org/10.1037/0893-3200.17.2.238

Berkman, L. F. (2009). Social epidemiology: Social determinants of health in the United States: Are we losing ground? *Annual Review of Public Health, 30*, 27–41. http://dx.doi.org/10.1146/annurev.publhealth.031308.100310

Berlinger, N., & Berlinger, A. (2017). Culture and moral distress: What's the connection and why does it matter? *AMA Journal of Ethics, 19*, 608–616. http://dx.doi.org/10.1001/journalofethics.2017.19.6.msoc1-1706

Bernal, G., & Sáez-Santiago, E. (2006). Culturally centered psychosocial interventions. *Journal of Community Psychology, 34*, 121–132. http://dx.doi.org/10.1002/jcop.20096

Bernard, J. D., Whittles, R. L., Kertz, S. J., & Burke, P. A. (2015). Trauma and event centrality: Valence and incorporation into identity influence well-being more than exposure. *Psychological Trauma: Theory, Research, Practice, and Policy, 7*, 11–17. http://dx.doi.org/10.1037/a0037331

Bersoff, D. N. (2014). Protecting victims of violent patients while protecting confidentiality. *American Psychologist, 69*, 461–467. http://dx.doi.org/10.1037/a0037198

Beutler, L. E., Rocco, F., Moleiro, C. M., & Talebi, H. (2001). Resistance. *Psychotherapy, 38*, 431–436. http://dx.doi.org/10.1037/0033-3204.38.4.431

Bhatia, A., & Gelso, C. J. (2017). The termination phase: Therapists' perspective on the therapeutic relationship and outcome. *Psychotherapy, 54*, 76–87. http://dx.doi.org/10.1037/pst0000100

Blake, P. (Writer), & Yaitanes, G. (Director). (2008). The itch [Television series episode]. In P. Attanasio, K. Jacobs, D. Shore, & B. Singer (Executive producers), *House, MD*. Santa Monica, CA: Heel & Toe Films.

Blanchard, M., & Farber, B. A. (2016). Lying in psychotherapy: Why and what clients don't tell their therapist about therapy and their relationship. *Counselling Psychology Quarterly,*

29, 90–112. http://dx.doi.org/10.1080/09515070.2015.1085365

Blum, M. C. (2015). Embodied mirroring: A relational, body-to-body technique promoting movement in therapy. *Journal of Psychotherapy Integration, 25,* 115–127. http://dx.doi.org/10.1037/a0038880

Bober, T., & Regehr, C. (2006). Strategies for reducing secondary or vicarious trauma: Do they work? *Brief Treatment and Crisis Intervention, 6,* 1–9. http://dx.doi.org/10.1093/brief-treatment/mhj001

Bohart, A. C. (2001). The evolution of an integrative experiential therapist. In M. R. Goldfried (Ed.), *How therapists change: Personal and professional reflections* (pp. 221–246). Washington, DC: American Psychological Association. http://dx.doi.org/10.1037/10392-013

Bond, C. F., & DePaulo, B. M. (2008). Individual differences in judging deception: Accuracy and bias. *Psychological Bulletin, 134,* 477–492. http://dx.doi.org/10.1037/0033-2909.134.4.477

Borckardt, J. J., Nash, M. R., Murphy, M. D., Moore, M., Shaw, D., & O'Neil, P. (2008). Clinical practice as natural laboratory for psychotherapy research: A guide to case-based time-series analysis. *American Psychologist, 63,* 77–95. http://dx.doi.org/10.1037/0003-066X.63.2.77

Bowleg, L. (2008). When Black + lesbian + woman ≠ Black lesbian woman: The methodological challenges of qualitative and quantitative intersectionality research. *Sex Roles, 59,* 312–325. http://dx.doi.org/10.1007/s11199-008-9400-z

Brennan, J. (2001). Adjustment to cancer—coping or personal transition? *Psycho-Oncology, 10,* 1–18. http://dx.doi.org/10.1002/1099-1611(200101/02)10:1%3C1::AID-PON484%3E3.0.CO;2-T

Briñol, P., Petty, R. E., & Wheeler, S. C. (2006). Discrepancies between explicit and implicit self-concepts: Consequences for information processing. *Journal of Personality and Social Psychology, 91,* 154–170. http://dx.doi.org/10.1037/0022-3514.91.1.154

Brockell, G. (2019). Bullies and black trench coats: The Columbine shooting's most dangerous myths. *The Washington Post.* Retrieved from https://www.washingtonpost.com/history/2019/04/19/bullies-black-trench-coats-columbine-shootings-most-dangerous-myths/

Bronfenbrenner, U. (1989). Ecological systems theory. *Annals of Child Development, 6,* 187–249.

Brown, G. K., Jeglic, E., Henriques, G. R., & Beck, A. T. (2006). Cognitive therapy, cognition, and suicidal behavior. In T. E. Ellis (Ed.), *Cognition and suicide: Theory, research, and therapy* (pp. 53–74). Washington, DC: American Psychological Association. http://dx.doi.org/10.1037/11377-003

Brown, N. R., Lee, P. J., Krslak, M., Conrad, F. G., Hansen, T. G. B., Havelka, J., & Reddon, J. R. (2009). Living in history: How war, terrorism, and natural disaster affect the organization of autobiographical memory. *Psychological Science, 20,* 399–405. http://dx.doi.org/10.1111/j.1467-9280.2009.02307.x

Bruehlman-Senecal, E., Ayduk, Ö., & John, O. P. (2016). Taking the long view: Implications of individual differences in temporal distancing for affect, stress reactivity, and well-being. *Journal of Personality and Social Psychology, 111,* 610–635. http://dx.doi.org/10.1037/pspp0000103

Buhs, E. S., Ladd, G. W., & Herald, S. L. (2006). Peer exclusion and victimization: Processes that mediate the relation between peer group rejection and children's classroom engagement and achievement? *Journal of Educational Psychology, 98,* 1–13. http://dx.doi.org/10.1037/0022-0663.98.1.1

Bump, P. (2017). 70 percent of White men in the U.S. are represented by a White man in the House. *Washington Post.* Retrieved from https://www.washingtonpost.com/news/the-fix/wp/2017/01/12/70-percent-of-white-men-in-the-u-s-are-represented-by-a-white-man-in-the-house/?utm_term=.218b581ed9ae

Burkard, A. W., & Knox, S. (2004). Effect of therapist color-blindness on empathy and attributions in cross-cultural counseling. *Journal of Counseling Psychology, 51,* 387–397. http://dx.doi.org/10.1037/0022-0167.51.4.387

Butler, C. (2015). Intersectionality in family therapy training: Inviting students to embrace the complexities of lived experience. *Journal of Family Therapy, 37,* 583–589. http://dx.doi.org/10.1111/1467-6427.12090

Cai, W., & Patel, J. K. (2019, May 11). A half-century of school shootings like Columbine, Sandy Hook and Parkland. *The New York Times.* Retrieved from https://www.nytimes.com/interactive/2019/05/11/us/school-shootings-united-states.html

Caldwell, L. D. (2009). Counseling with the poor, underserved, and underrepresented. In C. M. Ellis & J. Carlson (Eds.), *Cross cultural awareness and social justice in counseling* (pp. 283–300). New York, NY: Routledge/Taylor & Francis.

Candib, L. M. (2002). Truth telling and advance planning at the end of life: Problems with autonomy in a multicultural world. *Families, Systems, & Health, 20,* 213–228. http://dx.doi.org/10.1037/h0089471

Cantor, D. W. (1998). Achieving a Mental Health Bill of Rights. *Professional Psychology: Research and Practice, 29,* 315–316. http://dx.doi.org/10.1037/0735-7028.29.4.315

Cantor, D. W., & Fuentes, M. A. (2008). Psychology's response to managed care. *Professional Psychology: Research and Practice, 39,* 638–645. http://dx.doi.org/10.1037/0735-7028.39.6.638

Carew, J. (1994). *Ghosts in our blood: With Malcolm X in Africa, England, and the Caribbean.* Chicago, IL: Lawrence Hill Books.

Carey, K. B., Merrill, J. E., Walsh, J. L., Lust, S. A., Kalichman, S. C., & Carey, M. P. (2018). Predictors of short-term change after a brief alcohol intervention for mandated college drinkers. *Addictive Behaviors, 77,* 152–159. http://dx.doi.org/10.1016/j.addbeh.2017.09.019

Carkhuff, R. R. (1969). *Helping and human relations: A primer for lay and professional helpers.* New York, NY: Holt, Rinehart, & Winston.

Carmel, S., Granek, L., & Zamir, A. (2016). Influences of nationalism and historical traumatic events on the will-to-live of elderly Israelis. *The Gerontologist, 56,* 753–761. http://dx.doi.org/10.1093/geront/gnv031

Carney, L. M., & Park, C. L. (2018). Cancer survivors' understanding of the cause and cure of their illness: Religious and nonreligious appraisals of cancer and well-being. *Psycho-Oncology, 27,* 1553–1558. http://dx.doi.org/10.1002/pon.4691

Cashman, M., & Cushman, F. A. (in press). Learning from moral failure. In E. Lambert & J. Schwenkler (Eds.), *Becoming someone new: Essays on transformative experience, choice, and change.* New York, NY: Oxford University Press.

Chang, J., Chan, M., & Stern, O. (2008, February 2). To drink or not to drink: Pregnancy and alcohol. *Good Morning America.* Retrieved from http://abcnews.go.com/video/playerindex?id=4232465

Chen, S. W.-H., & Davenport, D. S. (2005). Cognitive–behavioral therapy with Chinese American clients: Cautions and modifications. *Psychotherapy: Theory, Research, Practice, Training, 42,* 101–110. http://dx.doi.org/10.1037/0033-3204.42.1.101

Clauss-Ehlers, C. S. (2008). Sociocultural factors, resilience, and coping: Support for a culturally sensitive measure of resilience. *Journal of Applied Developmental Psychology, 29,* 197–212. http://dx.doi.org/10.1016/j.appdev.2008.02.004

CNN.com. (2006). *Yates' confession.* Retrieved from http://transcripts.cnn.com/TRANSCRIPTS/0608/01/ng.01.html

Cokley, K. O., & Vandiver, B. (2011). Ethnic and racial identity. In J. Hansen & E. Altmaier (Eds.), *The Oxford handbook of counseling psychology* (pp. 291–325). New York, NY: Oxford University Press.

Constantino, M. J., Ametrano, R. M., & Greenberg, R. P. (2012). Clinician interventions and participant characteristics that foster adaptive patient expectations for psychotherapy and psychotherapeutic change. *Psychotherapy, 49,* 557–569. http://dx.doi.org/10.1037/a0029440

Contemporary Authors Online. (2003). Anna Michener. *Gale.* PEN: 0000131492

Cooper, A. A., Zoellner, L. A., Roy-Byrne, P., Mavissakalian, M. R., & Feeny, N. C. (2017). Do changes in trauma-related beliefs predict PTSD symptom improvement in prolonged exposure and sertraline? *Journal of Consulting and Clinical Psychology, 85,* 873–882. http://dx.doi.org/10.1037/ccp0000220

Cooper, S. (2019, May 15). Sandra Bland's sister: She died because officer saw her as "threatening Black woman," not human. *USA Today.* Retrieved from https://www.usatoday.com/story/opinion/policing/

spotlight/2019/05/13/sandra-bland-sister-police-brutality-policing-the-usa/1169559001/

Costanzo, M., & Krauss, D. (2017). *Forensic and legal psychology: Psychological science applied to law* (3rd ed.). New York, NY: Worth.

Coyne, A. E., Constantino, M. J., Westra, H. A., & Antony, M. M. (2019). Interpersonal change as a mediator of the within- and between-patient alliance-outcome association in two treatments for generalized anxiety disorder. *Journal of Consulting and Clinical Psychology, 87*, 472–483. http://dx.doi.org/10.1037/ccp0000394

Court TV (Producer). (1999). *Psychiatric assessment of Andrea Yates*. Retrieved from http://www.courttv.com/trials/yates/docs/psychiatric6.html [No longer available online]

Csikszentmihalyi, M. (2014). Learning, "flow," and happiness. In M. Csikszentmihalyi (Ed.), *Applications of flow in human development and education* (pp. 153–172). Dordrecht, The Netherlands: Springer. http://dx.doi.org/10.1007/978-94-017-9094-9_7

Culpin, I., Stapinski, L., Miles, O. B., Araya, R., & Joinson, C. (2015). Exposure to socioeconomic adversity in early life and risk of depression at 18 years: The mediating role of locus of control. *Journal of Affective Disorders, 183*, 269–278. http://dx.doi.org/10.1016/j.jad.2015.05.030

Cummings, J. P., Ivan, M. C., Carson, C. S., Stanley, M. A., & Pargament, K. I. (2014). A systematic review of relations between psychotherapist religiousness/spirituality and therapy-related variables. *Spirituality in Clinical Practice, 1*, 116–132. http://dx.doi.org/10.1037/scp0000014

Dale, R., & Vinson, D. W. (2013). The observer's observer's paradox. *Journal of Experimental & Theoretical Artificial Intelligence, 25*, 303–322. http://dx.doi.org/10.1080/0952813X.2013.782987

D'Amico, E. J., Houck, J. M., Hunter, S. B., Miles, J. N. V., Osilla, K. C., & Ewing, B. A. (2015). Group motivational interviewing for adolescents: Change talk and alcohol and marijuana outcomes. *Journal of Consulting and Clinical Psychology, 83*, 68–80. http://dx.doi.org/10.1037/a0038155

Daniels, J. A., Alva, L. A., & Olivares, S. (2002). Graduate training for managed care: A national survey of psychology and social work programs. *Professional Psychology: Research and Practice,*

33, 587–590. http://dx.doi.org/10.1037/0735-7028.33.6.587

D'Arrigo-Patrick, J., Hoff, C., Knudson-Martin, C., & Tuttle, A. (2017). Navigating critical theory and postmodernism: Social justice and therapist power in family therapy. *Family Process, 56*, 574–588. http://dx.doi.org/10.1111/famp.12236

Denno, D. W. (2003). Appendix 1. Time line of Andrea Yates' life and trial. *Duke Journal of Gender Law and Policy, 10*, 61–84.

DeRubeis, R. J., Siegle, G. J., & Hollon, S. D. (2008). Cognitive therapy versus medication for depression: Treatment outcomes and neural mechanisms. *Nature Reviews Neuroscience, 9*, 788–796. http://dx.doi.org/10.1038/nrn2345

Doherty-Sneddon, G., & Phelps, F. G. (2005). Gaze aversion: A response to cognitive or social difficulty? *Memory & Cognition, 33*, 727–733. http://dx.doi.org/10.3758/BF03195338

Dorociak, K. E., Rupert, P. A., Bryant, F. B., & Zahniser, E. (2017). Development of a self-care assessment for psychologists. *Journal of Counseling Psychology, 64*, 325–334. http://dx.doi.org/10.1037/cou0000206

Dumont, F. (2014). Introduction to 21st-century psychotherapies. In D. Wedding & R. J. Corsini (Eds.), *Current psychotherapies* (10th ed., pp. 1–17). Belmont, CA: Cengage.

Duncan, D. T., & Hatzenbuehler, M. L. (2014). Lesbian, gay, bisexual, and transgender hate crimes and suicidality among a population-based sample of sexual-minority adolescents in Boston. *American Journal of Public Health, 104*, 272–278. http://dx.doi.org/10.2105/AJPH.2013.301424

Dunkley, J., & Whelan, T. A. (2006). Vicarious traumatisation: Current status and future directions. *British Journal of Guidance & Counselling, 34*, 107–116. http://dx.doi.org/10.1080/03069880500483166

Dweck, C. J. (2006). *Mindset: The new psychology of success*. New York, NY: Ballantine Books.

Dybicz, P. (2012). The ethic of care: Recapturing social work's first voice. *Social Work, 57*, 271–280. http://dx.doi.org/10.1093/sw/sws007

Edmondson, D., Chaudoir, S. R., Mills, M. A., Park, C. L., Holub, J., & Bartkowiak, J. M. (2011). From shattered assumptions to weakened worldviews: Trauma symptoms signal anxiety buffer disruption.

Journal of Loss and Trauma, 16, 358–385. http://dx.doi.org/10.1080/15325024.2011.572030

Elliott, R., Bohart, A. C., Watson, J. C., & Greenberg, L. S. (2011). Empathy. *Psychotherapy, 48*, 43–49. http://dx.doi.org/10.1037/a0022187

Elliott, R., Bohart, A. C., Watson, J. C., & Murphy, D. (2018). Therapist empathy and client outcome: An updated meta-analysis. *Psychotherapy, 55*, 399–410. http://dx.doi.org/10.1037/pst0000175

Epston, D., & White, M. (1995). Termination as a rite of passage: Questioning strategies for a therapy of inclusion. In R. A. Neimeyer & M. J. Mahoney (Eds.), *Constructivism in psychotherapy* (pp. 339–354). Washington, DC: American Psychological Association. http://dx.doi.org/10.1037/10170-014

Eubanks, C. F., Burckell, L. A., & Goldfried, M. R. (2018). Clinical consensus strategies to repair ruptures in the therapeutic alliance. *Journal of Psychotherapy Integration, 28*, 60–76. http://dx.doi.org/10.1037/int0000097

Ewing, C. P. (2005). Judicial notebook: *Tarasoff* reconsidered. *Monitor on Psychology, 36*, 112.

Fadiman, A. (2012). *The spirit catches you and you fall down: A Hmong child, her American doctors, and the collision of two cultures.* New York, NY: Farrar, Straus & Giroux.

Farb, N. A., Irving, J. A., Anderson, A. K., & Segal, Z. V. (2015). A two-factor model of relapse/recurrence vulnerability in unipolar depression. *Journal of Abnormal Psychology, 124*, 38–53. http://dx.doi.org/10.1037/abn0000031

Farber, B. A., Suzuki, J. Y., & Lynch, D. A. (2018). Positive regard and psychotherapy outcome: A meta-analytic review. *Psychotherapy, 55*, 411–423. http://dx.doi.org/10.1037/pst0000171

Farnsworth, J. K., & Callahan, J. L. (2013). A model for addressing client–clinician value conflict. *Training and Education in Professional Psychology, 7*, 205–214. http://dx.doi.org/10.1037/a0032216

Faust, J., & Katchen, L. B. (2004). Treatment of children with complicated posttraumatic stress reactions. *Psychotherapy: Theory, Research, Practice, Training, 41*, 426–437. http://dx.doi.org/10.1037/0033-3204.41.4.426

Fisher, C. B., & Oransky, M. (2008). Informed consent to psychotherapy: Protecting the dignity and respecting the autonomy of patients. *Journal of Clinical Psychology, 64*, 576–588. http://dx.doi.org/10.1002/jclp.20472

Fisher, M. A., & the Center for Ethical Practice, Inc. (2008). Protecting confidentiality rights: The need for an ethical practice model. *American Psychologist, 63*, 1–13. http://dx.doi.org/10.1037/0003-066X.63.1.1

Folkman, S., & Moskowitz, J. T. (2004). Coping: Pitfalls and promise. *Annual Review of Psychology, 55*, 745–774. http://dx.doi.org/10.1146/annurev.psych.55.090902.141456

Fowers, B. J., & Davidov, B. J. (2006). The virtue of multiculturalism: Personal transformation, character, and openness to the other. *American Psychologist, 61*, 581–594. http://dx.doi.org/10.1037/0003-066X.61.6.581

Frank, J. D., & Frank, J. B. (1993). *Persuasion and healing: A comparative study of psychotherapy* (3rd ed.). Baltimore: Johns Hopkins Paperbacks.

Frankl, V. E. (1946/1984). *Man's search for meaning* (rev.). New York, NY: Washington Square Press.

Franklin, C., Zhang, A., Froerer, A., & Johnson, S. (2017). Solution focused brief therapy: A systematic review and meta-summary of process research. *Journal of Marital and Family Therapy, 43*, 16–30. http://dx.doi.org/10.1111/jmft.12193

Fraser, J. S., & Solovey, A. D. (2007). *Second-order change in psychotherapy: The golden thread that unifies effective treatments.* Washington, DC: American Psychological Association.

Frazier, P. A., Mortensen, H., & Steward, J. (2005). Coping strategies as mediators of the relations among perceived control and distress in sexual assault survivors. *Journal of Counseling Psychology, 52*, 267–278. http://dx.doi.org/10.1037/0022-0167.52.3.267

Friedlander, M. L., Escudero, V., & Heatherington, L. (2006). *Therapeutic alliances in couple and family therapy: An empirically informed guide to practice.* Washington, DC: American Psychological Association. http://dx.doi.org/10.1037/11410-000

Fuertes, J. N., Gelso, C. J., Owen, J. J., & Cheng, D. (2013). Real relationship, working alliance, transference/countertransference and outcome in time-limited counseling and psychotherapy. *Counselling Psychology Quarterly, 26*, 294–312. http://dx.doi.org/10.1080/09515070.2013.845548

Fukuyama, M. A., & Sevig, T. D. (1999). *Integrating spirituality into multicultural counseling.* Thousand Oaks, CA: Sage.

Gabriella. (2001, February). Interview with Eminem: It's lonely at the top. *NY Rock.* Retrieved from http://www.eminem.net/interviews/lonely_at_the_top/

Gandy, K. (2002, March 13). Yates verdict can serve as warning to prevent future tragedies. *National Organization for Women.* Retrieved from http://www.now.org/press/03-02/03-13a.html

Garcia, A. (2018). These are the only two owners of color in the NFL. *CNN Money.* Retrieved from https://money.cnn.com/2018/05/18/news/nfl-nba-mlb-owners-diversity/index.html

Gately, G. (2006, January 7). Miner's wife hopes prayers and Metallica will help him pull through. *New York Times,* Retrieved from http://www.nytimes.com/2006/01/07/national/07survivor.html?_r=1&n=Top%2fNews%2fNational%2fU.S.%20States%2c%20Territories%20and%20Possessions%2fWest%20Virginia

Gendlin, E. T., & Hendricks, M. (n.d.). Rap manual. In *Changes.* Unpublished manuscript, Chicago, IL.

George, L. S., & Park, C. L. (2016). Meaning in life as comprehension, purpose, and mattering: Towards integration and new research questions. *Review of General Psychology, 20,* 205–220.

Gilstrap, L. L. (2004). A missing link in suggestibility research: What is known about the behavior of field interviewers in unstructured interviews with young children? *Journal of Experimental Psychology: Applied, 10*, 13–24. http://dx.doi.org/10.1037/1076-898X.10.1.13

Ginzburg, K. (2004). PTSD and world assumptions following myocardial infarction: A longitudinal study. *American Journal of Orthopsychiatry, 74*, 286–292. http://dx.doi.org/10.1037/0002-9432.74.3.286

Glick, D., Keene-Osborn, S., Gegax, T. T., Bai, M., Clemetson, L., Gordon, D., & Klaidman, D. (1999, May 3). Anatomy of a massacre. *Newsweek, 153*, pp. 24–30.

The Global Deception Research Team. (2006). A world of lies. *Journal of Cross-Cultural Psychology, 37*, 60–74. http://dx.doi.org/10.1177/0022022105282295

Glosoff, H. L., & Kocet, M. M. (2005). Highlights of the 2005 *ACA Code of Ethics.* In G. R. Walz, J. C. Bleuer, & R. K. Yep (Eds.), *Vistas: Compelling perspectives on counseling 2006* (pp. 5–9). Alexandria, VA: American Counseling Association.

Gökbayrak, N. S., Paiva, A. L., Blissmer, B. J., & Prochaska, J. O. (2015). Predictors of relapse among smokers: Transtheoretical effort variables, demographics, and smoking severity. *Addictive Behaviors, 42*, 176–179. http://dx.doi.org/10.1016/j.addbeh.2014.11.022

Goldfried, M. R. (2002). A cognitive-behavioral perspective on termination. *Journal of Psychotherapy Integration, 12*, 364–372. http://dx.doi.org/10.1037/1053-0479.12.3.364

Goldfried, M. R. (2004). Integrating integratively oriented brief psychotherapy. *Journal of Psychotherapy Integration, 14*, 93–105. http://dx.doi.org/10.1037/1053-0479.14.1.93

Goldfried, M. R. (2007). What has psychotherapy inherited from Carl Rogers? *Psychotherapy: Theory, Research, Practice, Training, 44*, 249–252. http://dx.doi.org/10.1037/0033-3204.44.3.249

Goldfried, M. R. (2019). Obtaining consensus in psychotherapy: What holds us back? *American Psychologist, 74*, 484–496. http://dx.doi.org/10.1037/amp0000365

Goldsmith, L. P., Lewis, S. W., Dunn, G., & Bentall, R. P. (2015). Psychological treatments for early psychosis can be beneficial or harmful, depending on the therapeutic alliance: An instrumental variable analysis. *Psychological Medicine, 45*, 2365–2373. http://dx.doi.org/10.1017/S003329171500032X

Gollwitzer, P. M., & Sheeran, P. (2006). Implementation intentions and goal achievement: A meta-analysis of effects and processes. *Advances in Experimental Social Psychology, 38*, 69–119. http://dx.doi.org/10.1016/S0065-2601(06)38002-1

Gonzalez, J. S., Safren, S. A., Cagliero, E., Wexler, D. J., Delahanty, L., Wittenberg, E., . . . Grant, R. W. (2007). Depression, self-care, and medication adherence in type 2 diabetes: Relationships across the full range of symptom severity. *Diabetes Care, 30,* 2222–2227. http://dx.doi.org/10.2337/dc07-0158

Goode, J., Park, J., Parkin, S., Tompkins, K. A., & Swift, J. K. (2017). A collaborative approach to psychotherapy termination. *Psychotherapy, 54,* 10–14. http://dx.doi.org/10.1037/pst0000085

Gottlieb, M. C., Robinson, K., & Younggren, J. N. (2007). Multiple relations in supervision: Guidance for administrators, supervisors, and students. *Professional Psychology: Research and Practice, 38,* 241–247. http://dx.doi.org/10.1037/0735-7028.38.3.241

Gray, M. J., Maguen, S., & Litz, B. T. (2007). Schema constructs and cognitive models of Posttraumatic Stress Disorder. In L. P. Riso, P. L. du Toit, D. J. Stein, & J. E. Young (Eds.), *Cognitive schemas and core beliefs in psychological problems: A scientist–practitioner guide* (pp. 59–92). Washington, DC: American Psychological Association. http://dx.doi.org/10.1037/11561-004

Greenberg, D., & Wiesner, I. S. (2004). Jews. In A. M. Josephson & J. R. Peteet (Eds.), *Handbook of spirituality and worldview in clinical practice* (pp. 91–109). Arlington, VA: American Psychiatric Association.

Greenberg, L. (2008). Emotion and cognition in psychotherapy: The transforming power of affect. *Canadian Psychology, 49,* 49–59. http://dx.doi.org/10.1037/0708-5591.49.1.49

Greenberg, L. S., Elliot, R., Watson, J. C., & Bohart, A. C. (2001). Empathy. *Psychotherapy, 38,* 380–384. http://dx.doi.org/10.1037/0033-3204.38.4.380

Greenfield, P. M., Trumbull, E., Keller, H., Rothstein-Fisch, C., Suzuki, L., & Quiroz, B. (2006). Cultural conceptions of learning and development. In P. A. Alexander & P. H. Winne (Eds.), *Handbook of educational psychology* (pp. 675–692). Mahwah, NJ: Erlbaum.

Grosse Holtforth, M., & Castonguay, L. G. (2005). Relationship and techniques in cognitive-behavioral therapy–A motivational approach. *Psychotherapy, 42,* 443–455. http://dx.doi.org/10.1037/0033-3204.42.4.443

Grouzet, F. M. E., Kasser, T., Ahuvia, A., Dols, J. M. F., Kim, Y., Lau, S., . . . Sheldon, K. M. (2005). The structure of goal contents across 15 cultures. *Journal of Personality and Social Psychology, 89,* 800–816. http://dx.doi.org/10.1037/0022-3514.89.5.800

Gutheil, T. G., & Gabbard, G. O. (1993). The concept of boundaries in clinical practice: Theoretical and risk-management dimensions. *The American Journal of Psychiatry, 150,* 188–196. http://dx.doi.org/10.1176/ajp.150.2.188

Gutierrez, D., Fox, J., Jones, K., & Fallon, E. (2018). The treatment planning of experienced counselors: A qualitative examination. *Journal of Counseling & Development, 96,* 86–96. http://dx.doi.org/10.1002/jcad.12180

Gutierrez, I., & Park, C. L. (2015). Emerging adulthood, evolving worldviews: How life events impact college students' developing belief systems. *Emerging Adulthood, 3,* 85–97. http://dx.doi.org/10.1177/2167696814544501

Handelsman, M. M., Gottlieb, M. C., & Knapp, S. (2005). Training ethical psychologists: An acculturation model. *Professional Psychology: Research and Practice, 36,* 59–65. http://dx.doi.org/10.1037/0735-7028.36.1.59

Harriot, M. (2019). Redlining: The origin story of institutional racism. *The Root.* https://www.theroot.com/redlining-the-origin-story-of-institutional-racism-1834308539

Hart, J., Shaver, P. R., & Goldenberg, J. L. (2005). Attachment, self-esteem, worldviews, and terror management: Evidence for a tripartite security system. *Journal of Personality and Social Psychology, 88,* 999–1013. http://dx.doi.org/10.1037/0022-3514.88.6.999

Hawley, K. M., & Weisz, J. R. (2003). Child, parent, and therapist (dis)agreement on target problems in outpatient therapy: The therapist's dilemma and its implications. *Journal of Consulting and Clinical Psychology, 71,* 62–70. http://dx.doi.org/10.1037/0022-006X.71.1.62

Hays, J. R. (2002, May–June). State of Texas v. Andrea Yates. *National Psychologist, 11.* Retrieved from http://nationalpsychologist.com/articles/art_v11n3_3.htm

Heilbrun, K., & Kramer, G. M. (2005). Involuntary medication, trial competence, and clinical dilemmas: Implications of *Sell v. United States* for psychological practice. *Professional Psychology: Research and Practice, 36,* 459–466. http://dx.doi.org/10.1037/0735-7028.36.5.459

Heinonen, E., & Orlinsky, D. E. (2013). Psychotherapists' personal identities, theoretical orientations, and professional relationships: Elective affinity and role adjustment as modes of congruence. *Psychotherapy Research, 23,* 718–731. http://dx.doi.org/10.1080/10503307.2013.814926

Heintzelman, S. J., & King, L. A. (2014). Life is pretty meaningful. *American Psychologist, 69,* 561–574. http://dx.doi.org/10.1037/a0035049

Hensel, J. M., Ruiz, C., Finney, C., & Dewa, C. S. (2015). Meta-analysis of risk factors for secondary traumatic stress in therapeutic work with trauma victims. *Journal of Traumatic Stress, 28,* 83–91. http://dx.doi.org/10.1002/jts.21998

Hess, U., Cossette, M., & Hareli, S. (2016). I and my friends are good people: The perception of incivility by self, friends and strangers. *Europe's Journal of Psychology, 12,* 99–114. http://dx.doi.org/10.5964/ejop.v12i1.937

Hooley, J. M., & Miklowitz, D. J. (2017). Perceived criticism in the treatment of a high-risk adolescent. *Journal of Clinical Psychology, 73,* 570–578. http://dx.doi.org/10.1002/jclp.22454

Hoop, J. G., DiPasquale, T., Hernandez, J. M., & Roberts, L. W. (2008). Ethics and culture in mental health care. *Ethics & Behavior, 18,* 353–372. http://dx.doi.org/10.1080/10508420701713048

Horvath, A. O., Del Re, A. C., Flückiger, C., & Symonds, D. (2011). Alliance in individual psychotherapy. *Psychotherapy, 48,* 9–16. http://dx.doi.org/10.1037/a0022186

Hundt, N. E., Helm, A., Smith, T. L., Lamkin, J., Cully, J. A., & Stanley, M. A. (2018). Failure to engage: A qualitative study of veterans who decline evidence-based psychotherapies for PTSD. *Psychological Services, 15,* 536–542. http://dx.doi.org/10.1037/ser0000212

Hwang, W. C. (2016). Culturally adapting evidence-based practices for ethnic minorities and immigrant families. In N. Zane, G. Bernal, & F. T. L. Leong (Eds.), *Evidence-based psychological practice with ethnic minorities: Culturally informed research and clinical strategies* (pp. 289–309).

Washington, DC: American Psychological Association. http://dx.doi.org/10.1037/14940-014

Ibrahim, F. A. (1985). Effective cross-cultural counseling and psychotherapy: A framework. *The Counseling Psychologist, 13,* 625–638. http://dx.doi.org/10.1177/0011000085134006

Ivey, A. E., & Ivey, M. B. (2014). *Intentional interviewing and counseling: Facilitating client development in a multicultural society* (8th ed.). Belmont, CA: Brooks/Cole.

Janoff-Bulman, R. (1989). Assumptive worlds and the stress of traumatic events: Applications of the schema construct. *Social Cognition, 7,* 113–136. http://dx.doi.org/10.1521/soco.1989.7.2.113

Jennings, L., & Skovholt, T. M. (1999). The cognitive, emotional, and relational characteristics of master therapists. *Journal of Counseling Psychology, 46,* 3–11. http://dx.doi.org/10.1037/0022-0167.46.1.3

Jennings, L., Sovereign, A., Botorff, N., Mussell, M. P., & Vye, C. (2005). Nine ethical values of master therapists. *Journal of Mental Health Counseling, 27,* 32–47. http://dx.doi.org/10.17744/mehc.27.1.lmm8vmdujgev2qhp

Johnson, A., & Jackson Williams, D. (2015). White racial identity, color-blind racial attitudes, and multicultural counseling competence. *Cultural Diversity and Ethnic Minority Psychology, 21,* 440–449. http://dx.doi.org/10.1037/a0037533

Kahana, B., Harel, Z., & Kahana, E. (1998). Predictors of psychological well-being among survivors of the Holocaust. In J. Wilson, Z. Harel, & B. Kahana (Eds.), *Human adaptation to extreme stress* (pp. 171–192). New York, NY: Plenum.

Karno, M. P., & Longabaugh, R. (2005). Less directiveness by therapists improves drinking outcomes of reactant clients in alcoholism treatment. *Journal of Consulting and Clinical Psychology, 73,* 262–267. http://dx.doi.org/10.1037/0022-006X.73.2.262

Kasser, T. (2016). Materialistic values and goals. *Annual Review of Psychology, 67,* 489–514. http://dx.doi.org/10.1146/annurev-psych-122414-033344

Kassin, S., Fein, S., & Markus, H. R. (2017). *Social psychology* (10th ed.). Boston, MA: Cengage.

Kelly, R. E., Mansell, W., & Wood, A. M. (2015). Goal conflict and well-being: A review and hierarchical model of goal conflict, ambivalence, self-discrepancy and self-concordance. *Personality and Individual Differences, 85,* 212–229. http://dx.doi.org/10.1016/j.paid.2015.05.011

Kidd, S. M. (2006). *When the heart waits: Spiritual direction for life's sacred questions.* New York, NY: HarperOne.

Killian, K. D. (2008). Helping till it hurts? A multi-method study of compassion fatigue, burnout, and self-care in clinicians working with trauma survivors. *Traumatology, 14,* 32–44. http://dx.doi.org/10.1177/1534765608319083

Kim, B. S. K., Ng, G. F., & Ahn, A. J. (2005). Effects of client expectation for counseling success, client–counselor worldview match, and client adherence to Asian and European American cultural values on counseling process with Asian Americans. *Journal of Counseling Psychology, 52,* 67–76. http://dx.doi.org/10.1037/0022-0167.52.1.67

Kirsch, I. (2014). Antidepressants and the placebo effect. *Zeitschrift für Psychologie mit Zeitschrift für Angewandte Psychologie, 222,* 128–134. http://dx.doi.org/10.1027/2151-2604/a000176

Klug, H. J., & Maier, G. W. (2015). Linking goal progress and subjective well-being: A meta-analysis. *Journal of Happiness Studies, 16,* 37–65. http://dx.doi.org/10.1007/s10902-013-9493-0

Knapp, S., Gottlieb, M. C., & Handelsman, M. M. (2018). The benefits of adopting a positive perspective in ethics education. *Training and Education in Professional Psychology, 12,* 196–202. http://dx.doi.org/10.1037/tep0000195

Knapp, S., & Slattery, J. M. (2004). Professional boundaries in non-traditional settings. *Professional Psychology: Research and Practice, 35,* 553–558. http://dx.doi.org/10.1037/0735-7028.35.5.553

Knapp, S., Younggren, J. N., VandeCreek, L., Harris, E., & Martin, J. (2013). *Assessing and managing risk in psychological practice: An individualized approach* (2nd ed.). Rockville, MD: The Trust.

Knapp, S. J., VandeCreek, L. D., & Fingerhut, R. (2017). *Practical ethics for psychologists: A positive approach* (3rd ed.). Washington, DC: American Psychological Association. http://dx.doi.org/10.1037/0000036-000

Knox, S., Adrians, N., Everson, E., Hess, S., Hill, C., & Crook-Lyon, R. (2011). Clients' perspectives on therapy termination. *Psychotherapy Research, 21,* 154–167. http://dx.doi.org/10.1080/10503307.2010.534509

Kolden, G. G., Klein, M. H., Wang, C. C., & Austin, S. B. (2011). Congruence/genuineness. *Psychotherapy, 48,* 65–71. http://dx.doi.org/10.1037/a0022064

Kolmes, K., & Taube, D. O. (2014). Seeking and finding our clients on the Internet: Boundary considerations in cyberspace. *Professional Psychology: Research and Practice, 45,* 3–10. http://dx.doi.org/10.1037/a0029958

Koltko-Rivera, M. E. (2004). The psychology of worldviews. *Review of General Psychology, 8,* 3–58. http://dx.doi.org/10.1037/1089-2680.8.1.3

Kottler, J. A. (2004). *Introduction to therapeutic counseling: Voices from the field* (5th ed.). Pacific Grove, CA: Brooks/Cole.

Kouchaki, M., & Desai, S. D. (2015). Anxious, threatened, and also unethical: How anxiety makes individuals feel threatened and commit unethical acts. *Journal of Applied Psychology, 100,* 360–375. http://dx.doi.org/10.1037/a0037796

Lakin, J. L., & Chartrand, T. L. (2003). Using nonconscious behavioral mimicry to create affiliation and rapport. *Psychological Science, 14,* 334–339. http://dx.doi.org/10.1111/1467-9280.14481

Lamb, D. H., & Catanzaro, S. J. (1998). Sexual and nonsexual boundary violations involving psychologists, clients, supervisees, and students: Implications for professional practice. *Professional Psychology: Research and Practice, 29,* 498–503. http://dx.doi.org/10.1037/0735-7028.29.5.498

Lambert, M. J. (2015). Effectiveness of psychological treatment. *Resonanzen. E-Journal für Biopsycho-soziale Dialoge in Psychotherapie. Supervision und Beratung, 3,* 87–100.

Lambert, M. J., & Archer, A. (2006). Research findings on the effects of psychotherapy and their implications for practice. In C. D. Goodheart, A. E. Kazdin, & R. J. Sternberg (Eds.), *Evidence-based psychotherapy: Where practice and research meet* (pp. 111–130). Washington, DC: American Psychological Association. http://dx.doi.org/10.1037/11423-005

Lambert, M. J., Gregersen, A. T., & Burlingame, G. M. (2004). The Outcome Questionnaire—45. In M. E. Maruish (Ed.), *The use of psychological testing for treatment planning and outcome assessment* (3rd ed., pp. 191–234). Mahwah, NJ: Erlbaum.

Larsen, D. L., Attkisson, C. C., Hargreaves, W. A., & Nguyen, T. D. (1979). Assessment of client/patient satisfaction: Development of a general scale. *Evaluation and Program Planning, 2*, 197–207. http://dx.doi.org/10.1016/0149-7189(79)90094-6

Laudet, A. B., Magura, S., Vogel, H. S., & Knight, E. L. (2004). Perceived reasons for substance misuse among persons with a psychiatric disorder. *American Journal of Orthopsychiatry, 74*, 365–375. http://dx.doi.org/10.1037/0002-9432.74.3.365

Lazarus, A. A. (2002). How certain boundaries and ethics diminish therapeutic effectiveness. In A. A. Lazarus & O. Zur (Eds.), *Dual relationships and psychotherapy* (pp. 25–31). New York, NY: Springer.

Lee, R. E. (2009). "If you build it, they may not come": Lessons from a funded project. *Research on Social Work Practice, 19*, 251–260. http://dx.doi.org/10.1177/1049731508329416

Lee, S. Y., Park, C. L., & Hale, A. (2016). Relations of trauma exposure with current religiousness and spirituality. *Mental Health, Religion & Culture, 19*, 493–505. http://dx.doi.org/10.1080/13674676.2016.1207161

Lent, R. W. (2004). Toward a unifying theoretical and practical perspective on well-being and psychosocial adjustment. *Journal of Counseling Psychology, 51*, 482–509. http://dx.doi.org/10.1037/0022-0167.51.4.482

Lerner, M. J. (1980). The desire for justice and reactions to victims: Social psychological studies of some antecedents and consequences. In J. Macaulay & L. Berkowitz (Eds.), *Altruism and helping behavior* (pp. 205–229). New York, NY: Academic Press.

Lidén, M., Gräns, M., & Juslin, P. (2018). The presumption of guilt in suspect interrogations: Apprehension as a trigger of confirmation bias and debiasing techniques. *Law and Human Behavior, 42*, 336–354. http://dx.doi.org/10.1037/lhb0000287

Lilliengren, P., & Werbart, A. (2005). A model of therapeutic action grounded in the patients' view of curative and hindering factors in psychoanalytic psychotherapy. *Psychotherapy: Theory, Research, Practice, Training, 42*, 324–339. http://dx.doi.org/10.1037/0033-3204.42.3.324

Lindert, J., von Ehrenstein, O. S., Priebe, S., Mielck, A., & Brähler, E. (2009). Depression and anxiety in labor migrants and refugees—A systematic review and meta-analysis. *Social Science & Medicine, 69*, 246–257. http://dx.doi.org/10.1016/j.socscimed.2009.04.032

Lindhiem, O., Bennett, C. B., Orimoto, T. E., & Kolko, D. J. (2016). A meta-analysis of personalized treatment goals in psychotherapy: A preliminary report and call for more studies. *Clinical Psychology: Science and Practice, 23*, 165–176. http://dx.doi.org/10.1111/cpsp.12153

Liszcz, A. M., & Yarhouse, M. A. (2005). Same-sex attraction: A survey regarding client-directed treatment goals. *Psychotherapy: Theory, Research, Practice, Training, 42*, 111–115. http://dx.doi.org/10.1037/0033-3204.42.1.111

Lopez, S. J., & Snyder, C. R. (2003). The future of positive psychological assessment: Making a difference. In S. J. Lopez & V. R. Snyder (Eds.), *Positive psychological assessment: A handbook of models and measures* (pp. 461–468). Washington, DC: American Psychological Association.

López, S. R., Nelson Hipke, K., Polo, A. J., Jenkins, J. H., Karno, M., Vaughn, C., & Snyder, K. S. (2004). Ethnicity, expressed emotion, attributions, and course of schizophrenia: Family warmth matters. *Journal of Abnormal Psychology, 113*, 428–439. http://dx.doi.org/10.1037/0021-843X.113.3.428

LoSavio, S. T., Dillon, K. H., & Resick, P. A. (2017). Cognitive factors in the development, maintenance, and treatment of post-traumatic stress disorder. *Current Opinion in Psychology, 14*, 18–22. http://dx.doi.org/10.1016/j.copsyc.2016.09.006

MacKenzie, M. B., Abbott, K. A., & Kocovski, N. L. (2018). Mindfulness-based cognitive therapy in patients with depression: Current perspectives.

Neuropsychiatric Disease and Treatment, 14, 1599–1605. http://dx.doi.org/10.2147/NDT.S160761

Makover, R. B. (2016). *Treatment planning for psychotherapists: A practical guide to better outcomes.* Arlington, VA: American Psychiatric Publishing.

Malcolm X. (2015, February 20). By any means necessary. *The Washington Post.* Retrieved from https://www.washingtonpost.com/video/national/malcolm-xs-by-any-means-necessary-speech/2015/02/20/16fecd00-b955-11e4-bc30-a4e75503948a_video.html?utm_term=.3d9bc1105b86

Malcolm X., & Haley, A. (1964/1999). *The autobiography of Malcolm X.* New York, NY: Ballantine Books.

Marchese, D. (2017). In conversation: Eminem. *Vulture.* Retrieved from http://www.vulture.com/2017/12/eminem-in-conversation.html

Masland, S. R., & Hooley, J. M. (2015). Perceived criticism: A research update for clinical practitioners. *Clinical Psychology: Science and Practice, 22,* 211–222. http://dx.doi.org/10.1111/cpsp.12110

Mattos, L. A., Schmidt, A. T., Henderson, C. E., & Hogue, A. (2017). Therapeutic alliance and treatment outcome in the outpatient treatment of urban adolescents: The role of callous-unemotional traits. *Psychotherapy, 54,* 136–147. http://dx.doi.org/10.1037/pst0000093

May, R. (1967). *The art of counseling.* Nashville, TN: Abingdon.

McAdams, C. R., Chae, K. B., Foster, V. A., Lloyd-Hazlett, J., Joe, J. R., & Riechel, M. K. (2015). Perceptions of the first family counseling session: Why families come back. *Journal of Family Psychotherapy, 26,* 253–268. http://dx.doi.org/10.1080/08975353.2015.1097239

McGoldrick, M., Gerson, R., & Petry, S. (2020). *Genograms: Assessment and intervention* (4th ed.). New York, NY: W. W. Norton.

McIntosh, P. (1989, July–August). White privilege: Unpacking the invisible knapsack. *Peace and Freedom,* pp. 10–12.

Meissner, C. A., & Kassin, S. M. (2004). "You're guilty, so just confess!" Cognitive and behavioral confirmation biases in the interrogation room. In G. D. Lassiter (Ed.), *Interrogations, confessions, and entrapment* (pp. 85–106). New York, NY: Kluwer. http://dx.doi.org/10.1007/978-0-387-38598-3_4

Michalak, J., & Grosse Holtforth, M. (2006). Where do we go from here? The goal perspective in psychotherapy. *Clinical Psychology: Science and Practice, 13,* 346–365. http://dx.doi.org/10.1111/j.1468-2850.2006.00048.x

Michalak, J., Heidenreich, T., & Hoyer, J. (2004). Goal conflicts: Concepts, findings, and consequences for psychotherapy. In W. M. Cox & E. Klinger (Eds.), *Handbook of motivational counseling: Concepts, approaches, and assessment* (pp. 83–98). New York, NY: Wiley.

Michener, A. J. (1998). *Becoming Anna: The autobiography of a sixteen-year-old.* Chicago, IL: University of Chicago Press. http://dx.doi.org/10.7208/chicago/9780226524047.001.0001

Miller, R. B. (2005). Suffering in psychology: The demoralization of psychotherapeutic practice. *Journal of Psychotherapy Integration, 15,* 299–336. http://dx.doi.org/10.1037/1053-0479.15.3.299

Moeseneder, L., Ribeiro, E., Muran, J. C., & Caspar, F. (2019). Impact of confrontations by therapists on impairment and utilization of the therapeutic alliance. *Psychotherapy Research, 29,* 392–305.

Mohr, J. J., Weiner, J. L., Chopp, R. M., & Wong, S. J. (2009). Effects of client bisexuality on clinical judgment: When is bias most likely to occur? *Journal of Counseling Psychology, 56,* 164–175. http://dx.doi.org/10.1037/a0012816

Molnar, B. E., Sprang, G., Killian, K. D., Gottfried, R., Emery, V., & Bride, B. E. (2017). Advancing science and practice for vicarious traumatization/secondary traumatic stress: A research agenda. *Traumatology, 23,* 129–142. http://dx.doi.org/10.1037/trm0000122

Moore, L. E., Tambling, R. B., & Anderson, S. R. (2013). The intersection of therapy constructs: The relationship between motivation to change, distress, referral source, and pressure to attend. *American Journal of Family Therapy, 41,* 245–258. http://dx.doi.org/10.1080/01926187.2012.685351

Moos, R. H., & Moos, B. S. (2006). Rates and predictors of relapse after natural and treated remission from alcohol use disorders. *Addiction*, *101*, 212–222. http://dx.doi.org/10.1111/j.1360-0443.2006.01310.x

Morales, E., & Norcross, J. C. (2010). Evidence-based practices with ethnic minorities: Strange bedfellows no more. *Journal of Clinical Psychology*, *66*, 821–829. http://dx.doi.org/10.1002/jclp.20712

Mozdrzierz, G. J., Peluso, P. R., & Lisiecki, J. (2009). *Principles of counseling and psychotherapy: Learning the essential domains and nonlinear thinking of master practitioners*. New York, NY: Routledge.

Muder, D. (2007, Fall). Not my father's religion: Unitarian Universalism and the working class. *UU World*, *21*, 33–37.

Murphy, B. C., & Dillon, C. (2015). *Interviewing in action in a multicultural world* (5th ed.). Stamford, CT: Brooks/Cole.

National Association of Social Workers. (2017). *Code of ethics*. Retrieved from https://www.socialworkers.org/About/Ethics/Code-of-Ethics

National Center for Education Statistics. (2017). *Race/ethnicity of college faculty*. Retrieved from https://nces.ed.gov/fastfacts/display.asp?id=61

National Institute on Drug Abuse. (2012). *Principles of drug addiction treatment* (3rd ed.). Retrieved from https://d14rmgtrwzf5a.cloudfront.net/sites/default/files/podat_1.pdf

Nelson, M. L., Englar-Carlson, M., Tierney, S. C., & Hau, J. M. (2006). Class jumping into academia: Multiple identities for counseling academics. *Journal of Counseling Psychology*, *53*, 1–14. http://dx.doi.org/10.1037/0022-0167.53.1.1

Neville, H. A., Awad, G. H., Brooks, J. E., Flores, M. P., & Bluemel, J. (2013). Color-blind racial ideology: Theory, training, and measurement implications in psychology. *American Psychologist*, *68*, 455–466. http://dx.doi.org/10.1037/a0033282

News Conference With CEO of International Coal Group. (2006, January 4). *The New York Times*. Retrieved from https://www.nytimes.com/2006/01/04/national/news-conference-with-ceo-of-international-coal-group.html

Nolen-Hoeksema, S., Wisco, B. E., & Lyubomirsky, S. (2008). Rethinking rumination. *Perspectives on Psychological Science*, *3*, 400–424. http://dx.doi.org/10.1111/j.1745-6924.2008.00088.x

Norcross, J. C., Krebs, P. M., & Prochaska, J. O. (2011). Stages of change. *Journal of Clinical Psychology*, *67*, 143–154. http://dx.doi.org/10.1002/jclp.20758

Norcross, J. C., & Lambert, M. J. (2011). Evidence-based therapy relationships. In J. C. Norcross (Ed.), *Psychotherapy relationships that work: Evidence-based responsiveness* (2nd ed., pp. 3–22). New York, NY: Oxford University Press. http://dx.doi.org/10.1093/acprof:oso/9780199737208.003.0001

Norcross, J. C., & Lambert, M. J. (2018). Psychotherapy relationships that work III. *Psychotherapy*, *55*, 303–315. http://dx.doi.org/10.1037/pst0000193

Norcross, J. C., & VandenBos, G. R. (2018). *Leaving it at the office: A guide to psychotherapist self-care* (2nd ed.). New York, NY: Guilford Press.

Norcross, J. C., & Wampold, B. E. (2011a). Evidence-based therapy relationships: Research conclusions and clinical practices. *Psychotherapy*, *48*, 98–102. http://dx.doi.org/10.1037/a0022161

Norcross, J. C., & Wampold, B. E. (2011b). What works for whom: Tailoring psychotherapy to the person. *Journal of Clinical Psychology*, *67*, 127–132. http://dx.doi.org/10.1002/jclp.20764

Norcross, J. C., Zimmerman, B. E., Greenberg, R. P., & Swift, J. K. (2017). Do all therapists do that when saying goodbye? A study of commonalities in termination behaviors. *Psychotherapy*, *54*, 66–75. http://dx.doi.org/10.1037/pst0000097

O'Connor, K. (2005). Addressing diversity issues in play therapy. *Professional Psychology: Research and Practice*, *36*, 566–573. http://dx.doi.org/10.1037/0735-7028.36.5.566

Ohlheiser, A., & Philip, A. (2015, July 22). "I will light you up!": Texas officer threatened Sandra Bland with Taser during traffic stop. *The Washington Post*. Retrieved from https://www.washingtonpost.com/news/morning-mix/wp/2015/07/21/much-too-early-to-call-jail-cell-hanging-death-of-sandra-bland-suicide-da-says/

Olivera, J., Challú, L., Gómez Penedo, J. M., & Roussos, A. (2017). Client–therapist agreement in the termination process and its association with therapeutic relationship. *Psychotherapy*, *54*, 88–101. http://dx.doi.org/10.1037/pst0000099

O'Malley, S. (2004). *"Are you there alone"? The unspeakable crime of Andrea Yates*. New York, NY: Simon & Schuster.

Orlinsky, D. E., & Rønnestad, M. H. (2005). Career development: Correlates of evolving expertise. In D. E. Orlinsky & M. H. Rønnestad (Eds.), *How psychotherapists develop: A study of therapeutic work and professional growth* (pp. 131–142). Washington, DC: American Psychological Association.

Orlinsky, D. E., Rønnestad, M. H., Gerin, P., Davis, J. D., Ambühl, H., Davis, M. L., . . . Schröder, T. A. (2005). The development of psychotherapists. In D. E. Orlinsky & M. H. Rønnestad (Eds.), *How psychotherapists develop: A study of therapeutic work and professional growth* (pp. 3–13). Washington, DC: American Psychological Association.

Owen, J., Jordan, T. A., II, Turner, D., Davis, D. E., Hook, J. N., & Leach, M. M. (2014). Therapists' multicultural orientation: Client perceptions of cultural humility, spiritual/religious commitment, and therapy outcomes. *Journal of Psychology and Theology, 42*, 91–98. http://dx.doi.org/10.1177/009164711404200110

Owen, J., Tao, K. W., Drinane, J. M., Hook, J., Davis, D. E., & Kune, N. F. (2016). Client perceptions of therapists' multicultural orientation: Cultural (missed) opportunities and cultural humility. *Professional Psychology: Research and Practice, 47*, 30–37. http://dx.doi.org/10.1037/pro0000046

Owen, J., Tao, K. W., Imel, Z. E., Wampold, B. E., & Rodolfa, E. (2014). Addressing racial and ethnic microaggressions in therapy. *Professional Psychology: Research and Practice, 45*, 283–290. http://dx.doi.org/10.1037/a0037420

Oyserman, D., & Destin, M. (2010). Identity-based motivation: Implications for intervention. *The Counseling Psychologist, 38*, 1001–1043. http://dx.doi.org/10.1177/0011000010374775

Paniagua, F. A. (2014). *Assessing and treating culturally diverse clients: A practical guide* (4th ed.). London, England: Sage. http://dx.doi.org/10.4135/9781506335728

Park, C. L. (2010). Making sense of the meaning literature: An integrative review of meaning making and its effects on adjustment to stressful life events. *Psychological Bulletin, 136*, 257–301. http://dx.doi.org/10.1037/a0018301

Park, C. L. (2013). Religion and meaning. In R. F. Paloutzian & C. L. Park (Eds.), *Handbook of the psychology of religion and spirituality* (2nd ed., pp. 357–379). New York, NY: Guilford Press.

Park, C. L. (2016). Meaning making in the context of disasters. *Journal of Clinical Psychology, 72*, 1234–1246. http://dx.doi.org/10.1002/jclp.22270

Park, C. L. (2017a). Distinctions to promote an integrated perspective on meaning: Global meaning and meaning making processes. *Journal of Constructivist Psychology, 30*, 14–19. http://dx.doi.org/10.1080/10720537.2015.1119082

Park, C. L. (2017b). Meaning making and resilience. In U. Kumar (Ed.), *The Routledge international handbook of psychosocial resilience* (pp. 162–172). New York, NY: Routledge.

Park, C. L. (2017c). Spiritual well-being after trauma: Correlates with appraisals, coping, and psychological adjustment. *Journal of Prevention & Intervention in the Community, 45*, 297–307. http://dx.doi.org/10.1080/10852352.2016.1197752

Park, C. L. (2017d). Unresolved tensions in the study of meaning in life. *Journal of Constructivist Psychology, 30*, 69–73. http://dx.doi.org/10.1080/10720537.2015.1119083

Park, C. L., Currier, J., Harris, J. I., & Slattery, J. M. (2017). *Trauma, meaning, and spirituality: Translating research into clinical practice.* Washington, DC: American Psychological Association. http://dx.doi.org/10.1037/15961-000

Park, C. L., Edmondson, D., & Hale-Smith, A. (2013). Why religion? Meaning as motivation. In K. I. Pargament, J. J. Exline, J. Jones, & A. Mahoney (Eds.), *APA handbook of psychology, religion and spirituality* (pp. 157–171). Washington, DC: American Psychological Association.

Park, C. L., Edmondson, D., & Mills, M. A. (2010). Reciprocal influences of religiousness and global meaning in the stress process. In T. Miller (Ed.), *Coping with life transitions* (pp. 485–501). New York, NY: Springer.

Park, C. L., & Kennedy, M. C. (2017). Meaning violation and restoration following trauma: Conceptual overview and clinical implications. In E. Altmaier (Ed.), *Reconstructing meaning after trauma* (pp. 17–27). London, England:

Elsevier. http://dx.doi.org/10.1016/B978-0-12-803015-8.00002-4

Park, C. L., Riley, K. E., George, L., Gutierrez, I., Hale, A., Cho, D., & Braun, T. (2016). Assessing disruptions in meaning: Development of the Global Meaning Violation Scale. *Cognitive Therapy and Research, 40,* 831–846. http://dx.doi.org/10.1007/s10608-016-9794-9

Park, C. L., & Slattery, J. M. (2009). Including spirituality in case conceptualizations: A meaning system approach. In J. Aten & M. Leach (Eds.), *Spirituality and the therapeutic practice: A guide for mental health professionals* (pp. 121–142). Washington, DC: American Psychological Association. http://dx.doi.org/10.1037/11853-006

Partie, M. (2005, October). Flying back over the cuckoo's nest. *Therapeutic Options.* Retrieved from http://therops.net/node/26

Pedersen, P. B., Crethar, H. C., & Carlson, J. (2008). *Inclusive cultural empathy: Making relationships central in counseling and psychotherapy.* Washington, DC: American Psychological Association. http://dx.doi.org/10.1037/11707-000

Peter-Hagene, L. C., & Ullman, S. E. (2018). Longitudinal effects of sexual assault victims' drinking and self-blame on posttraumatic stress disorder. *Journal of Interpersonal Violence, 33,* 83–93. http://dx.doi.org/10.1177/0886260516636394

Petty, S. C., Sachs-Ericsson, N., & Joiner, T. E., Jr. (2004). Interpersonal functioning deficits: Temporary or stable characteristics of depressed individuals? *Journal of Affective Disorders, 81,* 115–122. http://dx.doi.org/10.1016/S0165-0327(03)00158-7

Pew Research Center. (2014). *Religious Landscape Study.* Retrieved from http://www.pewforum.org/religious-landscape-study/racial-and-ethnic-composition/

Phelps, R., Bray, J. H., & Kearney, L. K. (2017). A quarter century of psychological practice in mental health and health care: 1990–2016. *American Psychologist, 72,* 822–836. http://dx.doi.org/10.1037/amp0000192

Pinel, E. C., & Constantino, M. J. (2003). Putting self psychology to good use: When social and clinical psychologists unite. *Journal of Psychotherapy Integration, 13,* 9–32. http://dx.doi.org/10.1037/1053-0479.13.1.9

Pipes, R. B., Blevins, T., & Kluck, A. (2008). Confidentiality, ethics, and informed consent. *American Psychologist, 63,* 623–624. http://dx.doi.org/10.1037/0003-066X.63.7.623

Pitts, G., & Wallace, P. A. (2003). Cultural awareness in the diagnosis of attention deficit/hyperactivity disorder. *Primary Psychiatry, 10,* 84–88.

Pomerantz, A. M., & Handelsman, M. M. (2004). Informed consent revisited: An updated written question format. *Professional Psychology: Research and Practice, 35,* 201–205. http://dx.doi.org/10.1037/0735-7028.35.2.201

Pope, K. S. (2015). Record-keeping controversies: Ethical, legal, and clinical challenges. *Canadian Psychology, 56,* 348–356. http://dx.doi.org/10.1037/cap0000021

Pope, K. S., & Keith-Spiegel, P. (2008). A practical approach to boundaries in psychotherapy: Making decisions, bypassing blunders, and mending fences. *Journal of Clinical Psychology: In Session, 64,* 638–652. http://dx.doi.org/10.1002/jclp.20477

Pope, K. S., Keith-Spiegel, P., & Tabachnick, B. G. (1986). Sexual attraction to clients: The human therapist and the (sometimes) inhuman training system. *American Psychologist, 41,* 147–158. http://dx.doi.org/10.1037/0003-066X.41.2.147

Pope, K. S., Tabachnick, B. G., & Keith-Spiegel, P. (1988). Good and poor practices in psychotherapy: National survey of beliefs of psychologists. *Professional Psychology: Research and Practice, 19,* 547–552. http://dx.doi.org/10.1037/0735-7028.19.5.547

Pope, K. S., & Vasquez, M. J. T. (2016). *Ethics in psychotherapy and counseling: A practical guide* (5th ed.). Hoboken, NJ: Wiley.

Powell, D. N., & Karraker, K. (2019). Expectations, experiences, and desires: Mothers' perceptions of the division of caregiving and their postnatal adaptation. *Journal of Family Psychology, 33,* 401–411. http://dx.doi.org/10.1037/fam0000526

Price, J. L., MacDonald, H. Z., Adair, K. C., Koerner, N., & Monson, C. M. (2016). Changing beliefs about trauma: A qualitative study of cognitive processing therapy. *Behavioural and Cognitive Psychotherapy, 44*, 156–167. http://dx.doi.org/10.1017/S1352465814000526

Prochaska, J. O., & Norcross, J. C. (2010). *Systems of psychotherapy: A transtheoretical analysis* (7th ed.). Belmont, CA: Brooks/Cole.

Quintana, S. M. (2007). Racial and ethnic identity: Developmental perspectives and research. *Journal of Counseling Psychology, 54*, 259–270. http://dx.doi.org/10.1037/0022-0167.54.3.259

Reichenberg, L. W., & Seligman, L. (2016). *Selecting effective treatments: A comprehensive, systematic guide to treating mental disorders* (5th ed.). Hoboken, NJ: Wiley.

Richards, K. C., Campenni, C. E., & Muse-Burke, J. L. (2010). Self-care and well-being in mental health professionals: The mediating effects of self-awareness and mindfulness. *Journal of Mental Health Counseling, 32*, 247–264. http://dx.doi.org/10.17744/mehc.32.3.0n31v88304423806

Rieder, H., & Elbert, T. (2013). Rwanda—lasting imprints of a genocide: Trauma, mental health and psychosocial conditions in survivors, former prisoners and their children. *Conflict and Health, 7* (article 6), 1–13. http://dx.doi.org/10.1186/1752-1505-7-6

Rigazio-DiGilio, S. A., Ivey, A. E., Kunkler-Peck, K. P., & Grady, L. T. (2005). *Community genograms: Using individual, family and cultural narratives with clients.* New York, NY: Teachers College Press.

Rivas-Drake, D., Syed, M., Umaña-Taylor, A., Markstrom, C., French, S., Schwartz, S. J., Lee, R., & the Ethnic and Racial Identity in the 21st Century Study Group. (2014). Feeling good, happy, and proud: A meta-analysis of positive ethnic-racial affect and adjustment. *Child Development, 85*, 77–102. http://dx.doi.org/10.1111/cdev.12175

Roberts, B. W., & Robins, R. W. (2000). Broad dispositions, broad aspirations: The intersection of personality traits and major life goals. *Personality and Social Psychology Bulletin, 26*, 1284–1296. http://dx.doi.org/10.1177/0146167200262009

Robinson, K. (2002). *A single square picture.* New York, NY: Berkley.

Robinson, K., & Harris, A. L. (2013). Racial and social class differences in how parents respond to inadequate achievement: Consequences for children's future achievement. *Social Science Quarterly, 94*, 1346–1371. http://dx.doi.org/10.1111/ssqu.12007

Roche, T. (2002a, March 18). Andrea Yates: More to the story. *Time.* Retrieved from http://content.time.com/time/nation/article/0,8599,218445,00.html

Roche, T. (2002b, January 28). The Yates odyssey. *Time, 159*, 42–50.

Rogers, A. G. (1995). *A shining affliction: A story of harm and healing in psychotherapy.* New York, NY: Penguin Books.

Rogers, A. G. (2001, Winter). Alphabets of the night: Toward a poetics of trauma. *Radcliffe Quarterly*, pp. 20–23.

Rogers, C. R. (1992). The necessary and sufficient conditions of therapeutic personality change. *Journal of Consulting and Clinical Psychology, 60*, 827–832. (Original work published 1957) http://dx.doi.org/10.1037/0022-006X.60.6.827

Rosler, N., Cohen-Chen, S., & Halperin, E. (2017). The distinctive effects of empathy and hope in intractable conflicts. *Journal of Conflict Resolution, 61*, 114–139. http://dx.doi.org/10.1177/0022002715569772

Rozensky, R. H., Grus, C. L., Nutt, R. L., Carlson, C. I., Eisman, E. J., & Nelson, P. D. (2015). A taxonomy for education and training in professional psychology health service specialties: Evolution and implementation of new guidelines for a common language. *American Psychologist, 70*, 21–32. http://dx.doi.org/10.1037/a0037988

Rudd, T. (2014). *Racial disproportionality in school discipline.* Retrieved from http://kirwaninstitute.osu.edu/wp-content/uploads/2014/02/racial-disproportionality-schools-02.pdf

Rupert, P. A., & Baird, K. A. (2004). Managed care and the independent practice of psychology. *Professional Psychology: Research and Practice, 35*, 185–193. http://dx.doi.org/10.1037/0735-7028.35.2.185

Rupert, P. A., & Kent, J. S. (2007). Gender and work setting differences in career-sustaining behaviors and burnout among professional psychologists. *Professional Psychology: Research and Practice, 38*, 88–96. http://dx.doi.org/10.1037/0735-7028.38.1.88

Rupert, P. A., Miller, A. O., & Dorociak, K. E. (2015). Preventing burnout: What does the research tell us? *Professional Psychology: Research and Practice, 46,* 168–174. http://dx.doi.org/10.1037/a0039297

Ruybal, A. L., & Siegel, J. T. (2017). Increasing social support for women with postpartum depression: An application of attribution theory. *Stigma and Health, 2,* 137–156. http://dx.doi.org/10.1037/sah0000047

Ruybal, A. L., & Siegel, J. T. (2019). Attribution theory and reducing stigma toward women with postpartum depression: Examining the role of perceptions of stability. *Stigma and Health, 4,* 320–329. Advance online publication. http://dx.doi.org/10.1037/sah0000146

Saks, E. R. (2007). *The center cannot hold: My journey through madness.* New York, NY: Hyperion.

Samson, S. (2006, January 3). KY miners comment about WV mine explosion. *14News.com.* Retrieved from https://www.14news.com/story/4313743/ky-miners-comment-about-wv-mine-explosion/

Sanchez, R. (2000). *My bloody life: The making of a Latin King.* Chicago, IL: Chicago Review Press.

Sanchez, R. (2003). *Once a king, always a king: The unmaking of a Latin King.* Chicago, IL: Chicago Review Press.

Saxbe, D., Rossin-Slater, M., & Goldenberg, D. (2018). The transition to parenthood as a critical window for adult health. *American Psychologist, 73,* 1190–1200. http://dx.doi.org/10.1037/amp0000376

Schauer, M., Neuner, F., & Elbert, T. (2011). *Narrative exposure therapy: Short-term treatment for traumatic stress disorders.* Cambridge, MA: Hogrefe.

Schopp, R. F. (2001). *Competence, condemnation, and commitment: An integrated theory of mental health law.* Washington, DC: American Psychological Association. http://dx.doi.org/10.1037/10435-000

Schwartz, E. K., Docherty, N. M., Najolia, G. M., & Cohen, A. S. (2019). Exploring the racial diagnostic bias of schizophrenia using behavioral and clinical-based measures. *Journal of Abnormal Psychology, 128,* 263–271. http://dx.doi.org/10.1037/abn0000409

Schwartz, S. H., Cieciuch, J., Vecchione, M., Davidov, E., Fischer, R., Beierlein, C., . . .

Konty, M. (2012). Refining the theory of basic individual values. *Journal of Personality and Social Psychology, 103,* 663–688. http://dx.doi.org/10.1037/a0029393

Seligman, L. (2004). *Technical and conceptual skills for mental health professionals.* Upper Saddle River, NJ: Pearson.

Serran, G., Fernandez, Y., Marshall, W. L., & Mann, R. E. (2003). Process issues in treatment: Application to sexual offender programs. *Professional Psychology: Research and Practice, 34,* 368–374. http://dx.doi.org/10.1037/0735-7028.34.4.368

Shafranske, E. P. (2005). The psychology of religion in clinical and counseling psychology. In R. F. Paloutzian & C. L. Park (Eds.), *Handbook of the psychology of religion and spirituality* (pp. 496–514). New York, NY: Guilford Press.

Shaharabani Saidon, H., Shafran, N., & Rafaeli, E. (2018). Teach them how to say goodbye: The CMRA model for treatment endings. *Journal of Psychotherapy Integration, 28,* 385–400. http://dx.doi.org/10.1037/int0000127

Shapiro, J. P. (1995). Attribution-based treatment of self-blame and helplessness in sexually abused children. *Psychotherapy: Theory, Research, Practice, Training, 32,* 581–591. http://dx.doi.org/10.1037/0033-3204.32.4.581

Sherby, L. B. (2009). Considerations on counter-transference love. *Contemporary Psychoanalysis, 45,* 65–81. http://dx.doi.org/10.1080/00107530.2009.10745987

Shirk, S. R., Karver, M. S., & Brown, R. (2011). The alliance in child and adolescent psychotherapy. *Psychotherapy, 48,* 17–24. http://dx.doi.org/10.1037/a0022181

Shockley, K. M., Shen, W., DeNunzio, M. M., Arvan, M. L., & Knudsen, E. A. (2017). Disentangling the relationship between gender and work–family conflict: An integration of theoretical perspectives using meta-analytic methods. *Journal of Applied Psychology, 102,* 1601–1635. http://dx.doi.org/10.1037/apl0000246

Simms, J. (2017). Transformative practice. *Counselling Psychology Review, 32,* 46–56.

Slattery, J. M. (2004). *Counseling diverse clients: Bringing context into therapy.* Belmont, CA: Brooks/Cole.

Slattery, J. M. (2005). Preventing role slippage during work in the community: Guidelines for new psychologists and supervisees. *Psychotherapy: Theory, Research, Practice, Training, 42*, 384–394. http://dx.doi.org/10.1037/0033-3204.42.3.384

Slattery, J. M., & Knauss, L. (2018, December). Should I offer in-home therapy? *Pennsylvania Psychologist, 78*, 28–29.

Slattery, J. M., Knauss, L. K., & Kossmann, D. (2018, September). My client wants to text me! *Pennsylvania Psychologist, 78*, 24–25.

Slattery, J. M., & Park, C. L. (2011a). *Empathic counseling: Meaning, context, ethics and skill.* Belmont, CA: Brooks/Cole.

Slattery, J. M., & Park, C. L. (2011b). Meaning making and spiritually oriented interventions. In J. Aten, M. R. McMinn, & E. V. Worthington (Eds.), *Spiritually oriented interventions for counseling and psychotherapy* (pp. 15–40). Washington, DC: American Psychological Association. http://dx.doi.org/10.1037/12313-001

Slattery, J. M., & Park, C. L. (2012). Clinical approaches to discrepancies in meaning: Conceptualization, assessment, and treatment. In P. Wong (Ed.), *Human quest for meaning* (2nd ed., pp. 493–516). New York, NY: Erlbaum.

Smith, D., & Fitzpatrick, M. (1995). Patient-therapist boundary issues: An integrative review of theory and research. *Professional Psychology: Research and Practice, 26*, 499–506. http://dx.doi.org/10.1037/0735-7028.26.5.499

Snibbe, A. C., & Markus, H. R. (2005). You can't always get what you want: Educational attainment, agency, and choice. *Journal of Personality and Social Psychology, 88*, 703–720. http://dx.doi.org/10.1037/0022-3514.88.4.703

Snyder, T. A., & Barnett, J. E. (2006). Informed consent and the process of psychotherapy. *Psychotherapy Bulletin, 41*, 37–42.

Soman, D., & Cheema, A. (2004). When goals are counterproductive: The effects of violation of a behavioral goal on subsequent performance. *Journal of Consumer Research, 31*, 52–62. http://dx.doi.org/10.1086/383423

Starbranch, E. K. (1999). *Psychiatric assessment of Andrea Yates.* Court TV. Retrieved from http://www.courttv.com/trials/yates/docs/psychiatric1.html [No longer available online]

Stecker, T., Shiner, B., Watts, B. V., Jones, M., & Conner, K. R. (2013). Treatment-seeking barriers for veterans of the Iraq and Afghanistan conflicts who screen positive for PTSD. *Psychiatric Services, 64*, 280–283. http://dx.doi.org/10.1176/appi.ps.001372012

Steele, C. M. (1997). A threat in the air: How stereotypes shape intellectual identity and performance. *American Psychologist, 52*, 613–629. http://dx.doi.org/10.1037/0003-066X.52.6.613

Stith, S. M., Miller, M. S., Boyle, J., Swinton, J., Ratcliffe, G., & McCollum, E. (2012). Making a difference in making miracles: Common roadblocks to miracle question effectiveness. *Journal of Marital and Family Therapy, 38*, 380–393. http://dx.doi.org/10.1111/j.1752-0606.2010.00207.x

Strupp, H. H. (1996). Some salient lessons from research and practice. *Psychotherapy, 33*, 135–138. http://dx.doi.org/10.1037/0033-3204.33.1.135

Stüntzner-Gibson, D., Koren, P. E., & DeChillo, N. (1995). The Youth Satisfaction Questionnaire: What kids think of services. *Families in Society, 76*, 616–624. http://dx.doi.org/10.1177/104438949507601004

Substance Abuse and Mental Health Services Administration. (2017). *Behavioral Health Barometer: United States, Volume 4: Indicators as measured through the 2015 National Survey on Drug Use and Health and National Survey of Substance Abuse Treatment Services* (HHS Publication No. SMA-17-BaroUS-16). Rockville, MD: Author.

Substance Abuse and Mental Health Services Administration. (2018, July). Substance use and mental health issues among U.S.-born American Indians or Alaska Natives residing on and off tribal lands. *CBHSQ Data Review.* Retrieved from https://www.samhsa.gov/data/sites/default/files/cbhsq-reports/DRAIANTribalAreas2018/DRAIANTribalAreas2018.pdf

Sue, D. W. (2004). Whiteness and ethnocentric monoculturalism: Making the "invisible" visible. *American Psychologist, 59*, 761–769. http://dx.doi.org/10.1037/0003-066X.59.8.761

Sue, D. W. (2015). Therapeutic harm and cultural oppression. *The Counseling Psychologist,*

43, 359–369. http://dx.doi.org/10.1177/0011000014565713

Sue, D. W., Capodilupo, C. M., Torino, G. C., Bucceri, J. M., Holder, A. M. B., Nadal, K. L., & Esquilin, M. (2007). Racial microaggressions in everyday life: Implications for clinical practice. *American Psychologist, 62*, 271–286. http://dx.doi.org/10.1037/0003-066X.62.4.271

Sue, D. W., & Sue, S. (2016). *Counseling the culturally diverse: Theory and practice* (7th ed.). Hoboken, NJ: Wiley.

Sue, S. (1998). In search of cultural competence in psychotherapy and counseling. *American Psychologist, 53*, 440–448. http://dx.doi.org/10.1037/0003-066X.53.4.440

Swift, J. K., & Callahan, J. L. (2008). A delay-discounting measure of great expectations and the effectiveness of psychotherapy. *Professional Psychology: Research and Practice, 39*, 581–588. http://dx.doi.org/10.1037/0735-7028.39.6.581

Swift, J. K., & Callahan, J. L. (2011). Decreasing treatment dropout by addressing expectations for treatment length. *Psychotherapy Research, 21*, 193–200. http://dx.doi.org/10.1080/10503307.2010.541294

Swift, J. K., & Greenberg, R. P. (2012). Premature discontinuation in adult psychotherapy: A meta-analysis. *Journal of Consulting and Clinical Psychology, 80*, 547–559. http://dx.doi.org/10.1037/a0028226

Swift, J. K., & Greenberg, R. P. (2015). *Premature termination in psychotherapy: Strategies for engaging clients and improving outcomes.* Washington, DC: American Psychological Association. http://dx.doi.org/10.1037/14469-000

Swift, J. K., Greenberg, R. P., Tompkins, K. A., & Parkin, S. R. (2017). Treatment refusal and premature termination in psychotherapy, pharmacotherapy, and their combination: A meta-analysis of head-to-head comparisons. *Psychotherapy, 54*, 47–57. http://dx.doi.org/10.1037/pst0000104

Szczepanek, D. (2017). Ranking the 9 best (and only) female owners in sports. *Grandstand Central.* Retrieved from https://grandstandcentral.com/best-women-owners-pro-sports-37a32b603f18

Taft, C. T., Murphy, C. M., Musser, P. H., & Remington, N. A. (2004). Personality, interpersonal, and motivational predictors of the working alliance in group cognitive-behavioral therapy for partner violent men. *Journal of Consulting and Clinical Psychology, 72*, 349–354. http://dx.doi.org/10.1037/0022-006X.72.2.349

Taleb, N. N. (2010). *The black swan: The impact of the highly improbable.* New York, NY: Random House.

Taliaferro, L. A., & Muehlenkamp, J. J. (2017). Nonsuicidal self-injury and suicidality among sexual minority youth: Risk factors and protective connectedness factors. *Academic Pediatrics, 17*, 715–722. http://dx.doi.org/10.1016/j.acap.2016.11.002

Tambag, H., Turan, Z., Tolun, S., & Can, R. (2018). Perceived social support and depression levels of women in the postpartum period in Hatay, Turkey. *Nigerian Journal of Clinical Practice, 21*, 1525–1530.

Thériault, A., Gazzola, N., Isenor, J., & Pascal, L. (2015). Imparting self-care practices to therapists: What the experts recommend/Entrainer des pratiques d'auto-soin chez les thérapeutes: Recommandations des experts. *Canadian Journal of Counselling and Psychotherapy, 49*, 379–400.

Thomas, P. M. (2005). Dissociation and internal models of protection: Psychotherapy with child abuse survivors. *Psychotherapy: Theory, Research, Practice, Training, 42*, 20–36. http://dx.doi.org/10.1037/0033-3204.42.1.20

Thompson, M. N., Chin, M. Y., & Kring, M. (2019). Examining mental health practitioners' perceptions of clients based on social class and sexual orientation. *Psychotherapy, 56*, 217–228. http://dx.doi.org/10.1037/pst0000222

Triandis, H. C., & Gelfand, M. J. (1998). Converging measurement of horizontal and vertical individualism and collectivism. *Journal of Personality and Social Psychology, 74*, 118–128. http://dx.doi.org/10.1037/0022-3514.74.1.118

Trimble, J. E. (2007). Prolegomena for the connotation of construct use in the measurement of ethnic and racial identity. *Journal of Counseling*

Psychology, 54, 247–258. http://dx.doi.org/10.1037/0022-0167.54.3.247

Turchik, J. A., Karpenko, V., Ogles, B. M., Demireva, P., & Probst, D. R. (2010). Parent and adolescent satisfaction with mental health services: Does it relate to youth diagnosis, age, gender, or treatment outcome? *Community Mental Health Journal, 46*, 282–288. http://dx.doi.org/10.1007/s10597-010-9293-5

Twenty-First Century Books. (2008). *Malcolm X: A research site.* Retrieved from http://www.brothermalcolm.net/

Umaña-Taylor, A. J., Quintana, S. M., Lee, R. M., Cross, W. E., Jr., Rivas-Drake, D., Schwartz, S. J., . . . the Ethnic and Racial Identity in the 21st Century Study Group. (2014). Ethnic and racial identity during adolescence and into young adulthood: An integrated conceptualization. *Child Development, 85*, 21–39. http://dx.doi.org/10.1111/cdev.12196

U.S. Census Bureau. (2018). *Quick facts: United States.* Retrieved from https://www.census.gov/quickfacts/fact/table/US/PST045218

U.S. Department of Health and Human Services. (2014). *TIP 59: Improving cultural competence: A treatment improvement protocol.* Rockville, MD: Substance Abuse and Mental Health Administration.

Uwiringiyimana, S. (2017). *How dare the sun rise: Memoirs of a war child.* New York, NY: HarperCollins.

Vallacher, R. R., & Wegner, D. M. (2012). Action identification theory. In P. A. M. Van Lange, A. W. Kruglanski, & E. T. Higgins (Eds.), *Handbook of theories of social psychology* (pp. 327–348). Los Angeles, CA: Sage. http://dx.doi.org/10.4135/9781446249215.n17

van Baaren, R. B., Holland, R. W., Kawakami, K., & van Knippenberg, A. (2004). Mimicry and prosocial behavior. *Psychological Science, 15*, 71–74. http://dx.doi.org/10.1111/j.0963-7214.2004.01501012.x

Varner, F., & Mandara, J. (2013). Discrimination concerns and expectations as explanations for gendered socialization in African American families. *Child Development, 84*, 875–890. http://dx.doi.org/10.1111/cdev.12021

Vasquez, M. J., Bingham, R. P., & Barnett, J. E. (2008). Psychotherapy termination: Clinical and ethical responsibilities. *Journal of Clinical Psychology, 64*, 653–665. http://dx.doi.org/10.1002/jclp.20478

Verkuyten, M. (2016). Further conceptualizing ethnic and racial identity research: The social identity approach and its dynamic model. *Child Development, 87*, 1796–1812. http://dx.doi.org/10.1111/cdev.12555

Voronov, M., & Singer, J. A. (2002). The myth of individualism-collectivism: A critical review. *The Journal of Social Psychology, 142*, 461–480. http://dx.doi.org/10.1080/00224540209603912

Wade, N. G., Vogel, D. L., Liao, K. Y.-H., & Goldman, D. B. (2008). Measuring state-specific rumination: Development of the Rumination About an Interpersonal Offense Scale. *Journal of Counseling Psychology, 5*, 419–426. http://dx.doi.org/10.1037/0022-0167.55.3.419

Walker, E. R., Cummings, J. R., Hockenberry, J. M., & Druss, B. G. (2015). Insurance status, use of mental health services, and unmet need for mental health care in the United States. *Psychiatric Services, 66*, 578–584. http://dx.doi.org/10.1176/appi.ps.201400248

Walker, M., Jacobs, M. (Producers), & Crisp, D. (Director). (1992). *The clumsy counselor: Loaded remarks from the client's perspective* [Motion picture]. (Available from University of Leicester, P.O. Box 138, Maurice Shock Building, University Road, Leicester LE1 9HN)

Wampold, B. E. (2007). Psychotherapy: The humanistic (and effective) treatment. *American Psychologist, 62*, 855–873. http://dx.doi.org/10.1037/0003-066X.62.8.857

Wampold, B. E., & Imel, Z. E. (2015). *The great psychotherapy debate: The evidence for what makes psychotherapy work* (2nd ed.). New York, NY: Routledge. http://dx.doi.org/10.4324/9780203582015

Ward, S., Donovan, H., Gunnarsdottir, S., Serlin, R. C., Shapiro, G. R., & Hughes, S. (2008). A randomized trial of a representational intervention to decrease cancer pain (RIDcancerPain). *Health Psychology, 27*, 59–67. http://dx.doi.org/10.1037/0278-6133.27.1.59

Weaver, R. K. (2014). Compliance regimes and barriers to behavioral change. *Governance: An*

International Journal of Policy, Administration and Institutions, 27, 243–265. http://dx.doi.org/10.1111/gove.12032

Weinberger, J. (2014). Common factors are not so common and specific factors are not so specified: Toward an inclusive integration of psychotherapy research. *Psychotherapy, 51,* 514–518. http://dx.doi.org/10.1037/a0037092

Weiss, L. (2004). *Therapist's guide to self-care.* New York, NY: Brunner-Routledge. http://dx.doi.org/10.4324/9780203340110

Westmacott, R., & Hunsley, J. (2010). Reasons for terminating psychotherapy: A general population study. *Journal of Clinical Psychology, 66,* 965–977. http://dx.doi.org/10.1002/jclp.20702

Westmacott, R., & Hunsley, J. (2017). Psychologists' perspectives on therapy termination and the use of therapy engagement/retention strategies. *Clinical Psychology & Psychotherapy, 24,* 687–696. http://dx.doi.org/10.1002/cpp.2037

Westover, T. (2018). *Educated: A memoir.* New York, NY: Random House.

Wicks, R. J. (2008). *The resilient clinician.* New York, NY: Oxford University Press.

Williams, D. R., & Jackson, P. B. (2005). Social sources of racial disparities in health. *Health Affairs, 24,* 325–334. http://dx.doi.org/10.1377/hlthaff.24.2.325

Wise, E. H., & Barnett, J. E. (2016). Self-care for psychologists. In J. C. Norcross, G. R. VandenBos, D. K. Freedheim, & L. F. Campbell (Eds.), *APA handbook of clinical psychology: Education and profession* (pp. 209–222). Washington, DC: American Psychological Association. http://dx.doi.org/10.1037/14774-014

Worthington, R. L., Soth-McNett, A. M., & Moreno, M. V. (2007). Multicultural counseling competencies research: A 20-year content analysis. *Journal of Counseling Psychology, 54,* 351–361. http://dx.doi.org/10.1037/0022-0167.54.4.351

Wurm, S., Warner, L. M., Ziegelmann, J. P., Wolff, J. K., & Schüz, B. (2013). How do negative self-perceptions of aging become a self-fulfilling prophecy? *Psychology and Aging, 28,* 1088–1097. http://dx.doi.org/10.1037/a0032845

Yalom, I. D. (2003). *The gift of therapy: An open letter to a new generation of therapists and their patients.* New York, NY: HarperCollins.

Yates, R. (2004, January 18). *Are you there alone? A review.* Retrieved from http://www.yateskids.org/are_you_there_alone.php [No longer available online]

Yates, R. (n.d.). Welcome. Retrieved from http://www.yateskids.org/

Younggren, J. N., & Gottlieb, M. C. (2008). Termination and abandonment: History, risk, and risk management. *Professional Psychology: Research and Practice, 39,* 498–504. http://dx.doi.org/10.1037/0735-7028.39.5.498

Zachrisson, A. (2014). Ethical breaches and deviations of method in psychoanalysis: A heuristic model for the differentiation of boundary transgressions in psychoanalytic work. *International Forum of Psychoanalysis, 23,* 246–252. http://dx.doi.org/10.1080/0803706X.2013.781272

Zahniser, E., Rupert, P. A., & Dorociak, K. E. (2017). Self-care in clinical psychology graduate training. *Training and Education in Professional Psychology, 11,* 283–289. http://dx.doi.org/10.1037/tep0000172

Zaki, J., Bolger, N., & Ochsner, K. (2008). It takes two: The interpersonal nature of empathic accuracy. *Psychological Science, 19,* 399–404. http://dx.doi.org/10.1111/j.1467-9280.2008.02099.x

Zapf, P. A., Kukucka, J., Kassin, S. M., & Dror, I. E. (2018). Cognitive bias in forensic mental health assessment: Evaluator beliefs about its nature and scope. *Psychology, Public Policy, and Law, 24,* 1–10. http://dx.doi.org/10.1037/law0000153

Zarya, V. (2018, May 21). The share of female CEOs in the Fortune 500 dropped by 25% in 2018. *Fortune.* Retrieved from http://fortune.com/2018/05/21/women-fortune-500-2018/

Zilcha-Mano, S. (2017). Is the alliance really therapeutic? Revisiting this question in light of recent methodological advances. *American Psychologist, 72,* 311–325. http://dx.doi.org/10.1037/a0040435

Zillman, C. (2014). Microsoft's new CEO: One minority exec in a sea of white. *Fortune.* Retrieved from http://fortune.com/2014/02/04/microsofts-new-ceo-one-minority-exec-in-a-sea-of-white/

Zimbardo, P. G., & Boyd, J. N. (1999). Putting time in perspective: A valid, reliable individual-differences metric. *Journal of Personality and Social Psychology, 77,* 1271–1288. http://dx.doi.org/10.1037/0022-3514.77.6.1271

Zimmerman, G. L., Olsen, C. G., & Bosworth, M. F. (2000). A "stages of change" approach to helping patients change behavior. *American Family Physician, 61,* 1409–1416.

Zorn, E. (2015). Why, yes, Sandra Bland was "irritated." *Chicago Tribune.* Retrieved from https://www.chicagotribune.com/columns/eric-zorn/ct-bland-encinia-texas-suicide-zorn-perspec-0726-20150724-column.html

Zuckerman, E. (2019). *Clinician's thesaurus: The guide for writing psychological reports* (8th ed.). New York, NY: Guilford Press.

Zwebner, Y., Sellier, A.-L., Rosenfeld, N., Goldenberg, J., & Mayo, R. (2017). We look like our names: The manifestation of name stereotypes in facial appearance. *Journal of Personality and Social Psychology, 112,* 527–554. http://dx.doi.org/10.1037/pspa0000076

INDEX

A

Abandonment, 213
Academic achievement, 48
Acceptance
    clients' need to feel, 80
    as component of empathy, 8–9
Accepting (in termination), 215, 216
Accommodation, 25
Accurate empathy, 102–104
Achievable goals, 166–167
Action phase, 163–164, 194
Adaptive coping, 287
Adaptive stress, 281
Additive empathy, 102
ADHD (attention-deficit/hyperactivity disorder),
    151–152
Adjunctive services, 180
Adolescents, therapeutic alliance with, 73
Adoption, across cultures, 52–53
Advice, giving, 189
Affect, 256. *See also* Emotion(s)
    in clinical report, 261
    in mental status evaluation, 131–132
African Americans
    with ADHD, 151–152
    cultural context for, 48
    discrimination against, 57–58
    and group identities, 49
    group identity and world views of, 50
Agreeing with the client, 188
Alternative explanations, 149–151
Alternatives to therapy, 84
American Counseling Association, 247
American Nurses Association, 229
American Psychological Association (APA), 64, 217–218,
    228, 229, 276
Antidepressants, 13–14
APA. *See* American Psychological Association
APA Ethics Code. *See* Ethical Principles of Psychologists
    and Code of Conduct
Appearance, in mental status evaluation, 131
Appointments, 84

Approach goals, 165
Archer, A., 14
Asian Americans, 29, 48
Aspirational principles, 15, 228–229
Assertiveness, 10
Assessment(s), 143–156
    alternative explanations in, 149–151
    assumptions and values in clinical practice, 144–146
    considering culture and oppression in, 62–63
    countering observer biases in, 151–152
    critical thinking in, 148–149
    empathic, 17
    multiple assessment strategies, 138–140
    questions during, 115–117
    social psychological processes influencing, 146–147
    strengths and exceptions to problems in, 152–155
    three-dimensional, 113–118
Assimilation, 25
Assumptions, 144–146
Attention-deficit/hyperactivity disorder (ADHD), 151–152
Attribution, 32
Audience, considering the, 268
Authority, 29–30
Autonomy, 228–229, 239
Avoidance, reducing, 200–201
Avoidance goals, 165

B

Bad things happening, reasons for, 32–33
Bai, S., 154
Barnum statements, 263
Barriers to change, 172, 203–205
Barriers to communicating empathy, 92–93
Barriers to treatment, 195
Bartholomew, Saint, 212
Beck Depression Inventory (BDI), 182
Behavior(s)
    assessing explanations for, 149
    beliefs revealed by, 31
    as cause of bad events, 32
    changes in, due to situational meaning, 39
    in clinical report, 260, 261

influenced by time orientation, 36
interventions for changing, 194–197
nonverbal. *See* Nonverbal behaviors
Behavioral component, of prejudice, 58
Behavioral measures, 182
Behavioral model, of psychotherapy, 13, 135
Beliefs
conflicting, in goal-setting, 86–87
interventions for changing, 197–201
in meaning systems, 24
Benchley, Robert, 210
Beneficence, 218, 228
Benevolence, of the world, 31
Bernal, G., 50
Bersoff, D. N., 239
Bias(es)
of clinicians, 66
confirmation, 147
implicit, 148
observer, 151–152
trait negativity, 147
Bien educado, 42
Big picture, crises vs., 173–174
Billable hours, 242
Biological model, of psychotherapy, 13, 135
Black Legion, 118
Bland, Sandra, 45–47, 52, 60–61
Bloom's taxonomy of learning and goal statements, 167
Blumenfeld, Dr., 91–92
Blurred boundaries, 272–274
Bohart, A. C., 81
Bond, C. F., 149
Borchardt, J. J., 182
Boundaries, 272–274
Boundary crossings, 233–234, 248, 273
Boundary violations, 233, 234, 273
Brethnach, Sarah Ban, 74
Brom, Danny, 51
Brown, William Wells, 54
Buddha, 23
Budgetary restrictions, 242–243
Burnout, 274, 276, 277

C
Caine, Mark, 148
Cale, John, 81
California Supreme Court, 238
Calvin and Hobbes (comic strip), 181
Carver, Jeffrey A., 266
Case conceptualization, 50, 134–135
Case conferences, 147

Caskey, Rick, 33
CBCL (Child Behavior Checklist), 182
Challenging, of clients, 10
Change, 160–165
addressing obstacles to, 172
commitment to, 168, 171–172
expectancies for, 15
helping clients own their, 221–222
identifying/addressing barriers to, 203–205
introducing, as part of intervening, 192–194
in meaning systems, 25–28
skills to facilitate positive, 17
stages of, 161–165
therapeutic alliance as precondition to, 73–74
Change process, in clinical report, 261
Chen, S. W.-H., 29
Child Behavior Checklist (CBCL), 182
Children, therapeutic alliance with, 73
Chopra, Deepak, 92
Churchill, Winston, 6, 54
Cicero, 264
Clark, Alexander, 72
Client(s)
agreeing with, 188
contributions of, to treatment, 80–81
defining, 11
describing, in clinical report, 259–261
with different meaning systems than clinicians, 42–43
dimensions to consider when meeting, 50
feeling understood, 4
identifying, 169–170
reaction of, to termination, 213–214
sexual relationships with, 234, 273
summarizations generated by, 101
therapeutic alliance with new, 81–87
therapy-related lies told by, 104
working with, where they are, 171
Client-induced stress, 280–281
Client rights, 236–245
financial considerations with, 242–243
legal requirements, 236–241
and supervisory issues, 242–243
and time/energy limitations, 243–244
worksite requirements, 241–242
Client Satisfaction Questionnaire (CSQ), 181–182
Client variable, 14
Clinical assessment, 112. *See also* Assessment
Clinical reports, 253–270
contents of, 258–264
hypothetical example, 262
importance of writing in, 256–258

and observations, 255–256
    questions to address in, 258–261
    recommendations for, 266–269
    SOAP notes, 264–265
Clinical risk, 246–247
Clinician(s)
    assertiveness displayed by, 10
    attending to racial and ethnic identities, 55–56
    with different meaning systems than clients, 42–43
    empathy necessary for, 4
    multicultural, 61–66
    reaction of, to termination, 213
    role of, 11–12
    self-awareness of, 5
    working with clients with minority identity status, 61–62
Closed questions, 95, 97–99
Clumsy Counsellor (Walker et al.), 82
Cognition
    in clinical report, 260
    in mental status evaluation, 132
Cognitive component, of prejudice, 58
Cognitive model, of psychotherapy, 13, 135
Cognitive skills, 65–66
Collaboration
    empowered, 230
    encouraged by informed consent process, 83
    in goal setting, 169–175
    on treatment goals and methods, 85–87
Collectivism, 30, 42
Colorblind approaches, 62–63
Columbine Massacre, 154–155
Commitment, to change, 168, 171–172
Common factors, 12–15
Communication(s)
    content and process of, 11
    cultural considerations in, 66
    of empathy, 9–10, 92–93
    verbal. *See* Verbal communication
Comorbidity, 137
Compassion fatigue, 274–275, 288
Competence, 231–232
    in APA Ethics Code, 16
    emotional, 231, 247, 277–280
    fostering perceptions of, 82
    multicultural, 65, 87, 197, 212, 231
    technical, 231
Conclusions, drawing, 267
Confidentiality, 230, 232–233
    in APA Ethics Code, 16
    and duty to warn, 238–239

informed consent about, 84
    and mandated reporting, 236–237
Confirmation bias, 147
Conflicts of interest, in APA Ethics Code, 16
Confronting the client, 189
Confucius, 249, 285
Congo, 202
Consolidating (in termination), 214–215
Constantino, M. J., 108
Consultation, 214
Consumer Bill of Rights, 236
Contemplation phase, 162–163, 194, 195
Contemporary Authors Online, 107–108
Content
    of communications, 11
    cultural, in treatment, 50
    developing empathic understanding with, 79
    listening to, 77–79
Context, 111–141
    case conceptualizations, 134–135
    cultural, 47–48
    Malcolm X example, 118–133
    multiple assessment strategies, 138–140
    multiple perspectives, 136
    recognizing context, 112–113
    research and treatment decisions, 137–138
    for therapy, 50
    three-dimensional assessments, 113–118
Control
    in achievable and realistic goals, 166
    beliefs about, 34–35
    locus of, 34
Cooper, Sharon, 46
Copayments, 243
Coping, effective, 285–286
Corrective emotional experience, 86
Corsini, Raymond J., 111–112
Counseling, 11
Counselors, 4. *See also* Clinician(s)
Crises, big picture vs., 173–174
Crisp, D., 82
Critical thinking
    in assessments, 148–149
    by multicultural clinicians, 65–66
CSQ (Client Satisfaction Questionnaire), 181–182
Cultural adaptations, of psychotherapies, 61
Cultural competence, 63–65
Cultural context, 64
Cultural humility, 62
Cultural level, of oppression, 57

Culture, 45–68
  in assessment, 62–63, 137
  defining, 47–50
  ethnic and racial identity in treatment, 55–56
  and goal setting, 170
  impacts of group identity, 54–55
  and interpersonal relationships, 29
  and interpretation of nonverbal behaviors, 75–76
  and mental status evaluations, 132, 133
  and multicultural clinicians, 61–66
  multiple group identities, 51–54
  and oppression, 57–61
  seeing, 47–50, 52–54
  in therapy, 66–67
  and time orientation, 35–36
"CYA," 266
"CYCA," 266

D

Dalai Lama, 63–64, 108, 194, 236, 276
Dangers in providing empathic therapy, 272–277
  blurred boundaries, 272–274
  compassion fatigue, 274–275
  remaining vigilant to, 276–280
  vicarious traumatization, 275–276
Data, sensory, 255
Davenport, D. S., 29
Decision making, 245–249
Demographics, in clinical report, 259
Denial, of insight, 162
DePaulo, B. M., 149
Depression
  efficacy of psychotherapy in treatment of, 13–14
  social skill deficits concomitant with, 196
Description, of problem, 151
D'Evelyn, Thomas, 258
Didion, Joan, 256
Dietz, Park, 246
Differences, sensitivity to, 235–236
DiFranco, Ani, 151
Directiveness, 29
Directives, 189
Discharge summary, 222–223
Discrepancy, 79, 190–191, 199
Discrimination, 57–58
Disordered thinking, 132
Dodson, Fitzhugh, 175
Duty to warn, 238–239

E

Educated (Westover), 27
Egalitarian, 29

Emerson, Ralph Waldo, 4, 272
Eminem, 143–144
Emotion(s). *See also* Affect
  interventions for changing, 201–203
  negative, 201–202
  overtly displayed, 256
  restraint of strong, 48
Emotional competence, 231
Emotional component, of prejudice, 58
Empathic counseling, 16–17
Empathy, 3–18
  accurate, 102–104
  and clinicians, 11–12
  and common factors, 12–15
  communicating, 9–10
  components of, 6–10
  defining, 4–5
  and differing meaning systems, 42
  in ethical work, 15–16
  in model of empathic counseling, 16–17
Empowered collaboration, 230
Empowerment, 11, 229
Encinia, Brian, 45–47, 52, 60
Encouragers, 95, 99–100
Enmeshed families, 126
Environmental setting, 151
Epston, D., 222
Ethical acculturation model, 283–284
Ethical Principles of Psychologists and Code of Conduct (APA Ethics Code), 15–16, 217–218, 228, 229, 276
Ethical standards, 15, 229–236
Ethical work, 15–16
Ethics, 227–252
  and aspirational principles, 228–229
  and client rights, 236–245
  in decision making, 245–249
  ethical standards, 229–236
  personal vs. professional, 283–285
  positive approach to, 249–250
  and remaining vigilant, 276–277
  and termination of treatment, 217–219
Ethics codes, 16
Ethnic identity, 55–56
European Americans, 35–36, 145
Evaluation, of interventions, 205–206
Evaluation report, 139–140
Event-related stress, 281
Exceptions, to problems, 152–155
Expectancies for change, 15
Expectancy confirmation, 79
External locus of control, 34

External locus of responsibility, 34
Extratherapeutic events, 14
Extrinsic goals, 25
Eye contact, 75–76, 79

F

Facial expressions, 79
Fadiman, Anne, 86–87
Familism, 42
Family genogram, 126–128
Fatigue, compassion, 274–275, 288
Feedback, 189
Feelings, during treatment termination, 212–214.
    See also Emotion(s)
Fees, 84
Fidelity, 228, 229
Filial piety, 48
Financial considerations, 242–243
Fingerhut, R., 228
Finn, Charles, C., 104
Fixed mind-set, 164
Forced terminations, 219
Forensic interviews, 99
Frankl, Viktor, 33
Fraser, J. S., 80
Frequency, of problem, 151
Functional analysis, 153
Fundamental attribution error, 147
Future orientation, 36–37

G

Gabriella, 144
Gabriel-Rodriguez, Carmen D., 265, 266
Gandhi, Mohandas, 33
Garvey, Marcus, 118
Gatumba massacre, 202
Gendlin, E. T., 93
Generalizing, 213
Genuineness, 9
Goals
    in meaning systems, 24–25, 37–38
    treatment. *See* Treatment goals
Goal-setting, 165–175
    collaboration in, 86–87
    as collaborative process, 169–175
    good goals, 165–169
Goal statements, 175–176
Good, doing, 228. *See also* Beneficence
Gottlieb, M. C., 247, 284
Grant, Robert R., 283
Grosse Holtforth, M., 168

Group identity
    defining, 47
    and differences within groups, 48–49
    impacts of, 54–55
    multiple, 51–54
Groupthink, 147
Growth mind-set, 164

H

Haldol, 240
Handelsman, M. M., 284
Harm, avoiding, 228. *See also* Nonmaleficence
Harmony, 48
Harris, Eric, 154–155
Hatfield, Ben, 32
Health, questions for monitoring professional and
    personal, 279–280
Health services, 58–59
Healthy lifestyle, 287
Helper, Dr. (pseudonym), 227–229, 245, 248–249, 283
Hendricks, M., 93
Hierarchical structure, 48
Hilt, Jeanine, 87
Hmong people
    collaboration with, 86–87
    goal setting with, 170
    time orientation of, 35
Holland, 51
Holocaust, 49
Home ownership, 57–58
Hope, need for, 108–109
Hopefulness, 9
House (television program), 83
Hubbard, Elbert, 102
Hwang, W. C., 67
Hypotheses, 255–256, 267

I

Identity
    beliefs about, 33–34
    of clients, 50
    ethnic, 55–56
    group. *See* Group identity
    minority identity status, 61–62
    multiple, 51–54, 137
    personal vs. professional, 282–283
    racial, 54–56
    sexual, 170
Implementation intentions, 176
Implicit biases, 148
Individualism, 30

Individual level, of oppression, 57
Inferences, 148–150, 255
Information
    excluding irrelevant, 268
    multiple sources of, 136
    sources of, 30–31
Information giving (verbal influencing skill), 189
Informed consent, 83–85, 229–230
    in APA Ethics Code, 16
Initial session, informed consent in, 230
Insight
    denial of, 162
    in mental status evaluation, 132
Institutional level, of oppression, 57
Integrity, 228
Intensity, of problem, 151
Internalized homophobia, 51
Internal locus of control, 34
Internal locus of responsibility, 34
Interpersonal bonds, having, 286
Interpersonal harmony, 48
Interpersonal level, of oppression, 57
Interpersonal presentation and behavior,
    in clinical report, 260–261
Interpersonal relationships, 29–30
Interpreting (verbal influencing skill), 189
Intersectionality, 52
Interventions, 187–207
    for changing behaviors, 194–197
    for changing beliefs, 197–201
    for changing emotions, 201–203
    cultural adaptations of, 61
    evaluations of, 205–206
    goals, values, and beliefs in, 39–40
    identifying and addressing barriers to change, 203–205
    processes in, 188–194
    scale for rating the effectiveness of, 206
    in treatment plans, 175–176
Interviewer–client relationship, 131
Intrinsic goals, 25, 167–168
Introducing change, 192–194
Intrusive thoughts, 200
Irrelevant information, excluding, 268
Ivey, A. E., 188
Ivey, M. B., 188

J
Jacobs, M., 82
Jennings, L., 288–289
Jewish people, 48, 51
Joining, 73, 81
Jones, D'Ja (pseudonym), 101–102, 253–258, 262–265

Judgment, in mental status evaluation, 132
Jung, Carl G., 8
Just-world theory, 32, 60

K
Kalil (pseudonym), 160, 169
Kassin, S. M., 149
Keith-Spiegel, P., 234, 245
Kellogg, Marjorie, 205
Kennedy, John F., 169
Kennedy, Patrick J., 11
Kidd, Sue Monk, 160–161
King, Kay, 112
King, Martin Luther, Jr., 9
King Leo (pseudonym), 159–160, 169
Klebold, Dylan, 154–155
Knapp, S. J., 228, 246, 284, 286
Koltko-Rivera, M. E., 28
Korea, 52–53
Kottler, J. A., 117
Krishnamurti, Jiddu, 188

L
Lambert, M. J., 14
Language
    of clients, 50
    cues in, 105–106
    in mental status evaluation, 132
Lapse, 164
Latin Kings, 159
Latinx
    cultural values and norms for, 42
    goal setting with, 170
    sensitivity to differences with, 235
    time orientation of, 35
Law & Order (television program), 246
Lee, Harper, 28
Lee, Lia, 86–87
Lee family, 86–87, 153
Legal requirements, 236–241
Lent, R. W., 170
Lesbian, gay, bisexual, and transgender (LGBT) people,
    49–50
LGBT (lesbian, gay, bisexual, and transgender) people,
    49–50
Life experience, 5
Lifestyle, healthy, 287
Lil Loco. *See* Sanchez, Reymundo
Listening
    and acceptance, 9
    by clinicians, 11–12

nonverbal skills for, 74–80
as part of intervening, 188–189
and therapeutic alliance, 73
in working with clients with minority identity status, 62
Liszcz, A. M., 170
Little, Earl, 118
Little, Louise, 118, 119
Little, Malcolm. *See* X, Malcolm
Little, Wilfred, 119
Littleton, Colorado, 154
Locus of control, 34
Locus of responsibility, 34
Long-term goals, 165, 176
Loss, feelings of, 213
Lying, in therapy, 104

M

Machismo, 42
Maintaining (in termination), 215–216
Maintenance phase, 164
Majority culture, 52
Maladaptive beliefs, 12
Maladaptive coping, 287
Maladaptive stress, 281
Malcolm X. *See* X, Malcolm
Mal educado, 42
Managed care, 210–211
Mandated reporting, 236–238
Marchese, D., 143–144
"marginalization" stance, 284
Marianisma, 42
May, Rollo, 197
McCloskey, Robert, 80
McCloy, Anna, 32
McCloy, Randal, 33–34
Meanings, developing new, 197–199
Meaning system(s), 21–44
    clients and clinicians with different, 42–43
    components of, 24–25
    construction of, 6
    in context of therapy, 28–37
    defining, 23–24
    global, 28, 39, 43
    in goal setting, 174–175
    situational meanings informed by, 39–42
    stability and change in, 25–28
    values and goals in, 37–38
Measurable goals, 165–166
Medical treatment, collaboration in, 86–87
Meditation, 200–201
Mehl, Eric, 98

Meissner, C. A., 149
Memory, in mental status evaluation, 132
Mencken, H. L., 138
Mental health care system, 107–108
Mental status evaluation, 131–133
Meta-analysis, 72
Metaphors
    cultural, 67
    meaningful to clients, 50
    understanding clients with, 105–106
    using, in goal setting, 174–175
Michalak, J., 168
Michener, Anna, 71–72, 107–108
Microaggressions, 58, 63
Microskills, 93, 95
Mindfulness meditation, 200–201
Minimal encouragers, 95, 99
Minority identity status, 61–62
Miracle question, 168
Mirroring, 75, 105
Mood
    in clinical report, 261
    in mental status evaluation, 131–132
Muder, Doug, 21–22
Multicultural clinicians, 61–66
    cognitive skills of, 65–66
    cultural competence of, 63–65
    defining, 64
Multicultural competence, 231
Multicultural model, of psychotherapy, 13, 135
Multiple assessment strategies, 138–140
Multiple hypotheses, 267
Multiple identities, 51–54, 137
Multiple relationships, 233–234
    in APA Ethics Code, 16

N

Narrative exposure therapists, 113
National Organization of Women (NOW), 134
Native Americans, 35, 49
Negative emotions, 201–202
Nichols, Ralph, 77
Nike, 161
Nin, Anaïs, 144
Nonmaleficence, 228
Nonverbal behaviors
    communicating values with, 37–38
    culture and interpretation of, 75–76
    to develop empathic understanding, 79
    difficulties in understanding, 76–77
    interpretations of, 38
    and therapeutic alliance, 73

Nonverbal listening skills, 74–80
Norcross, J. C., 61, 162, 194, 195
Normalization, 189
Normal termination, 211
Norman, Jessye, 243
NOW (National Organization of Women), 134

O

Objectivity, in writing, 266
Observations, 148, 255–256
Observer biases, 151–152
Observer's paradox, 151
Omissions, in clients' communication, 106
Open questions, 95, 97–99
Oppression, 57–63
Outcome Questionnaire—45 (OQ–45), 182
Owen, J., 56

P

Pagels, Heinz, 247
Palmer, Parker, 282
Paralanguage, 79
Paraphrases, 94–96
Parenting, 145
Pascal, Blaise, 24
Past orientation, 36–37
Past tense, using, 258
Pederson, Paul, 61
Personal identity, 282–283
Personalismo, 42, 235
Personal space, 79
Person-centered model, of psychotherapy, 13, 135
Person-first language, 268
Physical appearance, in clinical report, 259
Pinel, E. C., 108
Poddar, Prosenjit, 238
Police brutality, 60
Pope, K. S., 234, 245, 249
Positive change, 17
Positive ethics, 249–250
Positive group identities, 55
Postpartum depression and psychosis, 138
Posttraumatic growth, 26
Posture, 79
Precontemplation phase, 162, 194–195
Prejudice, 58
Premature termination, 63, 211–212
Preparation phase, 163
Presentation, in clinical report, 260
Present orientation, 36–37
Present tense, using, 258–269

Privilege, 57, 59–60
Problems
    and meaning systems, 34–35
    strengths and exceptions to, 152–155
    treatment goals fitting, 170
Problem-solving, 34–35
Pro bono clients, 242
Process, 11, 78
Prochaska, J. O., 162, 194, 195
Productivity, 36
Professional development, 288
Professional identity, 282–283
Progress notes, 242
Proofreading, 259
Psychoanalytic model, of psychotherapy, 135
Psychodynamic model, of psychotherapy, 13
Psychosocial history, 114–118, 121–125
Psychotherapy, 11
    common models of, 13
    cultural adaptations of, 61
    models of, 15
Punctuality, 36

Q

Questions
    to address in clinical reports, 258–261
    appropriate for forensic interviews, 99
    for assessment phase, 115–117
    miracle, 168
    for monitoring professional and personal health,
        279–280
    open, 95, 97–99
    referral, 113, 257, 259
    scaling, 181

R

Racial identity, 54–56
Racism, 46, 118–120
Realistic goals, 166–167
Record keeping, 258
Redlining, 57–58
Referral questions, 113, 257, 259
Reflection of feeling, 95, 96
Reframing, 189, 192, 193
Refugees, working with, 204
Relapse, 13, 164
Relapse prevention, 216–217
Relationships
    interpersonal, 29–30
    interviewer–client, 131
    multiple, 16, 233–234
    sexual, with clients, 234, 273

therapeutic, 72
tracking changes in, 106
Religion
  and African Americans, 50
  explaining trauma with, 33
  role of, in clinicians' life, 23
  and social experiences, 21–22
Remen, Rachel Naomi, 275
Reporting, mandated, 236–238
Research, 137–138
Resilience, 125
Resnick, Phillip, 3–4, 240
Resolving (in termination), 215, 216
Respect
  attitude of, 235
  in clinical reports, 268
  uncritical agreement vs., 42–43
Respeto, 42
Responsibility, 34–35
Restraint, of strong emotion, 48
Risk management, 219–221, 246–247
Robinson, Katy (Kim Ji-yun), 52–54
Rogers, Annie G., 91–92, 105–106
Rogers, Carl, 8–9, 12, 102
Role models, having, 287
Rosenzweig, Saul, 14
Ruminations, 200
Rwanda, 202

S
Saeed, Dr., 240, 246, 283
Sáez-Santiago, E., 50
Safety
  for treatment, 81–82
  of the world, 31
Sago mining disaster, 32
Saks, Elyn, 209–211, 213–214, 218, 223
Samson, S., 33
Sanchez, Reymundo (Lil Loco), 39–41, 159–160, 169
Satisfaction questionnaires, 181–182
Savant, Marilyn vos, 176
Scaling questions, 181
Schneider, Beth (pseudonym), 201
Schutz, Susan Polis, 217
Schwarzenegger, Arnold, 152
Schweitzer, Albert, 15, 54, 228
Secondary victimization, 276
Self-awareness
  of beliefs, 24
  of clinicians, 5
  of personal biases, 66
  of privilege, 59

Self-blame, 32
Self-care, 271–290
  and dangers in providing empathic therapy, 272–277
  defining, 272
  and effective coping, 285–286
  and personal vs. professional ethics, 283–285
  and personal vs. professional identity, 282–283
  preventing stress-related problems, 286–289
  scale for assessing level of, 278
  stressors for clinicians, 274–281
Self-disclosure, 189
Self-efficacy, 35, 164, 173, 199
Self-examination, 63
Self-fulfilling prophecy, 152
Self-induced stress, 281
Seneca, Lucius Annaeus, 165
Sensitivity to differences, 235–236
Sensory data, 255
Sensory observations, 148
Serran, G., 205
Services, need for, 180–181
Session objective, in SOAP notes, 264, 265
Sexual identity, 170
Sexual relationships with clients, 234, 273
Sharing your understanding, 189–191
Short-term goals, 165, 176
Simpatía, 42
Singer, J. A., 30
Situational meanings, 39–42
Skovholt, T. M., 288–289
Slattery, Jeanne, 101–102, 253–254
Slip, in stages of change, 164
SMART-IC (specific, measurable, achievable, realistic, time-bounded, intrinsic, and committed) model, 165–169
SOAP notes, 264–265
Social justice, 228
Social psychological processes, 146–147
Social skill deficits, 196
Social support, 286
Socioeconomic status, 145
Solovey, A. D., 80
Sources of information, 30–31
Specific goals, 165–166
Speech
  in clinical report, 260
  in mental status evaluation, 132
Spirituality
  and coping, 287
  role of, in clinicians' life, 23
Spontaneity, 36
Stability, of meaning systems, 25–28

Stages, of change, 161–165
Starbranch, E. K., 240
States, 6
Stith, S. M., 168
Strength-based reports, 263–264, 266
Strengths
 assessment of, in Malcolm X example, 120
 in assessments, 152–155
 attending, in treatment plans, 176–179
 in goal setting, 172–173
 in timelines, 131
Stressors (for clients)
 assessment of, in Malcolm X example, 125
 in timelines, 129
Stressors (for clinicians), 274–281
 adaptive vs. maladaptive responses to, 281, 287
 client-induced stress, 280–281
 compassion fatigue, 274–275
 coping with, 285–286
 event-related stress, 281
 preventing problems related to, 286–288
 self-induced stress, 281
 vicarious traumatization, 275–276
 work environment stress, 281
Subjectivity, of mental status evaluations, 132, 133
Subtractive empathy, 102
Succinct, being, 266
Sue, D. W., 57, 58, 61, 62, 66
Sue, S., 57
Suicidal clients
 assessments of, 99
 mandated reporting with, 237
Summarizations, 95, 100–101
Supervisory issues, 242–243
Supports, assessment of, 120
Suske, Linda, 113
Symptoms, in clinical report, 259
Systemic oppression, 57

T

Tao, K. W., 56
Tarasoff, Tatiana, 238
Tarasoff v. Regents of the University of California, 238–239
Technical competence, 231
Temporal distancing, 36
Tense, choice of grammatical, 258–269
Terentius, 16
Termination of treatment, 209–224
 balancing opposing reactions to, 216
 clinicians' and clients' feelings during, 212–214
 discharge summary, 222–223

 ethical considerations during, 217–219
 forced terminations, 219
 goals for ending treatment well, 214–217
 helping clients own their change, 221–222
 normal vs. premature, 210–212
 and relapse prevention, 216–217
 risk management during, 219–221
Thatcher, Margaret, 29
Theoretical viewpoints, 134–135
Therapeutic alliance, 71–89
 clients' contributions to treatment, 80–81
 as common factor, 14
 defining, 72–74
 with new clients, 81–87
 nonverbal listening skills, 74–80
Therapeutic relationship, 72
Therapists. *See* Clinician(s)
Therapy
 culture in, 66–67
 informed consent about, 84
 lying in, 104
 meaning systems in context of, 28–37
 questions to assess, 115–117
 reasons for entering, 39
Therapy models, 12, 13, 15
Thompson, J. P., 240
Thoughts, intrusive, 200
Three-dimensional assessments, 113–118
Time-bounded goals, 167
Time limitations, 243–244
Timeline, 129–131
Time orientation, 35–37
Tolkien, J. R. R., 136, 137
Touch
 and culture, 76
 as nonverbal behavior, 79
Trait negativity bias, 147
Traits, 6
Transfer, 213
Trauma
 and beliefs about identity, 33–34
 beliefs changed by, 32
 effect of, on meaning systems, 26
 reasons for occurrence of, 32–33
 vicarious traumatization, 275–276
Trauma and Meaning (video), 101
Traumatization, vicarious, 275–276
Treatment
 clients' contributions to, 80–81
 collaboration on, 85–87
 research and decisions about, 137–138

Treatment goals
    collaboration on, 85–87
    defined, 165
    fitting problems, 170
Treatment plans, 175–183
    defined, 175
    revisiting, 181–183
    writing, 175–181
Trenchcoat Mafia, 154
Triage, 195
Triangles, in genograms, 126
Triggers, to problem behaviors, 164
Tutsi, 202
Txiv neeb (shaman), 86

U

Unconditional positive regard, 8–9
Uncritical agreement, respect vs., 42–43
Underrepresentation, 59
Understanding
    as component of empathy, 6–8
    in goal setting, 171
    of others, 104–108
    sharing your, 189–191
    strategies for sharing, 93–102
Uwiringiyimana, Agathe, 202
Uwiringiyimana, Sandra, 202–203

V

Validation, need for, 108–109
Validity, 131
Values
    of Asian Americans, 48
    in clinical practice, 144–146
    communicating nonverbally, 37–38
    competing, 26
    in meaning systems, 24, 37–38
    personal vs. professional, 284
VandeCreek, L. D., 228
Verbal communication, 91–110
    accurate empathy in, 102–104
    barriers to, 92–93
    to develop empathic understanding, 79
    and need for validation and hope, 108–109
    strategies for sharing understanding, 93–102
    strategies for understanding others, 104–108

Verbal influencing skills, 189
Verbal underlining, 79
Vicarious traumatization, 275–276
Viewpoints, considering different, 105
Voronov, M., 30

W

Walker, M., 82
Waller, Sukey, 87
Wampold, B. E., 61, 64
Warn, duty to, 238–239
Weaknesses, 120, 176–179
Weill, Sanford I., 180
Weinberger, J., 15
Weiss, L., 280
Well-being, 217
Westover, Tara, 26–28, 31
White, M., 222
"Why, Yes, Sandra Bland Was 'Irritated'" (Zorn), 60
Word choice, 79, 105–106
Work environment stress, 281
Work–personal life balance, 287
Worksite requirements, 241–242
Writing, importance of, 256–258

X

X, Malcolm, 118–133, 137, 139–140

Y

Yalom, I. D., 113
Yalom, Irvin, 7
Yarhouse, M. A., 170
Yates, Andrea, 3–4, 98, 134, 135, 137, 239–241, 246
Yates, Rusty, 239
YAVIS (young, attractive, verbal, intelligent, successful) clients, 61
Younggren, J. N., 247
Youth Satisfaction Questionnaire (YSQ), 181–182

Z

Ziglar, Zig, 214
Zimbardo, Philip, 146
Zorn, Eric, 60–61
Zyprexa, 240

Jeanne M. Slattery, PhD, is a professor of psychology at Clarion University. She is passionate about teaching and helping students learn to become more empathic and respectful clinicians. She has also written *Trauma, Meaning, and Spirituality: Translating Research Into Clinical Practice* and *Counseling Diverse Clients: Bringing Context Into Therapy.* She is a licensed psychologist with a small private practice and primarily works with adults and children with a history of trauma and mood and anxiety disorders. She lives in Clarion, Pennsylvania. Visit her website (https://jeannemslattery. wordpress.com) to learn more about her work.

Crystal L. Park, PhD, is a professor of clinical psychology at the University of Connecticut, Storrs. Her research focuses on coping with stressful events, particularly on the making of meaning in the context of traumatic events and life-threatening illnesses. This work is conducted with cancer survivors, patients with congestive heart failure, and military veterans. She also conducts research in integrative medicine, with a specific focus on yoga. At UConn, she maintains an active research lab and teaches health psychology at both the graduate and undergraduate levels. She lives in the lovely village of Mystic. Visit her website (https://spiritualitymeaningandhealth.uconn.edu) to learn more about her work.